AUTHENTIC ASSESSMENT FOR EARLY CHILDHOOD INTERVENTION

The Guilford School Practitioner Series

EDITORS

STEPHEN N. ELLIOTT, PhD
Vanderbilt University

JOSEPH C. WITT, PhD
Louisiana State University, Baton Rouge

Recent Volumes

Authentic Assessment for Early Childhood Intervention: Best Practices
STEPHEN J. BAGNATO

Patterns of Learning Disorders:
Working Systematically from Assessment to Intervention
DAVID J. WODRICH and ARA J. SCHMITT

Assessment for Intervention: A Problem-Solving Approach
RACHEL BROWN-CHIDSEY, Editor

Individualized Supports for Students with Problem Behaviors:
Designing Positive Behavior Plans
LINDA M. BAMBARA and KEE KERN

Think First: Addressing Aggressive Behavior in Secondary Schools
JIM LARSON

Academic Skills Problems Workbook, Revised Edition
EDWARD S. SHAPIRO

Academic Skills Problems: Direct Assessment and Intervention,
Third Edition
EDWARD S. SHAPIRO

ADHD in the Schools, Second Edition:
Assessment and Intervention Strategies
GEORGE J. DuPAUL and GARY STONER

Helping Schoolchildren Cope with Anger:
A Cognitive-Behavioral Intervention
JIM LARSON and JOHN E. LOCHMAN

Child Abuse and Neglect: The School's Response
CONNIE BURROWS HORTON and TRACY K. CRUISE

Traumatic Brain Injury in Children and Adolescents:
Assessment and Intervention
MARGARET SEMRUD-CLIKEMAN

Authentic Assessment for Early Childhood Intervention

BEST PRACTICES

◆ ◆ ◆

Stephen J. Bagnato

◆

Foreword by Rune J. Simeonsson

THE GUILFORD PRESS
New York   London

Library of Congress Cataloging-in-Publication Data
Bagnato, Stephen J.
    Authentic assessment for early childhood intervention : best practices / by Stephen
J. Bagnato.
        p. ; cm.—(The Guilford school practitioner series)
    Includes bibliographical references and index.
    ISBN-13: 978-1-59385-474-4 (hardcover : alk. paper)
    ISBN-10: 1-59385-474-9 (hardcover : alk. paper)
    1. Developmental disabilities—Diagnosis. 2. Developmentally disabled children—
Psychological testing. 3. Children with mental disabilities—Psychological
testing. 4. Preschool children—Psychological testing. 5. Psychological tests for
children. 6. Child development—Testing. I. Title. II. Series.
    [DNLM: 1. Child Development. 2. Psychological Tests. 3. Child,
Preschool. 4. Developmental Disabilities—diagnosis. WS 105.5.E8 B147a 2007]
    RJ135.B342 2007
    618.92′8588—dc22

                                                            2007006524

About the Author

◆

Stephen J. Bagnato, EdD, is a developmental school psychologist and Professor of Pediatrics and Psychology at the University of Pittsburgh School of Medicine. Dr. Bagnato is a core faculty member for Developmental Psychology Interdisciplinary Training at the UCLID Center at the University of Pittsburgh, a Maternal and Child Health Bureau leadership education institute in neurodevelopmental disabilities. He is Director of Early Childhood Partnerships (ECP) at Children's Hospital of Pittsburgh. ECP is an innovative university–hospital–community consultation and research collaborative that promotes the use of "best practices" and advancements in the evidence base in early childhood intervention. Within ECP, Dr. Bagnato directs the Pennsylvania satellite of the TRACE Center for Excellence in Early Childhood Assessment, a 5-year initiative funded by the Office of Special Education Programs to research and establish the evidence base for promising early childhood assessment practices (see *www. uclid.org* for details on ECP core programs and initiatives).

In over 30 years of research, Dr. Bagnato has specialized in authentic curriculum-based assessment and program evaluation research strategies for young children at developmental risk and with neurodevelopmental disabilities. He has authored over 120 research and applied publications in the fields of early intervention, early childhood education, school psychology, developmental disabilities, and developmental neuropsychology. He has received numerous professional research awards from the National Brain Injury Research Association and the American Psychological Association (Division 16) and was the 2001 recipient of the University of Pittsburgh Chancellor's Distinguished Public Service Award for his activities in ECP. His latest publications include the third edition of the widely used resource text *LINKing Assessment and Early Intervention: An Authentic Curriculum-Based Approach* (1997, Brookes) and the *Temperament and Atypical Behavior Scale* (TABS); *Early Childhood Indicators of Developmental Dysfunction* (2000, Brookes).

Dr. Bagnato provides consultation and training to state agencies in early childhood intervention "best practices," challenging and atypical behaviors, authentic assessment in early childhood, and authentic program outcome evaluation research.

Foreword

♦

Authentic is the adjective used in this book to frame the central activity of assessment in early childhood intervention. Clearly this word can be defined in a number of ways and convey a variety of meanings. A definition of *authentic* that may be well suited to its use in this volume is "worthy of acceptance because of accuracy" (*Merriam-Webster's Collegiate Thesaurus*, 1988, p.57). Synonyms for *authentic* identified in the same source include such words as *convincing, credible,* and *trustworthy* and refer also to words such as *accurate, factual, reliable, sound,* and *valid.*

In this book, *authentic assessment* is defined as "the developmentally appropriate alternative to conventional tests and testing practices." The first chapter begins by defining the need for authentic assessment in the context of professional standards of the field. This is followed by the rationale for authentic assessment as an alternative to the mismeasurement of children using conventional, norm-referenced instruments. Stephen Bagnato has characterized authentic assessment as the "systematic record of developmental observation over time by families and knowledgeable caregivers about the naturally occurring competencies of young children in daily routines" (Bagnato & Yeh-Ho, 2006). Developmental theory and recognition of the mediating role of the environment are seen as foundational for authentic assessment. The authentic approach offers flexibility in that it can accommodate a number of different assessment strategies, including testing without tests, the use of curriculum-based assessment, clinical judgment, and functional behavioral assessment. Furthermore, it recognizes the significance of assessing the individuality of each child's behavioral style as a factor defining the child's performance.

The importance of authentic assessment is reinforced by the fact that it addresses legal and procedural requirements governing the field, with particular reference to the eight standards identified in the Division for Early Childhood's Recommended Practices and Guidelines (Sandall, McClean, & Smith, 2000). The primacy of a developmental perspective and the recognition of the central role of the family were two unifying principles serving as the basis for the standards. With reference to authentic assessment, the standards of *utility, equity,* and *congruence* are consistent with the fundamental goal of ensuring that the assessment yields information that is useful and valid for intended purposes. Adherence to the standards of *authenticity* and *sensitivity* requires that the measures and tools used for assessment do in fact capture information about the child that is as accurate and precise as possible. Finally, the standards of *acceptability, convergence,* and *collaboration* relate to authentic assessment understood as a shared endeavor of both primary caregivers and professionals.

Although authentic assessment, as defined in this book, is framed as an alternative to conventional tests and testing practices in early childhood intervention, authenticity (in the fullest sense of the word) should in fact characterize all forms of assessment practice. This premise is supported by a comparison of the standards for assessment with the synonyms and related words associated with the word *authentic,* cited earlier as meaning "worthy of acceptance because of accuracy." In particular, the words *trustworthy, valid, reliable, factual,* and *accurate* can be used to link the concept of authentic assessment as advanced in this book to the professional standards for the field.

Assessment addressing the standards of *acceptability* and *equity* can be seen as authentic to the extent to which it is *trustworthy.* Characteristics that make assessment trustworthy are sensitivity to individual differences and acceptance by parents and professionals. The standards of *utility* and *congruence* are likely to be met by assessment which is *valid.* In this case, assessment is authentic when it fulfills intended purposes, such as screening, characterizing levels of functioning, defining intervention priorities, monitoring progress, and evaluating outcomes. Assessment is also valid when there is assurance of a match between the reference sample and the child being assessed. Assessment that is *reliable* relates to the standards of *convergence* and *collaboration.* These standards are addressed when parents and professionals are involved in shared efforts across activities and time to obtain the best picture of the child's abilities and skills. For the standard of *sensitivity,* authenticity is addressed by assessment that is *factual* in nature. Specifically, assessment must have a sufficient level of factual detail to capture small gradients of change in children characterized by very early or significantly delayed development. Finally, the standard of *authenticity* itself is met by assessment that is carried out in environments common to the child in order to optimize the picture of the child. In this context, assessment has to be *accurate* to be authentic. Assessment that is accurate is geared to the child's level and carried out with materials and in a manner consistent with the child's lived experience. Instead of taking the form of imposing demands on the child to play games structured by adults, assessment shifts to observing and joining the games and play of the child.

This volume presents a strong rationale for assessment that is authentic as defined by compatibility with the eight standards of practice in the field of early childhood intervention. As such, it offers an important resource for applying the principles of authenticity to dimensions of assessment practice. Its conceptual grounding in developmental theory, the significance of environmental factors, and the focus on assessment of function are consistent with contemporary views of human development and disability. A timely coincidence with its publication is the approval of the *International Classification of Functioning, Disability and Health, Version for Children and Youth* (ICF-CY; World Health Organization, 2006). A limitation of most assessment tools and methods in the past has been the lack of an integrated framework of health and distinctions among dimensions of functioning. By providing a classification of distinct domains of body functions, body structures, activities and participation, and environmental factors, the ICF-CY offers a common language with which to define and document the assessment. To this end, the goals and practices of authentic assessment advanced in this volume can be furthered on behalf of young children.

RUNE J. SIMEONSSON, PhD
School Psychology Program
University of North Carolina at Chapel Hill

REFERENCES

Bagnato, S. J., & Yeh-Ho, H. (2006). High stakes testing of preschool children: Violation of professional standards for evidence-based practice in early childhood intervention. *KEDI Journal of Educational Policy, 3,* 23–43.

Sandall, S., McClean, M. E., & Smith, B. J. (2000). *DEC recommended practices in early intervention/early childhood special education.* Longmont, CO: Sopris West.

Merriam-Webster's collegiate thesaurus. (1988). Springfield, MA: Merriam-Webster.

World Health Organization. (2006). *International classification of functioning, disability and health, version for children and youth.* Geneva, Switzerland: Author.

Preface

◆

In 1991, the forerunner of the current text was published—*Assessment for Early Intervention: Best Practices for Professionals.* I cowrote the book with my long-time colleague John T. Neisworth. John and I have conducted research in early childhood intervention for over 25 years and published interesting and, we hope, influential articles and books on early childhood measurement. John is now Professor Emeritus at Penn State. Although his name does not appear on this revision and expansion of our original work, his invaluable contribution and spirit are ever-present in the current book—*Authentic Assessment for Early Childhood Intervention: Best Practices.*

Since the publication of the original book 16 years ago, there have been noteworthy—even extraordinary—advances in early childhood intervention. Federal and state policies now require assessment and evaluation of all young children enrolled in various types of programs: Early Head Start, Head Start, early care and education, as well as early intervention. A second noteworthy change is the full inclusion of children with developmental delays and disabilities in regular early childhood program settings, including family child care. Third, professional organizations devoted to the education and treatment of young children have published "best-practice" standards. In particular, the National Association for the Education of Young Children (NAEYC) and the Division for Early Childhood of the Council for Exceptional Children have provided remarkably similar guidelines for programs, instruction, and assessment. Fourth, current philosophy and practices sanctioned by both professional standards and an emerging evidence base emphasize the importance of *authentic assessment* for designing developmentally appropriate objectives and for reporting program progress.

For too long, assessment materials and methods have been based on a psychometric model that produces disability labeling, numbers, and "cut-off scores" that have the illusion of precision but that neither guide instruction nor track progress within a child's program. "From this perspective, it can be said that much of contemporary developmental psychology [early childhood assessment] is the science of the strange behavior of children in strange situations with strange adults for the briefest possible periods of time" (Bronfenbrenner, 1977). Standardized methods, based on children with typical development, have been forced upon children with atypical sensory, motor, language, affective, and cultural characteristics. There is great irony when the use of assessment as a tool for educational and therapeutic efforts actually results in thwarting and confusing such efforts.

Unlike traditional assessment, *authentic assessment* captures evidence of children's everyday skills displayed in everyday routines. Parents and professionals who use authentic assessment can appraise a child's current functional capabilities, design goals and objectives, and monitor and report progress of meaningful skills in real environments. Authentic assessment provides much more representative, genuine, and "true" appraisal of the capabilities and needs of all children.

We hope and trust that this new version of our text, with its emphasis on authentic assessment, will be helpful in your training and practice as you strive to help young children and families through the use of best professional practices. To this end, the book includes three new features in each chapter: *Best-Practice Issues, Best-Practice Guidepoints.* and *Best-Practice Evidence. Issues* are questions posed at the beginning of each chapter that serve to stimulate thought and indicate chapter content. *Guidepoints* at the end of each chapter summarize important take-home points for practices that are professionally sanctioned as well as those that have a research base. *Evidence* contains references for works cited in the text as well as additional suggested reading.

REFERENCE

Bronfenbrenner, U. (1977). Toward an experimental ecology of human development. *American Psychologist, 32*, 513–530.

Contents

◆

Best-Practice Evidence   75

CHAPTER 4   **What Are the Best Contexts**   78
             for Authentic Assessment?

             Best-Practice Issues   78
             Definition and Features   78
             The Importance of Developmental Context
                 for Authentic Assessment   80
             Considerations in Staging Authentic Assessments for Preschool
                 Children in Analogue Contexts   83
             Best-Practice Guidepoints   95
             Best-Practice Evidence   97

CHAPTER 5   **Can Professionals "Test without Tests"**   98
             for Authentic Assessment?
             with RICHARD LeVAN

             Best-Practice Issues   98
             Adventures in Assessment   99
             Preschoolers and Tests   100
             Sampling Developmental Skills   101
             Shopping for Skills: An Assessment Analogue   102
             Sampling Strategies   104
             Clarence: The Adventure Continues   107
             Activity-Based Assessment in Early Childhood Intervention:
                 Operationalizing Shopping for Skills   109
             Best-Practice Guidepoints   113
             Best-Practice Evidence   115

CHAPTER 6   **How Does Authentic Curriculum-Based**   117
             Assessment Work?

             Best-Practice Issues   117
             Definition of Authentic Curriculum-Based Assessment   119
             Purposes of Curriculum-Based Assessment   119
             Benefits of a Developmental Curriculum   120
             Developmental Curricula   121
             Selecting Developmental or Functional Curricula   126
             Two Types of Authentic Curriculum-Based Assessment   131
             Authentic Assessment for Intervention Using
                 Curriculum-Embedded Scales   133
             Sequence of Steps for Curriculum-Based Assessment   135
             Best-Practice Guidepoints   138
             Best-Practice Evidence   139

CHAPTER 7   **Can Clinical Judgments Guide Parent–Professional**   142
             Team Decision Making for Early Intervention?
             with EILEEN McKEATING-ESTERLE

             Best-Practice Issues   142
             Clinical Judgment: Operational Definition
                 and Historical Context   144

CHAPTER 1

◆ ◆ ◆

What Are the Professional Standards for Assessment of Preschool Children?

◆

BEST-PRACTICE ISSUES

◆ Can parents contribute reliable and valid assessment information about their children?

◆ Is high-stakes testing a recommended practice in early childhood?

◆ Why are natural observations the preferred way to gather child performance information?

◆ Should assessment and instruction be related?

◆ Is it all right to "teach to the test" in early childhood intervention?

◆ Are standardized, norm-referenced tests to be used predominantly in early childhood?

Professionals and families have promoted some notable changes in assessment for young children with disabilities since the early 1980s. Yet, these changes are meager in comparison to fundamental transformations witnessed in early intervention/early childhood special education (EI/ECSE): use of natural settings, developmentally appropriate practices and family-centered methods. In this respect, assessment for early intervention has been *delayed* in its own development. Materials that are family friendly

---

and that link assessment and teaching seem critical to early intervention; however, few changes have occurred in the process, style, and methods of assessment to complement inclusion or developmentally appropriate and family-centered practices (Neisworth & Bagnato, 2004).

Assessment is a pivotal event for families and their children; assessment results are used to include children in specialized interventions that can change their developmental destinies. Beyond the eligibility determination or *gatekeeping* purpose, assessment also is critical for program planning, monitoring (formative) progress, and for program (summative) evaluation. Given the importance of assessment, it is understandable that the materials and procedures for early childhood assessment are contentious. The professional literature, newsletters of parent organizations, and, indeed, the pages read by hearing officers, illustrate the assessment struggle.

The Recommended Practices included in this chapter emerged from focus groups and are supported by the literature. In addition, they reflect the ideas and experiences of many professionals and families with whom I have collaborated over several years. The practices also echo many suggestions and concerns of other professional standards, including those of the National Association for the Education of Young Children (NAEYC) and the National Association of Early Childhood Specialists in State Department of Education (NAECSSDE) (2003; see also Appendix B); the National Association of School Psychologists (NASP; Thomas & Grimes, 2002), the American Speech–Language–Hearing Association (ASHA; 1990), and the Association for Childhood Education International (ACEI; Perrone, 1991). Previously, I proposed a definition for early childhood assessment that is consistent with the recommendations reported in this chapter:

> Early childhood assessment is a flexible, collaborative decision-making process in which teams of parents and professionals repeatedly revise their judgments and reach consensus about the changing developmental, educational, medical, and mental health service needs of young children and their families. (Bagnato & Neisworth, 1991, p. xi).

GUIDING PRINCIPLES

The professionals and parents who participated in this effort repeatedly expressed two concerns. First, as principal stakeholders, parents and family members must play a vital and indispensable role in assessment from beginning to end. Second, assessment methods and materials must accommodate children's developmental and disability-specific characteristics. Because of the importance of these concerns, they are presented separately.

Parents as Partners

As professionals, we are committed to working with parents and others who know and care about the child. It is true, of course, that there can be obstacles to effective family participation. Families may be overwhelmed by their child's possible diagnosis and may be intimidated by jargon and differences in educational levels. Cultural differences, language barriers, and work, health, schedule, and transportation difficulties also can make collaboration difficult.

In addition to my legal and ethical responsibilities to partner with parents, there are sound professional and practical reasons for doing so. First, families provide valuable authentic and longitudinal information about their child that is not otherwise available (Diamond & Squires, 1993). Further, family members provide needed information about their circumstances and the possible impact on the child. More active involvement of parents in their child's program appears to be related to greater developmental progress (Ramey & Ramey, 1998). Not an isolated or perfunctory recommendation, parents as partners is a dominant theme that runs across all phases of the assessment and intervention sequence.

Developmental Appropriateness

Organizations representing young children (e.g., NAEYC, ACEI) have for some time advocated approaches and materials that match children's interests and developmental status. Early childhood professionals oppose the use of school-age demands and practices with children who are neither developmentally prepared for nor benefit from such imposition. Conventional standardized norm-referenced assessment materials and tasks are very often seen as entirely wrong even for use with children of typical development (Perrone, 1991). The *inappropriateness* of such materials and demands becomes greatly exacerbated when considering young children with special needs (Bagnato, Neisworth, & Munson, 1997):

> Assessment of infants and preschoolers remains dominated by restrictive methods and styles that place a premium on inauthentic, contrived developmental tasks; that are administered by various professionals in separate sessions using small, unmotivating toys from boxes or test kits; staged at a table or on the floor in an unnatural setting; observed passively by parents; interpreted by norms based solely on typical children; and used for narrow purposes of classification and eligibility determination. (p. 69)

The styles, methods, and content of assessment must become compatible with, rather than at odds with, the behavior and interests of young children. A fundamental precept of developmentally appropriate practice is that teaching and assessment must take place in the child's *natural context* rather than being decontextualized (Bagnato & Neisworth, 2000):

> A developmental approach presumes a more whole-child view. Many developmental areas are sampled and child differences, from time to time, are highlighted so that the child's previous performance serves as the baseline for monitoring progress. Professionals use a flexible approach in choosing toys that are motivating for the child and are often the child's own. They are responsive to the fact that young children rarely sit still at tables or respond on command to typical structured tasks. A developmental approach acknowledges that professionals must adjust their own language, behavior, and expectations to the young child's level of developmental maturity. A more familiar play-based approach is used that does not force conformance to standardized procedures that are at odds with the typical behavior of young children. (p. 1)

New directions and professional standards for early childhood assessment must reflect eight critical qualities: assessment must be useful, acceptable, authentic, collaborative, convergent, equitable, sensitive, and congruent (Bagnato & Neisworth, 1999).

Utility

Assessment must be useful to accomplish the multiple and interrelated purposes of early care and education and early intervention. Assessment is critical for detecting possible problems and, through intervention, averting later more intractable and complex difficulties. Children must be able to access programs through flexible eligibility determination processes; assessment is crucial for planning individualized interventions, for monitoring progress through regular repeated assessments, and for documenting the impact of quality programs. Above all, assessment must have treatment validity—there must be an essential similarity or linkage among program goals, individual child objectives, and the developmental competencies that are assessed. Materials and methods of assessment must help families and professionals to identify instructional objectives and methods for helping.

Acceptability

The methods, styles, and materials for assessment must be mutually agreed upon by families and professionals. The objectives and methods suggested by assessment must be considered worthwhile and acceptable. Further, assessment should detect changes in behavior that are noticeable to caregivers in the home and early childhood environments. This standard of acceptability is an aspect of the wider construct usually referred to as social validity.

Authenticity

Contrived tasks and materials as well as unfamiliar people and circumstances are not optimal for true appraisals of what children really know and do. Tabletop testing with tiny little toys is often a task dreaded by the child, parents, and, indeed, the professional!

Psychometric items typically do not sample useful curricular content that could guide intervention. Observing children perform in their natural settings offers authentic information that is much more descriptive of the child. Rating scales, direct observation, curriculum-based checklists, and caregiver interview inventories are useful in helping professionals obtain a realistic appraisal of the child's strengths and intervention priorities.

Collaboration

Assessment methods and styles should promote teamwork among families and professionals. Parents and other family members are central partners in the assessment of their children; assessment materials should be chosen and used because they are written in understandable, family-friendly, jargon-free language to which anyone can respond. Assessment must promote the concept of parent–professional decision making in which *tests do not make decisions—people do*. Curriculum-based assessment can be used as a unifying approach that invites input from multiple team members, including family members.

Convergence

Functional, reliable, valid information on the status and progress of children can be obtained when typical behavior in everyday routines is observed repeatedly by several individuals—teachers, other professionals, and parents. Differences in such data are important to highlight so that areas of needed change or special emphasis in programming can be underscored. The pooling (convergence) of several perspectives (family, professional) provides a better information base.

Equity

Assessment must accommodate individual differences. The principle of equity is recognized (and mandated) as essential for instructional materials. For example, one would not use standard print material with children of low vision. Materials can be chosen that allow the child to demonstrate capabilities through several different response modes by using materials that can be changed in a flexible manner. When materials and procedures accommodate a child's sensory, response, affective, and cultural characteristics they are equitable. Conventional materials have been standardized with children of typical development; to force fit these materials to atypical children violates not only the standards of equity and developmental appropriateness, but common sense.

Sensitivity

Professionals and families must be given the opportunity to use assessment materials that sample evidence of progressively more complex skill development so that even the smallest increment of change can be detected and celebrated. Children with more severe delays and impairments especially need assessment that is sensitive to small increments of progress. Many conventional instruments do not include a sufficient number of items to make possible sensitive measurement of progress.

Congruence

Materials must be designed for, and field validated with, the very children who will be assessed, including those with typical development and those with varying degrees of mild to severe disabilities. Early intervention, specifically, and early childhood education, generally, require specialized materials that address the emerging talents of young children at play in various home- and center-based educational settings. Early childhood assessment materials and methods must be developed specifically for infants, toddlers, and preschool children and match the style and interests typical of young children.

ORGANIZATION OF THE PRACTICES

The Recommended Practices in assessment are organized around five statements. They reflect the issues just discussed and include the following: (1) professionals and families collaborate in planning and implementing assessment; (2) assessment is individualized and appropriate for the child and family; (3) assessment provides useful information for intervention; (4) professionals share information in respectful and useful ways; and (5) professionals meet legal and procedural requirements and Recommended Practices guidelines. Two central themes or dimensions inform all of the practices: (1) family members are partners in assessment; and (2) materials and practices must be developmentally appropriate.

BEST-PRACTICE GUIDEPOINTS
Division of Early Childhood (DEC)
Recommended Practices and Examples: Assessment

♦ **Professionals and families collaborate in planning and implementing assessment.**

A1. Professionals provide families with easy access by phone or other means for arranging initial screening and other activities.
Example:
- *The family is provided a phone number or e-mail address that will always be answered promptly by a knowledgeable person.*

A2. Professionals ensure a single point of contact for families throughout the assessment process.
Example:
- *From the very first contact with a family, one team member is identified to serve as coordinator (i.e., the single point of contact) for all assessment activities from referral to the initiation of services.*

A3. Families receive a written statement of program philosophy regarding family participation in assessment planning and activities.
Examples:
- *A brochure or written statement about family involvement in assessment is provided to families.*
- *A staff member verbally explains the philosophy of assessment when the brochure or written statement is provided and clarifies any questions the family may have.*

A4. Professionals meet and collaborate with families to discuss family preferences and reach consensus about the process, methods, materials, and situations of assessment that will meet the child's needs best.
Examples:
- *Families and professionals jointly plan the specifics of the assessment including the location, time of day, and strategies for assessment.*
- *Professionals are careful to incorporate culturally and linguistically appropriate procedures into the plans.*

A5. Professionals solicit information from families regarding the child's interests, abilities, and specials needs.
Examples:
- *The team plans which assessments to use only after obtaining information from the family about what the child typically does and what the child likes to do.*
- *The team asks for and utilizes family suggestions for favorite toys, activities, and accommodations to use in the assessment.*

A6. Professionals review, with parental consent, agency information about the child and family.

Example:

- *The service coordinator requests and the team reviews records of the child's birth history and medical history, and information from other agencies.*

A7. Professionals and families identify team members and the team assessment style to best fit the needs and goals of the child and family.
Examples:

- *It is decided that the occupational therapist, speech–language pathologist, early childhood special educator, and family members will conduct the assessment using a transdisciplinary play-based model.*

- *The physical therapist and early childhood special educator make a home visit to assess the child in a familiar setting and in the context of familiar activities.*

A8. Families participate actively in assessment procedures.
Example:

- *The child's mother observes as the team assesses her daughter and answers questions about what the child typically does at home.*

A9. Families choose their roles in the assessment of their children (e.g., assistant, facilitator, observer, assessor).
Examples:

- *Families may choose to watch the assessment, to serve as an informant, to participate by interacting with the child, or to provide support to the child by staying nearby. Prior to the day of the assessment, a professional explains what each role entails so that families can choose which they wish to assume and will know what to expect on the assessment day.*

- *Family members observe the assessment activities and comment on their child's performance.*

- *Family members make a list of the words their child understands.*

- *A family member helps the child eat a snack while the occupational therapist observes the child's chewing and swallowing abilities.*

A10. With each family's agreement, professionals help families identify resources, concerns, and priorities related to their child's development.
Examples:

- *In meetings prior to the development of the individualized family service plan (IFSP) or individualized education plan (IEP), families share their concerns and priorities for their child as well as the resources available to help them with their child's development.*

- *The early interventionist shares checklists of possible needs and resources for the family to use.*

A11. Professionals, families, and other regular caregivers work as equal team members for purposes of assessment (i.e., give equal priority to family/caregiver's observations and reports, discuss assessment results, reach consensus about the child's needs and programs).
Example:

- *At the team meeting, the parent, early interventionist, speech–language pathologist, and physical therapist all identify current functioning and areas of need for the child. All information is considered in the assessment process rather than viewing some information as more "correct" than other information.*

A12. Program administrators encourage the use of assessment procedures that ensure consultation and collaboration among families and professionals (e.g., the whole team discusses qualitative and quantitative information and negotiates consensus to make decisions).
Example:

- *The assessment team has an agreed upon model of teaming and consensus building that is followed.*

♦ **Assessment is individualized and appropriate for the child and family.**

A13. Professionals use multiple measures to assess child status, progress, and program impact and outcomes (e.g., developmental observations, criterion/curriculum-based interviews, informed clinical opinion, and curriculum-compatible norm-referenced scales).
Example:

- *Available measures include observations, criterion curriculum-based instruments, interviews, curriculum-compatible norm-referenced scales, informed clinical opinion, and work samples.*

A14. Professionals choose materials and procedures that accommodate the child's sensory, physical, responsive, and temperamental differences.
Examples:

- *The child uses her augmentative communication device and adaptive equipment when her progress is assessed by the team.*
- *The child uses eye gaze to indicate choices on an assessment of receptive vocabulary.*

A15. Professionals rely on materials that capture the child's authentic behaviors in routine circumstances.
Examples:

- *Assessment includes observation of the child's engagement in familiar activities in his typical environment rather than only behavior in contrived situations.*
- *The assessment is conducted in the classroom the child currently attends.*
- *Family members identify the child's favorite toys and these are used for assessment activities.*
- *A family member and the child look at picture books together while the speech therapist records the child's communication skills.*

A16. To design IFSP/IEP goals and activities, professionals seek information directly from families and other regular caregivers using materials and procedures that the families themselves can manage.

Examples:

- *Families provide information about potential learning opportunities for their child that occur in daily routines and that are feasible given the other demands of the family.*
- *Families choose to complete a questionnaire or checklist to help identify goals and learning activities.*
- *Assessment for program planning includes strategies for gaining information from families and other caregivers so that the IFSP/IEP goals pertain to the child's natural environment.*

A17. Professionals assess children in contexts that are familiar to the child.
Examples:

- *The professional observes the child in his usual early care and education.*
- *A family member reports that the child has some challenging behaviors in the early evening. The professional schedules a home visit at that time to try to understand the issues and potential solutions.*

A18. Professionals assess a child after they have become familiar to him or her.
Examples:

- *The assessment team members spend time with the child in play or in an informal activity to establish familiarity prior to assessment.*
- *Individuals who are familiar with and to the child are identified as members of the assessment team.*

A19. Professionals gather information from multiple sources (e.g., families, professional team members, agencies, service providers, other regular caregivers).
Examples:

- *The teacher and the babysitter make a list of the words the child uses, says, signs, or gestures.*
- *The occupational therapist observes the child playing with toys in the classroom and then sets up a few testing items to clarify the child's performance.*
- *The child's physician, early care and education providers, babysitter, extended family members, and religious school teacher are also asked for input.*

A20. Professionals assess the child's strengths and needs across all developmental and behavioral dimensions.
Examples:

- *The team completes all sections of the curriculum-referenced instrument even though stated concerns are only in one domain.*
- *The team assesses a child across all developmental domains (i.e., social, motor, communication, adaptive, sensory, and cognitive) and all behavioral dimensions (e.g., temperament, problem solving, and self-regulation).*

♦ Assessment provides useful information for intervention.

A21. Families and professionals assess the presence and extent of atypical child behavior that may be a barrier to intervention and progress.
Example:
- *The team assesses the occurrence of problematic atypical behavior, challenging behavior, and self-stimulation in naturally occurring routines and activities throughout the day.*

A22. Professionals use functional analysis of behavior to assess the form and function of challenging behaviors.
Examples:
- *Over a couple of days, the team members identify what happens just before and after they observe challenging behaviors (e.g., crying, hitting, throwing objects) by the child. They discuss whether the behavior is meant to obtain attention, avoid a specific activity, or serve another function. Then the team plans strategies to reduce the behavior and evaluate their hypothesis.*
- *For a week, the child's mother and father write down what happens right before the child's tantrums and what happens afterward. The early interventionist reviews these notes with them, and they form a "best guess" about the purpose or function of the tantrumming behavior. Based on this information, the early interventionist helps the parents develop a plan for reducing the occurrence of the child's tantrums.*

A23. Program supervisors, in concert with the EI/ECSE team, use only those measures that have high treatment validity (i.e., that link assessment, individual program planning, and progress evaluation).
Examples:
- *The team uses curriculum-based instruments that link directly to the curriculum.*
- *Assessment tools used are those that provide information that directly assists with program planning.*

A24. Professionals assess not only immediate mastery of a skill, but also whether the child can demonstrate the skill consistently across other settings and with other people.
Examples:
- *The team assesses whether new words learned at home are also used in the caregiving setting.*
- *The team assesses the child's ability to walk in the classroom, on the playground, to and from the car, and so forth.*

A25. Professionals appraise the level of support that a child requires in order to perform a task.
Examples:
- *The team assesses whether or not a child can request juice independently or with varying amounts of help.*

- *The team assesses whether the infant lifts her head on her own in response to interesting sounds or sights.*
- *Professionals access the level of prompting, environmental modification, or reinforcement required for a child to consistently demonstrate a skill.*

A26. Professionals choose and use scales with sufficient item density to detect even small increments of progress (especially important for children with more severe disabilities).
Example:

- *A curriculum-based instrument has too few items to demonstrate progress of a child over time, so the team breaks down items on the measure into smaller steps to make progress more apparent.*

A27. Professionals and families rely on curriculum-based assessment as the foundation or "mutual language" for team assessments.
Example:

- *In conducting an evaluation to determine eligibility for special education, the team uses a curriculum-based instrument in addition to a norm-referenced instrument.*

A28. Professionals conduct longitudinal, repeated assessments in order to examine previous assumptions about the child, and to modify the ongoing program.
Examples:

- *The team completes the curriculum-based measure twice per year for each child.*
- *Teachers collect weekly data on a child's fine motor objectives.*
- *Family members and early care and education providers keep track of what the child eats to monitor caloric intake for a child who has trouble gaining weight.*

A29. Professionals report assessment results in a manner that is immediately useful for planning program goals and objectives.
Examples:

- *The team uses a curriculum-based measure in which items become learning objectives.*
- *The team report describes the child's needs and suggests learning activities.*

♦ **Professionals share information in respectful and useful ways.**

A30. Professionals report assessment results so that they are understandable and useful for families.
Examples:

- *Reports are translated into the dominant language of the family.*
- *Reports use minimal technical jargon and include definitions of terms if needed.*
- *Reports give specific information about the child's abilities and needs rather than just scores or developmental ages.*

A31. Professionals report strengths as well as priorities for promoting optimal development.
Example:
- *Team members always take the time to include information about a child's areas of strength in their reports as well as discussing areas of need.*

A32. Professionals report limitations of assessments (e.g., questions of rapport, cultural bias, and sensory/response requirements).
Examples:
- *Team members report the results of an assessment with caution due to the child's physical impairment, which may have prevented a valid assessment.*
- *The team decides that an assessment should be conducted in the child's dominant language as well as in English so that a comparison of the results can be made.*

A33. Professionals write reports that contain findings and interpretations regarding the interrelatedness of developmental areas (e.g., how the child's limitations have affected development; how the child has learned to compensate).
Examples:
- *A child who is visually impaired may currently be demonstrating a delay in vocabulary development due to his inability to see objects and people around him.*
- *A child whose speech is delayed may not be able to express all that she knows.*

A34. Professionals organize reports by developmental/functional domains or concerns rather than by assessment device.
Example:
- *The physical therapist, early interventionist, and speech–language pathologist write their report by organizing all of their information together by developmental domain.*

A35. Families have adequate time to review reports, ask questions, or express concerns before the team uses the information for decision making.
Example:
- *In advance of the team meeting, information is shared and family members are provided the opportunity to ask questions or express concerns with at least one member of the team.*

A36. Family members may invite other individuals to evaluation meetings or meetings to discuss children's performance or progress.
Example:
- *In preparation for the evaluation meeting, the service coordinator asks the family if they would like to invite anyone to attend. Those invited may include other family members, friends, spiritual advisors, or other professionals.*

♦ **Professionals meet legal and procedural requirements and meet Recommended Practice guidelines.**

A37. Professionals inform families about state EI/ECSE rules and regulations regarding assessment.
Example:

- *Written information about state regulations is given to families prior to the eligibility assessment in written form or through other formats. The family has the opportunity to talk with a team member about the regulations if there are questions.*

A38. Professionals, when required by regulations to apply a diagnosis, employ measures and classification systems that are designed and developmentally appropriate for infants and young children.
Example:

- Assessment teams have guidance from their state that makes disability categories appropriate for young children.

A39. Psychologists rely on authentic measures of early problem-solving skills (instead of traditional intelligence tests) that link directly to program content and goals and that sample skills in natural, rather than contrived, circumstances (e.g., play-based).
Examples:

- *The assessment team always includes an authentic measure of child functioning in assessment to determine eligibility.*
- *The psychologist observes the child in her early education setting as part of the assessment process.*

A40. Professionals, when appropriate, choose those norm-referenced measures that are developed, field validated, standardized, and normed with children similar to the child being assessed.
Example:

- *The assessment team is careful to choose instruments that are appropriate to each child rather than always using the same instruments for every child.*

A41. Professionals monitor child progress based on past performance as the referent rather than on group norms.
Examples:

- *The assessment team considers assessment information from at least three points in time to monitor child progress.*
- *Rather than comparing a child's performance on an instrument to other children at the same age, the team analyzes the child's rate of development in relation to his previous rate of development.*

A42. Professionals defer a definitive diagnosis until evaluation of the child's response to a tailored set of interventions.
Example:

- The assessment team is cautious about identifying a category of disability for a child on the basis of one assessment only and has the option of using a "developmental delay" category so that services may be provided. More information will be learned about the child during intervention.

A43. Program administrators provide supervisory support for team members to enable them to maintain ethical standards and recommended practices. Examples:

- *In-service opportunities are provided for team members so they can maintain the skills necessary for appropriate assessment.*

- *Team members are encouraged to complete quality assessments. The need to complete assessments quickly is not allowed to compromise the quality of those assessments.*

A44. Professionals and families conduct an ongoing (formative) review of the child's progress at least every 90 days in order to modify instructional and therapeutic strategies. Example:

- *The team has review meetings scheduled every three months to review child progress and plan needed changes if identified.*

A45. Professionals and families assess and redesign outcomes to meet the ever changing needs of the child and family. Example:

- *A child's mother is returning to work, necessitating changes in the service plan. The team makes the needed changes to the intervention plan as requested by the family.*

A46. Professionals and families assess the child's progress on a yearly (summative) basis to modify the child's goal plan. Example:

- *The team summarizes the child's progress in preparation for the annual meeting to revise the IFSP or IEP.*

BEST-PRACTICE EVIDENCE

American Speech–Language–Hearing Association. (1990). *Guidelines for practices in early intervention*. Rockville, MD: Author.

Bagnato, S. J., & Neisworth, J. T. (1991). *Assessment for early intervention: Best practices for professionals*. New York: Guilford Press.

Bagnato, S. J., & Neisworth, J. T. (1999). Collaboration and teamwork in assessment for early intervention. *Child and Adolescent Psychiatric Clinics of North America, 8*(2), 347–363.

Bagnato, S. J., & Neisworth, J. T. (2000, Spring). Assessment is adjusted to each child's developmental needs. *Birth through 5 Newsletter, 1*(2), 1.

Bagnato, S. J., Neisworth, J. T., & Munson, S. M. (1997). *LINKing assessment and early intervention: An authentic curriculum-based approach*. Baltimore: Brookes.

Diamond, K., & Squires, J. (1993). The role of parental report in the screening and assessment of young children. *Journal of Early Intervention, 17*(2), 107–115.

National Association for the Education of Young Children (NAEYC) and National

Association of early Childhood Specialists in State Departments of Education (NAECSSDE). (2003). *Early childhood curriculum, assessment, and program evaluation: Building an effective, accountable system in programs for children birth through age eight.* Washington, DC: Author.

Neisworth J. T., & Bagnato, S. J. (2004). The mis-measure of young children: The authentic assessment alternative. *Infants and Young Children, 17*(3), 198–212.

Perrone, V. (1991, Spring). On standardized testing. *Childhood Education, 67*(3), 132–142.

Ramey, C. T., & Ramey, S. L. (1998). Early intervention and early experience. *American Psychologist, 53*(2), 109–120.

Suen, H. K., Lu, C. H., & Neisworth, J. T. (1993). Measurement of team decision making through generalizability theory. *Journal of Psychoeducational Assessment, 11*(2), 120–132.

Thomas, A., & Grimes, J. (2002). *Best practices in school psychology* (4th ed.). Washington, DC: National Association of School Psychologists.

CHAPTER 2

♦ ♦ ♦

How Can Authentic Assessment Prevent the Mismeasure of Young Children?

♦

BEST-PRACTICE ISSUES

♦ Why must conventional tests and testing practices be abandoned in early childhood intervention?

♦ What is the primary justification and purpose of assessment in early childhood intervention?

♦ Do published professional standards encourage and require authentic assessment?

♦ Can professionals and parents observe and record examples of problem-solving behavior in natural settings?

♦ Why are natural or analogue contexts preferred over clinical contexts for early childhood assessment?

♦ Can professionals use authentic assessment to accomplish both eligibility determination and program planning/program evaluation?

Measurement in early care and education, and early intervention, particularly, continues to be dominated by the use of conventional, norm-referenced testing practices to the detriment of young children. Conventional tests have been neither developed for nor field-validated on infants, toddlers, and preschoolers with developmental disabilities.

Thus, contrary to professional wisdom in the fields, conventional tests have no evidence base for use in early childhood intervention. Nevertheless, the accountability movement in education embodied in No Child Left Behind legislation continues to promote the use of conventional tests that yield distorted results for young children with special needs.

It is long overdue for our interdisciplinary fields to *abandon decontextualized testing practices* and to champion the use of measurement techniques that capture authentic portraits of the naturally occurring competencies of young exceptional children in everyday settings and routines—the natural developmental ecology for children.

In this chapter, I present the "authentic assessment alternative" to the mismeasure of young children.[1] I review the purposes for assessment in early childhood intervention; issues related to conventional testing; eight standards for professional "best practices"; a rationale and examples of the process and methods for authentic assessment; and guidepoints for implementing authentic assessment in action.

*   *   *

People have been testing and measuring other people for centuries. History is replete with examples of theories on and approaches to testing, diagnosing, labeling, and sorting people. Measurement has been conducted more often for the benefit of the assessor; certainly the history of racial and ethnic devaluation and relegation illustrates the complicity of (mis)measurement in justifying and validating social biases. I refer primarily to the attempts to assess personal qualities, often vaguely defined, such as character, morality, criminality, talent, and, of course, intelligence. As Gould (1981) asserts, "There are . . . few injustices deeper than the denial of an opportunity to strive or ever hope by a limit imposed from without, but falsely identified as lying within" (p. 28). Misrepresenting children through mismeasuring them denies children their rights to beneficial expectations and opportunities.

Given our history of mismeasurement, it seems crucial to look closely at what I advance as accurate and worthwhile assessment with young children, especially with the impending reauthorization of the Individuals with Disabilities Act (IDEA) and the ongoing implementation of No Child Left Behind. I contend that much of conventional early childhood measurement, the methods and materials I studied in graduate school, has been used to diagnose, label, and sort young children, based largely on inference and theory, and has resulted in questionable placements and service delivery.

---

[1] In tribute to the writings of Stephen J. Gould (1981).

I want to make five points very clear so that there is no misunderstanding about my beliefs about early childhood measurement and the implications of those beliefs:

1. Measurement in early childhood and in early intervention, particularly, continues to be dominated by conventional norm-referenced testing practices to the detriment of young children.
2. Conventional norm-referenced tests of development, intelligence, and psychoeducational functioning have been neither developed for, nor field-validated on, young children with developmental disabilities; thus, they have no evidence base in early childhood.
3. Conventional, laboratory-based testing procedures are decontextualized from children's natural, everyday routines and thus fail to capture the "true" functional capabilities of young children of varied ability levels.
4. Conventional testing must be abandoned within the early childhood fields for every purpose including screening, eligibility determination, program planning, progress monitoring, and, notably, program evaluation outcomes research.
5. Only authentic or other alternative, observational assessment forms that meet current recommended practice standards of the Division for Early Childhood of the Council for Exceptional Children (DEC; Neisworth & Bagnato, 2005) and the National Association for the Education of Young Children (NAEYC; Bredekamp & Copple, 1997) and are embodied in the eight standards discussed below should be promoted in the early childhood fields (e.g., Head Start, early intervention, early care and education).

To set the stage for my description of an alternative to conventional testing, I have organized this article into four major sections: (1) purposes for assessment, (2) issues related to conventional testing, (3) guidelines for recommended practices, and (4) the authentic assessment alternative.

WHY DO WE ASSESS YOUNG CHILDREN?

When children are thriving, with no evident problems, assessment is rarely attempted. Of course, routine screening programs and research projects involve assessment of children with typical development, as do accountability efforts to track child achievement. Yet, assessment becomes important or "high stakes" when problems are suspected or predicted. Thus, the specific purposes of assessment apply to children who have suspected or evident developmental delays and/or disabilities. Within early intervention, I recognize four assessment purposes: (1) screening and eligibility determination, (2) individualized program planning, (3) child progress monitoring, and (4) program evaluation.

Screening

Early detection of developmental problems can result from referrals by parents, teachers, or physicians or communitywide screening efforts. Screening is a relatively rapid method for selecting those children who should receive more detailed assessment. Such rapid methods are socially useful because of the economy of time, effort, and cost, but are subject to error—false negatives and false positives. Clearly, false negatives (i.e., indications of "no problem") when a problem really exists are the real issue. These instances will not be afforded up-close assessment, and children's problems will go unrecognized.

Eligibility

According to the current system, children who need early intervention services and supports must be evaluated and declared eligible before special help can be delivered. Eligibility determination refers to this assessment process. Although varying across states, criteria for eligibility are based on the extent of a child's test-identified deviation from norms for typical development. Ordinarily, cutoff scores are used to make decisions about the need for services. At best, eligibility testing documents disability rather than capability and so is a grossly incomplete look at the child. More serious, however, are the several aspects of the conventional testing approach to measurement that contradict recommended practices (to be discussed).

Program Planning and Progress Monitoring

Measurement plays an important role in outlining the child's individual plan of instruction and therapy. The plan should be based on a range of information about the child's strengths and needs. The child's developmental progress based on his or her individual plan should be recorded to guide instruction and detect change. Again, conventional measures do not sample curricular content and thus are insensitive to the gains that children evidence in a program. For this reason, much controversy surrounds the testing of children in Head Start and prekindergarten programs using conventional tests whose content is incompatible with curricula and whose testing approach is counter to typical early childhood behavior.

Program Evaluation

The quality and impact of the child's program should be clear if program evaluation is done effectively. Periodic feedback to teachers, parents, and staff is important for program modifications. Certainly, the importance of accountability driven by state and federal mandates underscores the critical role of program evaluation. Again, linkages between assessment content and instructional content are essential to reveal program outcomes and impact.

WHAT IS "CONVENTIONAL TESTING"?

Throughout this article I refer to "conventional" testing and the authentic assessment alternative. For purposes of this chapter, I describe key aspects of conventional testing. These features will be referred to as I present the authentic alternative.

First, conventional tests are *standardized*. The materials provided as stimuli to the tested child are held constant across all children. Many tests come with their own "kit" of toys, blocks, and pictures that are shown to children. Sometimes, although a kit may not be provided, detailed descriptions of test materials are offered so that the tester can purchase standard materials. In either case, the requirement is that all children be tested with the same materials, providing "a level playing field." Clearly, use of standard materials eliminates problems related to variance that might result from differences in the materials. "Point to the picture of the dog" might be more or less difficult depending on the size, color, and quality of the pictures. How the child is to respond to the test items is also typically standardized. Pointing, saying, stacking, and picking up items are often specified in the instructions to children.

Many useful assessment and instructional materials that I use are standardized, and that need not necessarily be a problem. For example, many curriculum packages come with a set of instructions on how to use the materials, recommendations on teaching, and information how to assess progress. Standardization can be "tight" or "loose." Curriculum materials are typically loosely standardized so that they can be adapted to a variety of child differences. Conventional testing, however, is almost always tightly standardized to prevent variance due to differences in materials and administration procedures. What the tester says is scripted, as well as the sequence of items. There may even be requirements regarding seating, table, and room conditions. Of course, all testers are to "establish rapport," but the criterion for "rapport" is not specified, nor typically attainable in the testing situation. Tight standardization makes sense within the psychometric approach, because control of testing conditions is required for making normative comparisons. To conclude that a 4-year-old child is one standard deviation below the normative average for her age, I must be confident that the deviation is due to the child's responding, and not to nonstandard testing conditions. Likewise, I cannot coach a child to have the "right answers," because that would obviously distort the meaning of the score and norm comparison. The problems avoided by tight standard-ization are acknowledged when seen from the psychometric perspective and tradition. The central issue, however, is that the standardization *is tai-lored to and for children of typical development*, and use of such standard materials and procedures with children of diverse special needs makes little psychometric or common sense.

A second hallmark of conventional tests is the procedure for *item selection*. Items are derived through a series of steps in which initial pool of potential items is reduced until "acceptable" items are identified. The goal of the item selection process is to identify items that discriminate between age (or diagnostic) groups. Usually, a criterion is set where an item is accepted if, for example, 80% of 4-year-olds in the norming sample pass it, but only 20% of 3-year-olds pass it. The items distilled in this way are con-sidered "good discriminators." If a child can show the skill or answer the question, then inferences are made concerning capabilities not on the test, per se, but represented by the item. The usual outcome of this distillation process, however, is the selection of items that involve nonfunctional skills that I would not want to teach. Standing on one foot, stringing beads, and stacking four blocks may separate age groups but would not be in any functional curriculum. These special items must be "kept secret" and used only for testing. Teaching to the test (not that the items are worth teaching) is clearly taboo because that would destroy any validity or normative com-parisons the test might offer. The characteristics and requirements of con-ventional, psychometrically based testing do indeed create dilemmas for those who must assess children with special needs, and who seek useful information for making worthwhile decisions.

Finally, both the item selection and standardized administration proce-dures result in restricted *sampling* of children's authentic behaviors. Profes-sionals who do research certainly recognize the critical role of sampling. We make inferences based on samples; we may make generalizations beyond the sample to a population to the extent that the sample is unbiased and representative. When we assess a child's developmental or behavioral status, we wish, of course, to make inferences about that child's function-ing beyond the particular assessment items and situation. We may consider assessment as an attempt to obtain a fair sample of behaviors that will per-mit us to make inferences concerning that child's population of perfor-mances. Both the content of the sample and the sampling plan (how assess-ment items are selected) come into play for enabling valid inferences. "Even if our conclusion concerns only one individual, . . . the measurements we have taken are only a sample of all that might be made, and in assigning particular values to the measured magnitudes we are making an inference, based on that sample, of what other measurements would yield" (Kaplan, 1964).

At the heart of authentic assessment is the issue of sampling behavior. In authentic assessment, we observe and/or obtain reports about the child's performances in and across natural settings and occasions. Appraisal of the child's developmental skills *as practiced in the child's real environments* cannot be done through "testing" by a stranger at a table with flashcards, blocks, and beads. Clearly, such conventional testing ignores the crucial requirement for valid sampling of behavior that enables inferences about the presence, absence, fluency, and utility of skills. Use of psychometrically selected items administered in decontextualized settings results in biased samples of the child's functioning—samples that often yield results far different from how the child really behaves.

WHAT ARE THE PROFESSIONAL STANDARDS FOR EARLY CHILDHOOD ASSESSMENT?

Many interdisciplinary professional organizations have published best practice "white papers" on assessment and intervention in early childhood. Among these are the National Association of School Psychologists; the American Speech–Language–Hearing Association; and the American Occupational Therapy Association. Yet, the most prominent and extensive professional standards regarding assessment and intervention in early childhood are published by three major early childhood organizations: the DEC (Sandall, McLean, & Smith, 2000); the NAEYC (Bredekamp & Copple, 1997); and the Head Start Bureau (2001).

Over the past decade, I have collaborated with numerous professionals in the field to develop and field-validate the DEC Assessment Standards (Neisworth & Bagnato, 2000). The 46 DEC standards, as part of this process, have been categorized into 10 overarching standards to guide developmentally appropriate assessment. The 10 standards that I summarize below are based on two fundamentals. First, assessment contexts, content, and procedures must be developmentally appropriate (i.e., be harmonious with and responsive to the interests, capabilities, and realities of early childhood). The imposition of school-age practices (themselves questionable) is at odds with the characteristics of all young children, with typical or atypical development.

The second fundamental element for early childhood assessment is sincere and active cooperation with parents (or primary caregivers). When parents are genuine (not perfunctory) team members, we are able to gather information not otherwise available (e.g., sleep patterns, social skill/difficulties in community settings, and toileting behavior). Additionally, information provided by parents may challenge professional data. When information discrepancies exist, additional collaborative assessment is needed, rather than a presumption of parent bias. These two fundamentals, developmental appropriateness and parent–professional partnerships, provide not only the values basis, but also a pragmatic basis for making authentic assessment feasible. Below are the 10 major standards (see Table 2.1).

TABLE 2.1. Ten Developmentally Appropriate
Practice (DAP) Assessment Standards

1.	Utility	Usefulness for intervention
2.	Acceptability	Social worth and agreement
3.	Authenticity	Natural methods and contexts
4.	Equity	Adaptable for special needs
5.	Sensitivity	Fine measurement gradations
6.	Convergence	Synthesis of ecological data
7.	Collaboration	Parent–professional teamwork
8.	Congruence	Special design/field validation/ evidence base
9.	Technology	Portable, computer-based observations, recordings, and reporting
10.	Outcomes	Assessed content aligned to state/federal outcome benchmarks

Utility

That assessment should be useful seems self-evident, yet much professional time and effort goes into testing that has little or no use. Often, professionals are required to use materials and procedures that just do not make sense, given the child and situation. Numbers, scores, percentiles, and standard deviations are generated that simply do not inform instruction or guide intervention.

Assessment can, however, be useful in several ways. First, assessment can help us to identify functional objectives and goals for child and family. Second, assessment can sometimes inform us as to a child's preferred ways or styles of learning and interacting. Third, assessment can be useful in tracking and summarizing progress. In brief, assessment, when appropriately done, can tell us what to teach (content/curriculum), how to teach (methods), and whether objectives are being reached (monitoring/accountability).

Acceptability

Sometimes the content or methods of assessment may not be acceptable. There may be items or testing demands that run counter to ethnic or cultural preferences or practices. Item content may also sample events and things not typically encountered by children or their families, yet used to gauge cognitive status. Assessment is acceptable when professionals and parents agree on its content and methods and when information generated by it portrays socially detectable and socially valued competencies.

Authenticity

When assessment is authentic, it yields information about functional behavior in children's typical/natural settings—what they really know and do. The pitfalls of conventional testing—the unfamiliar adult, unrealistic test demands, and nonfunctional item content distilled through psychometric item selection—are avoided. Information gathered in authentic settings, within the child's own developmental ecology, often provides us with a very different picture of strengths and needs.

Equity

Federal law, ethics, and common sense require us to accommodate individual differences in instruction. I certainly would not use the same materials or expect the same responses from a child with typical hearing and a child who is deaf. I would, of course, provide alternate ways to communicate and alternative materials. I would try to provide equitable instruction. Children with significant sensory, motor, affective, and/or cultural differences are not to be expected to relate to the standard "one size fits all" instructional materials and procedures.

What about equity in assessment? Conventional testing, as discussed earlier, requires strict adherence to standardized procedures. All children, regardless of their differences, must be administered test items in the same way as the items were administered to children in the standardization group. And who is in the standardization groups? Recall that the standardization group in almost all cases is composed exclusively of children with typical development. These children can point, speak, sit, listen, explain, and tolerate a stranger in ways that children with special needs might not. In fact, children with significant problems are excluded from standardization samples. What is wrong with this picture? The procedures are developed for a smooth administration with "standard children," but we do not typically need to assess these children. When we are forced to use standard procedures with "nonstandard" children, we have a dilemma: if one does not accommodate for differences, the child is penalized and results are questionable at best; if one alters the procedures, one has "violated standardization"! The crucial issue here is that conventional testing has built-in contradictions; it is not equitable, nor can it be. This issue is "high stakes" when testing "intelligence" or progress within an intervention program.

Sensitivity

Materials that are more sensitive provide more items within an age or skill range. More items permit greater precision for estimating child status and for tracking progress. As an example, a developmental or functional sequence of items related to communication skills will be more sensitive if it includes 100 instead of only 10 items. Some materials designed for assessment of more severe impairments must be sensitive in order to gauge minimal functioning and detect small increments of change. Many conventional tests are unsuitable for planning or progress monitoring, especially tests based on traits or constructs, such as intelligence tests; they do not offer adequate item density for detecting change. The need for program accountability argues for the use of tools that can detect intervention-related progress, in other words, assessment that is sensitive.

Convergence

Because teamwork is essential for gathering a wide base of information, we need materials that enable us to pool or to converge information. Materials facilitate convergence when professionals from multiple disciplines, as well as parents, can use them. Many new materials provide ways to gather information from multiple sources and to pool evidence. Minimal jargon, friendly formats, and ease of use and reporting are factors that make information convergence more possible. Discipline-specific tools are, of course, needed and are often important for close-up assessment of specific problems in early childhood education. Such discipline-specific materials are typically not easily converged with other information, and require "translation" for other professionals, and certainly for parents. Curriculum-based assessment tools, on the other hand, are often usable by various professionals, allowing easy pooling of observations.

Collaboration

Authentic assessment requires teamwork; it is simply neither feasible nor sensible for one person to observe and record child functioning across developmental domains, across several everyday settings, and over several occasions. Working in union with assessment partners allows us to assemble authentic information for worthwhile decision making. Finally, I enable parent collaboration when I offer the ways and means for significant parent input. Some assessment materials, for example, provide parent-friendly versions for child appraisal, or I can make available video cameras or other ways to facilitate parent participation.

Congruence

This final standard is actually one that, if followed, offers some guarantee of equity, technical adequacy, and a valid evidence base. Congruence refers to the similarity between the children employed during a test's development and the children whom you wish to assess. Many new (and some older) materials include children with specific special needs. Clearly, a scale or curriculum designed and developed for children with visual impairments would be a smart choice to use with such children. Some materials can be employed with children who have either typical or impaired vision when suggested and alternative administration procedures and items are provided and permitted. When selecting assessment materials, then, it is important to learn about the characteristics of the children involved in the development and field testing of the materials. When the child you are to assess is similar to children employed in the development of the materials, you can be somewhat assured that administration procedures will be suitable. Congruence requires that the assessment measure be developed for and field validated on children with special needs. When a measure is congruent, it demonstrates a clear evidence base in research.

Technology

Work to replace archaic paper-and-pencil tests and contrived test kits with more modern technologies; incorporate diverse forms of portable computer devices as essential supports to implement authentic observational assessments; new technologies include Palm Pilots loaded with the observational assessment items and rubrics, miniaturized videotaping capabilities, and web-based interfaces for in-situ data entry, profiling, analysis, and archiving.

Outcomes

Align assessment content with overarching school and government standards, indicators, and benchmarks of the expected competencies for early learning and school success; map assessed content to the ultimate state education early learning standards so that there exists an essential similarity among sampled and predicted behaviors for early school success; children's progress and success should be determined by their acquisition of the overarching expected performance standards of their school or state rather than their performance on test-derived content, especially if the test content is nonfunctional and noncurricular.

WHAT IS THE AUTHENTIC ASSESSMENT ALTERNATIVE?

Authentic Assessment refers to the systematic recording of developmental observations over time by familiar and knowledgeable caregivers about the naturally occurring competencies of young children in daily routines.
—BAGNATO AND YEH HO (2006)

Authentic assessment is a deliberate plan for investigating the natural behavior of young children. Information is captured through direct observation and recordings, interviews, rating scales, and observed samples of the natural or facilitated play and daily living skills of children.

There are four major differences between authentic assessment and conventional testing: where it's done, what is assessed, how it's done, and who does it. First, a crucial distinction is the *context* (the "where") for assessment. Authentic assessment relies on information that can be obtained only in the child's natural environments. These environments are the ongoing, daily routines and typical circumstances of the child. Examples of natural environments are children at play in their own preschools, at home during bath time, at child care, in the supermarket, and at church. This contrasts with the decontextualized, contrived arrangements that characterize conventional, psychometric practices. Conventional testing environments typically employ a clinic or "laboratory" setting such as testing rooms of schools or hospital examination rooms. As pointed out, conventional testing focuses upon standardized item content (the "what") and has little instructional use. By contrast, items for authentic assessment are real behaviors that have functional importance to children and their progress (e.g., getting across the room, communicating wants and needs, selecting an apple rather than a pear, and figuring out how a toy works). Note that these are all competencies that are worthwhile, teachable, and socially valued. Field validation and norming of assessment instruments for individuals with disabilities must emphasize the standardization of the *function rather than form* of the behavior under examination. Conventional testing records the child's narrow response to standardized objects and procedures and does not permit accommodations for special needs (the "how"). Authentic assessment relies on natural observations of the child's response to daily routines; in this context, the child can demonstrate competency in any way possible. The child who is blind can show object permanence by exploring the environment tactilely in search of a hidden toy; authentic assessment does not require the child to show only the narrow response of finding and seeing a hidden toy under a standard cup.

Authentic content invites teaching because the items are precursive to or are part of the curriculum. With a functional approach, the playing field for documenting capabilities becomes level and noninferential. Conventional psychometric items are not building blocks for future competency, and psychometric procedures prohibit "teaching to the test," and thus are insensitive to functional progress and outcomes.

Only specific professionals, often psychologists, are permitted to conduct traditional, psychometric testing (the "who"). These professionals are often not integral members of a child's program and are most probably strangers to the children. In most cases, these unfamiliar professionals administer tests as individuals rather than as true team members. On the other hand, authentic assessment depends upon the observations of familiar adults in the child's life to provide convergent data on real-life functioning. An array of family members, babysitters, teachers, and interdisciplinary professionals form a team that knows the child well and works to help the child.

Research Support for the Authentic Alternative

Bagnato, Suen, Brickley, Smith-Jones, and Dettore (2002) published a longitudinal study of the developmental impact and outcomes of an early childhood intervention model for children in high-risk communities. An "authentic assessment and program evaluation" model was employed with 1,350 children over a 3-year period of intervention to profile child progress. The Developmental Observation Checklist System (DOCS; Hresko, 1994) was modified so that over 125 early care and education providers could use it to record natural observations of child skills in everyday classroom routines. A weekly mentoring system was employed to teach the providers the specifics of conducting quarterly child assessments that would inform classroom learning activities, communications with parents, and documentation of child progress. The results of the 3-year study demonstrated the feasibility, utility, and validity of the authentic assessment methodology and the efficacy of the program.

In an article designated as the 1995 "Best Research Article" by Division 16 of the American Psychological Association, Bagnato and Neisworth (1995) documented the extent to which traditional tests of intelligence and development were inappropriate and failed to accomplish early intervention purposes for eligibility determination and assessment in the actual daily activities of over 250 preschool psychologists in 33 states working with over 7,000 children. In summary, the national survey research demonstrated that nearly 60% of the children would have been declared "untestable" if the psychologists had followed procedures in the test manuals. Major reasons for the child's inability to respond to the tests included behavior at odds with test requirements, lack of language, poor motor skills, poor social skills, and lack of attention and other self-control behaviors. On average, psychologists followed their state requirements to use traditional tests by devoting about 90 minutes to each testing, achieving "untestable" results. After futile effort, however, these expert psychologists were able to work with their teams to declare over 90% of the children eligible for early intervention services by using alternative and authentic measures to guide their decisions; the appropriate measures used included parent observations and reports, curriculum-based assessments by teachers and providers, play-based assessments, and observations of behavior at home or in the preschool. Clearly, both the required standardized tests and inflexible state regulations served as barriers to appropriate evaluations.

Studies demonstrate that the reliability and validity of assessments and associated decision making for children with disabilities are increased when parents and team members are involved (Briggs, 1997; Suen, Logan, Neisworth, & Bagnato, 1995; Suen, Lu, Neisworth, & Bagnato, 1993). The message of the research is "two heads are indeed better than one" when assessing the status and progress of young children with special needs. Using generalizability analysis techniques, the researchers demonstrated that each assessor added a unique dimension to the final assessment "portrait" for each child. Having additional members on the team was essential to accurate diagnosis, while single-member assessments tended to be unreliable and unrepresentative. Similarly, parent congruence with professional assessments should not be required, nor expected; because parents add information from natural contexts about important, often neglected, aspects of functioning (e.g., sleep routines, play with friends, interactions with grandparents, self-care skills, social and self-regulatory skills with familiar people).

Performance-based or authentic assessment has also been studied for children in kindergarten and the early primary grades (Meisels et al., 2002; Meisels, Bickel, Nicholson, Xue, & Atkins-Burnett, 2001). The results of these studies demonstrate clearly that ongoing teacher assessments of children's learning within the school curriculum that are structured by a type of curriculum-based instrument accurately identify and predict those children who will perform well and those who are at risk. In addition, the curriculum-based assessment (CBA) instrument (Work Sampling System) enhanced teaching, improved learning through feedback, and boosted scores on conventional group accountability tests of achievement.

The *TRACE Center for Excellence in Early Childhood Assessment* is a multicenter initiative funded by the U.S. Department of Education, Office of Special Education Programs, to conduct research on the evidence base for early childhood assessment practices. I am a co-investigator in TRACE and director of the Pennsylvania satellite through my Early Childhood Partnerships program (see *www.uclid.org*). Carl J. Dunst and Carol M. Trivette serve as co-directors and principal investigators of the TRACE Center. The new TRACE center unites researchers at the four satellite locations of the Puckett Institute (Asheville, North Carolina) with colleagues at Children's Hospital of Pittsburgh and the UCLID Center at the University of Pittsburgh, the Institute for Family-Centered Care (Bethesda, Maryland), the Family, Infant and Preschool Program (Morganton, North Carolina), and Mission St. Joseph's Health System (St. Louis, Missouri).

The 5-year grant will enable the national researchers at the four satellite centers to study and promote the use of the most beneficial and promising practices for identifying and evaluating infants, toddlers, and preschoolers who have or are at risk for disabilities or delays. Literature reviews and targeted studies to establish the evidence base are being conducted currently on a variety of topics including clinical judgment, team assessment models, authentic versus conventional measurement, Child Find, eligibility determination criteria, and validity of the "delay" concept.

TRACE researchers will collaborate with state and federal government officials to determine how regulatory policies and professional standards can be refined to enhance the use of effective early childhood assessments to identify young children with special needs and to better plan their programs and track their progress.

A CONTINUUM OF MEASUREMENT CONTEXTS

To organize and illustrate differences among assessment approaches, I offer a continuum of measurement contexts (see Table 2.2). The continuum encompasses four categories: (1) clinical, (2) simulated, (3) analogue, and (4) natural. Each category is discussed below.

Clinical

The most decontextualized measurement practices are traditional psychometric tests such as the Stanford–Binet Intelligence Scale (Thorndike, Hagen, & Sattler, 2003), the Wechsler Preschool and Primary Scale of Intelligence (Wechsler, 2002), and similar materials, including achievement and knowledge tests and personality measures. "Clinical" refers to highly scripted examiner behavior and the recording of highly scripted or "tested" child behavior in laboratory-like settings. Clinical settings ("where") are the most contrived circumstances and bear virtually no resemblance to the natural environments in which young children typically function.

TABLE 2.2. Continuum of Measurement Contexts

	Decontextualized			Contextualized
	Clinical	Simulated	Analogue	Natural
Where?	Laboratory situations	Replica situations	Everyday routines	Everyday routines
What?	Standard responses to standard stimuli	On-demand behaviors	Prompted natural behaviors	Spontaneous behaviors
How?	Psychometric tests	Structured tests and/or observation schedules	Direct observation; parent report; interview	Direct observation; parent report; interview
Who?	Certified/licensed professionals	Certified/licensed professionals	Professionals and caregivers	Professionals and caregivers

It is important to emphasize that administering a measure such as the Stanford–Binet in the child's home or preschool classroom does not make the testing more natural or authentic. The act of using the test in the child's everyday settings merely disrupts the flow of the child's natural activity and the contextual supports for behavior. In addition, such measures do not meet the eight standards for developmentally appropriate assessment previously discussed, especially the requirement for parent participation in the assessment. Previous studies and position statements (Bagnato & Neisworth, 1995; Neisworth & Bagnato, 1994) demonstrate clearly that traditional intelligence tests in use by even specially trained preschool psychologists fail to accomplish the major purposes of assessment for early intervention.

Simulated

We are all familiar with the use of testing rooms and clinics where more familiar, typical arrangements are introduced in order to make the environment less threatening. In this approach, concessions are made in favor of the natural environment, but they are often of a token nature. There is a soft rug on the floor, the testing table and chair are child-size, perhaps there is even a sofa or comfortable easy chair for the parent, and so forth. In general, the attempt is to have the office or clinic vaguely resemble a child's natural or typical environment. Many pediatric wards, for example, are now decorated to resemble a playful day care environment, with colorful walls (instead of the sterile white walls of the past), posters, and toys. Certainly, simulated arrangements are an improvement over the cold and intimidating circumstances that so often are imposed on children and their parents. Knowing what we do about behavior, we all should be clear that the closer the simulation, the greater the chance that typical behavior will be evidenced (i.e., enhanced generalization). As noted, however, simulation is often minimal, and the unfamiliarity of the setting and the testing demands trumps any efforts to make child and parents "feel at home." Drawbacks in the location of the testing situation, often at a testing room off the classroom, clinic, office, or even hospital, are certainly hard to overcome. Further, the time of day for the testing appointment is often driven by administrative convenience and contradicts the child's typical schedule and circumstances. The unfamiliarity of the person doing the assessment is supposedly diminished by "establishing rapport," but how and when that is achieved is not clear, and rarely a concern for the busy professional. A "simulated rapport" is about all that one can hope for in these circumstances.

The materials presented to the child may be modified, again in an attempt to approach the child's natural circumstances. Perhaps the child's toy is substituted for a toy in the testing kit; perhaps the child's friends' names are used in the questioning. Children are prompted to show a skill, or to play with objects provided by the tester.

Increasingly, revisions of standardized instruments are including recommendations for more flexible administration and the use of more child-friendly materials (popular toys). Nevertheless, the materials seldom permit too much variance from "standardized administration," that is, procedures standardized with children of typical development. These and other adjustments are attempted in recognition of the advantages of observing child behavior in context—but such efforts fall far short of observing and recording a child's real behavior in real settings. Arena assessment procedures and the Bayley Scales of Infant Development (Bayley, 1993) are examples of simulated assessment practices.

Analogue

Analogue practices involve arranging circumstances in the child's natural settings in order to increase the likelihood of occurrences of typical behavior. Daily settings are the contexts ("where") for analogue assessments, but behavior is prompted or motivated by the choice of toys and materials in these settings to create increased occasions for it to be observed. Sometimes, analogue arrangements reduce the need for protracted observation. Analogue assessments, use developmental observations as the preferred mode ("how") of examining and recording the display of these prompted play skills. Assessments associated with the analogue practices include the Communication and Symbolic Behavior Scales—Developmental Profile (Prizant & Wetherby, 2002), the DOCS, and Transdisciplinary Play-Based Assessment (Linder, 1999).

Natural

Assessment practices that are natural in character are distinguished in three ways. The "what" (content) refers only to naturally occurring behaviors; the "where" (context) refers to natural environments, namely, the child's everyday circumstances. Finally, the "how" refers to natural observations of the play and learning behaviors of children. Examples of natural or authentic assessment methods include functional behavior assessment and direct observation and recording of behavior. Also, studies have validated the utility of the DOCS (Hresko, 1994) for authentic assessments in early childhood program outcomes research (Bagnato, 2002; Bagnato et al., 2002). Natural or authentic assessments are the most contextualized practices on the continuum. Authentic assessments in the natural context include the Pediatric Evaluation of Disability Inventory (PEDI) and the Ages and Stages Questionnaire (ASQ).

THE AUTHENTIC ASSESSMENT ADVANTAGE

Early childhood specialists can use the continuum of measurement contexts as a guide to materials and practices. I contend that *context* is the major criterion regarding the evidence-based validity of authentic assessment practices over traditional psychometric testing. Researchers and policy makers have begun to recognize the overriding importance of context. The President's Commission on Special Education advanced recommendations to dramatically alter the purpose and activities of assessment (National Academy of Sciences, 2002). Referring to significant failures in appropriately identifying and assessing the needs of minority children and individuals with learning disabilities and other serious developmental disabilities, the National Academy of Sciences (NAS) stated that "while an IQ test may provide supplemental information, no IQ test should be required, and the results should not be the primary criterion on which eligibility rests . . . *the committee regards the effort to assess students' decontextualized potential or ability as inappropriate and scientifically invalid* [italics mine]" (p. 8). The committee recommended more authentic alternatives including structured team decision-making processes, and the observational recording of changes in the child's skill acquisition during participation in tailored interventions with individualized instructional modifications.

WHAT ARE GUIDELINES FOR AUTHENTIC ASSESSMENT IN ACTION?

It is one thing to propose a conceptual model for the authentic assessment alternative to conventional testing, but quite another to demonstrate how it can be put into action. In the following paragraphs, I discuss considerations and recommendations regarding how authentic assessment can be implemented in real-life circumstances.

• *Share assessment responsibilities with a team.* Assessment in early childhood must be a team enterprise, especially for children with serious disabilities. Professionals in early intervention must be committed to the worth and advantages of sharing assessment duties with parents, other important caregivers in the child's life (e.g., grandparents, babysitters), and various interdisciplinary team members. Teachers and child care providers are perhaps the most important sources of information about child performance, along with the parents.

• *Conduct assessment over time.* Professionals often wonder how they can do authentic assessments when they require time to observe the naturally occurring behaviors of young children with disabilities, some of whom have limited and inconsistent skill repertoires. I recommend that the team consider using a combination of natural and analogue practices to capture child capabilities; moreover, the assessment can be spread over a 15- to 30-day time frame for multiple children when conducting assessments for eligibility determination. In this way, multiple observers can use the same or similar observational measures such as the DOCS (Hresko, 1994) and the PEDI (Haley, Coster, Ludlow, Haltiwanger, & Andrellos, 1992) to record spontaneous and/or prompted behaviors across several everyday settings.

• *Become the "orchestrator" of authentic assessments across people, contexts, and occasions.* The team leader can frame his or her primary role as that of the orchestrator of authentic assessments and a facilitator of parent–professional decision-making. The assessment process can be organized so that everyone's role in collecting unique or corroborative information about child capabilities and needs is clear. Similarly, an organized assessment process can ensure that comprehensive and representative information on child performance is collected across several people, situations, and times. Parents can observe and record unique information about the child's self-care, temperament, play, and sleep habits at home and with relatives and friends.

• *Match the team assessment model to the child.* The advantages of interdisciplinary and transdisciplinary styles of teamwork for early intervention have been explored previously (Bagnato & Neisworth, 1991; Briggs, 1997). Similarly, the incompatibility of the multidisciplinary approach for early childhood has been documented. I recommend that early intervention teams use a process of collaborative decision making to determine the style of teamwork that is preferred by both parents and the involved professionals and that matches the functional needs of the child. For example, authentic assessments in an analogue context can be completed for a child with cerebral palsy by having the teacher, physical therapist, and parent prompt play behaviors in the home or classroom, and by observing how the child communicates, plays with toys, and moves about in natural activities.

• *Rely on parent judgments and observations.* Despite best practices and regulations, many professionals are still leery about relying on parent information, suspicious that it is biased and unreliable. In fact, however, parent involvement in the assessment process offers important information about the child's emerging skills, other subtle and inconsistently expressed attributes, and descriptions of critical aspects of temperament or behavioral style. As parents partner with professionals over a longer time period, trust develops and their developmental observations become more mutually attuned.

• *Select a common instrument to unify interdisciplinary and interagency teamwork.* Interdisciplinary professionals on a team can choose a common measure such as a curriculum-based instrument to unify the work of the team in the assessment process. A system such as the Assessment,

Evaluation, and Programming System (AEPS; Bricker, Cripe, & Slentz, 2003) enables professionals and parents to survey all aspects of development and behavior in an organized manner while focusing on a common core of functional objectives for both assessment and programming. In addition, I recommend that agencies responsive for implementing early intervention services facilitate transition and planning partly through the use of a common authentic assessment tool like the AEPS or other such scales.

• *Employ jargon-free materials.* Esoteric professional jargon prevents clear communication among parents and professionals. The use of assessment tools with clear content and objectives (i.e., "finds the correct toy at the bottom of a toy box," "lets you know what he means," or "uses eyes and hands together") allows all team members, including parents, to understand and agree on objectives.

• *Use sensitive instruments to gauge child progress.* Most often, conventional measures of intelligence and development lack the sensitivity to profile the status and progress of children with significant functional limitations. These scales lack a sufficient density of items at lower levels (e.g., floors); their normative samples do not include children with disabilities and thus generate standard scores, which do not describe lower functional levels (e.g., lowest attainable score is 50).

Team members can choose authentic curriculum-based measures that have been field validated on children with disabilities and have the needed equity and sensitivity features. Various techniques can be used to score and profile child status and progress, including graduated scoring options (1–7 scale) to capture the stimulus conditions under which performance is enhanced, ratio quotients, functional ages, growth curves, goal attainment scaling, and hierarchies of skill acquisition (Bagnato, Neisworth, & Munson, 1997).

• *Use technology to facilitate authentic assessments and progress or program evaluations.* Increasingly, teams are using various forms of technology to conduct authentic assessments in an efficient way. Videotaping of the child's and parent's interactive behaviors at home or in the community is a common way for a team representative to capture functional information for view by the entire team. Such video samples can be recorded on DVDs to compare past performance and observable progress that is indisputable.

Computer software packages enable interdisciplinary teams to conduct an itemized performance analysis of data on individual children and groups on authentic assessment instruments. These programs (e.g., Bagnato, 2002) not only generate individualized goals and learning experiences to be infused into daily care and education routines but can also profile developmental growth curves from authentic assessment data. Analyses can be performed on the archived data to document child progress, intervention outcomes, and program impact for teachers, parents, community stakeholders, and funding and oversight agencies.

CONCLUSIONS

Early childhood education and intervention have become national priorities. The humanitarian as well as cost benefits of early intervention are increasingly recognized, resulting in renewed political attention and financial support. Assessment plays a pivotal role in the design, delivery, and evaluation of early childhood intervention programs. Use of decontextualized conventional testing must be abandoned in favor of in-context authentic assessment. Observation and reporting of actual achievement, rather than inferences about competence based on global trait-based testing, provide real evidence of real child progress and program impact. The time has come for measurement that brings professionals and parents together; that directly informs intervention; and that enables professionals to record functional child progress and to document the success of programs. We must promote assessment that serves the social and humanitarian interests of children, professionals, and those who fund and support the education of all young children, especially those who are most vulnerable.

BEST-PRACTICE GUIDEPOINTS

♦ Abandon the use of conventional tests and testing practices with young children, particularly those with disabilities.

♦ Use authentic assessment methods and procedures to accomplish all early childhood intervention purposes, including eligibility determination.

♦ Eliminate tabletop testing procedures with contrived test kits.

♦ Share assessment responsibilities with a team of parents/caregivers and professionals working together.

♦ Conduct assessments over time rather than in one session.

♦ Orchestrate assessments across several people, places, and times.

♦ Use an assessment style that is acceptable to parents, matched to the child's needs, and likely to provide optimal information on functional capabilities.

♦ Learn to rely on parent information as another crucial source of information about child functioning guided by the use of jargon-free materials.

♦ Within a program, select a common curriculum-based instrument to unify interdisciplinary and interagency teamwork.

♦ Select instruments that have some "universal" attributes and can sensitively monitor child progress.

♦ Incorporate portable, computer-based technologies to make assessments more natural, efficient, and practical.

BEST-PRACTICE EVIDENCE

Bagnato, S. J. (2002). *Quality early learning: Key to school success.* Pittsburgh: Early Childhood Partnerships, Children's Hospital of Pittsburgh and the Heinz Endowments.

Bagnato, S. J., & Neisworth, J. T. (1991). *Assessment for early intervention: Best practices for professionals.* New York: Guilford Press.

Bagnato, S. J., & Neisworth, J. T. (1995). A national study of the social and treatment "invalidity" of intelligence testing in early intervention. *School Psychology Quarterly, 9*(2), 81–102.

Bagnato, S. J., Neisworth, J. T., & Munson, S. M. (1997). *LINKing assessment and early intervention: An authentic curriculum-based approach.* Baltimore: Brookes.

Bagnato, S. J., Suen, H., Brickley, D., Smith-Jones, J., & Dettore, E. (2002). Child developmental impact of Pittsburgh's Early Childhood Initiative (ECI): First-phase authentic evaluation research. *Early Childhood Research Quarterly, 17*(4), 559–580.

Bagnato, S. J., & Yeh-Ho, H. (2006). High-stakes testing of preschool children: Viola standards for professional and evidence-based practice. *International Journal of Korean Educational Policy, 3*(1), 23–43.

Bayley, N. (1993). *Bayley Scales of Infant Development—2nd edition.* San Antonio, TX: Psychological Corporation.

Bredekamp, S., & Copple, C. (1997). *Developmentally appropriate practice in early childhood programs* (rev. ed.). Washington, DC: National Association for the Education of Young Children.

Bricker, D., Cripe, J., & Slentz, K. (2003). *Assessment, Evaluation, and Programming System (AEPS).* Baltimore: Brookes.

Briggs, M. H. (1997). *Building early intervention teams.* Gaithersburg, MD: Aspen.

Fowler, O. S., & Fowler, L. N. (1855). *The illustrated self-instructor in phrenology and physiology.* New York: Fowler & Wells.

Gould, S. J. (1981). *The mismeasure of man.* New York: Norton.

Haley, S. M., Coster, W. J., Ludlow, L. H., Haltiwanger, J. T., & Andrellos, P. J. (1992). *Pediatric Evaluation of Disability Inventory.* Boston: PEDI Research Group.

Head Start Bureau. (2001). *Head start program performance standards and other regulations.* Washington, DC: U.S. Department of Health and Human Services, Administration on Children, Youth, and Families.

Hresko, W. (1994). *Developmental Observation Checklist System.* Austin, TX: PRO-ED.

Kaplan, A. (1964). *The conduct of inquiry.* San Francisco: Chandler.

Linder, T. (1999). *Transdisciplinary play-based assessment.* Baltimore: Brookes.

Meisels, S. J., Atkins-Burnett, S., Xue, Y., Nicholson, J., Bickel, D., & Son, S. (2002). Creating a system of accountability: The impact of instructional assessment on elementary children's achievement test scores. *American Educational Research Journal, 39*(1), 3–25.

Meisels, S. J., Bickel, D., Nicholson, J., Xue, Y., & Atkins-Burnett, S. (2001). Trusting teacher judgments: A validity study of a curriculum-embedded performance assessment in kindergarten to grade 3. *American Educational Research Journal, 38*(1), 73–95.

National Academy of Sciences. (2002). *NAS/NRC Report on minority students in special education*. Washington, DC: National Research Council/National Academy of Sciences.

Neisworth, J. T., & Bagnato, S. J. (1994). The case against intelligence testing in early intervention. *Topics in Early Childhood Special Education, 12*(11), 1–20.

Neisworth, J. T., & Bagnato, S. J. (2004). The mismeasure of young children: The authentic assessment alternative. *Infants and Young Children, 17*(4), 198–212.

Neisworth, J. T., & Bagnato, S. J. (2005). DEC recommended practices: Assessment. In S. Sandall, M. L. Hemmeter, B. J. Smith, & M. E. McLean (Eds.), *DEC recommended practices: A comprehensive guide for practical application in early interventional/early childhood special education* (pp. 45–61). Longmont, CO: Sopris West.

Prizant, B., & Wetherby, A. (2002). *The Communication and Symbolic Behavior Scales— Developmental Profile*. Baltimore: Brookes.

Sandall, S., McLean, M. E., & Smith, B. J. (2000). *DEC recommended practices in early intervention/early childhood special education*. Longmont, CO: Sopris West.

Suen, H. K., Logan, C. R., Neisworth, J. T., & Bagnato, S. J. (1993). Measurement of team decision-making through generalizability theory. *Journal of Psychoeducational Assessment, 11*, 120–132.

Suen, H. K., Lu, C. H., Neisworth, J. T., & Bagnato, S. J. (1993). Parent–professional congruence: Is it necessary? *Journal of Early Intervention, 19*(3), 243–252.

Thorndike, R. L., Hagen, E. P., & Sattler, J. M. (2003). *Stanford–Binet Intelligence Scale—4th Edition: Professional manual*. Itasco, IL: Riverside.

Wechsler, D. (2002). *Wechsler Preschool and Primary Scale of Intelligence—3rd Edition: Professional manual*. San Antonio, TX: Psychological Corporation.

CHAPTER 3

◆ ◆ ◆

What Are the Foundations for Authentic Assessment of Typical and Atypical Early Development?

◆

BEST-PRACTICE ISSUES

◆ Why is an understanding of principles of development important for assessment of young children if we use standardized scales?

◆ Do infants who are blind have object permanence?

◆ How does interaction with the environment promote early development for children with special needs?

◆ How common are attention problems and overactive behavior in early development?

◆ Can infants and toddlers show self-control behaviors?

◆ Why should IQ tests not be used with preschoolers who have cerebral palsy?

Young children develop abilities and learn skills through a universal set of principles and operations. Research in early childhood intervention strives to operationalize those principles so that professionals and parents can understand young children more sensitively and can plan treatment programs more effectively. Many early intervention programs merge two sets of principles and methods to promote gains for infants and preschoolers with delays and disabilities: *developmental* and *behavioral*. A combined *developmental–behavioral approach* recognizes that children's capabilities emerge in an invariant, sequential manner that is directly linked with neurophysiological factors. However, developmental capabilities, particularly for children with disabilities, emerge only when specific environmental opportunities to practice, learn, and generalize these skills in interaction with others are provided. Thus, various early intervention programs hold that developmental principles provide the *content* (e.g., developmental curricula and toys) of their program whereas behavioral principles provide the *methods* of teaching complex patterns of skills. This chapter reviews two topics relating to infant and early childhood development: (1) principles and assumptions within a developmental approach, and (2) typical and atypical patterns of development in infants and young children.

PRINCIPLES AND ASSUMPTIONS
OF A DEVELOPMENTAL PERSPECTIVE

Development is an orderly and sequential process of increasing refinement of the child's neurological, sensorimotor, and cognitive-behavioral capabilities. However, development is not an isolated process or series of events that occurs only *within* the child. Rather, it is the outcome of the child's continuous interactions with people and events in the immediate environment. These reciprocal interactions are important opportunities for the child to activate and practice emerging abilities. Developmental perspectives that stress the crucial importance of the child's environmental transactions for promoting progress are called *developmental interactionist* theories. Principles and characteristics of typical and atypical development within these theories are summarized in Table 3.1 and discussed more broadly in the following sections:

Active

Development used to be viewed narrowly as the result of the impact of environmental and/or innate biological factors. In contrast, child development specialists today emphasize that each child is an active agent in promoting his or her own course of progress. Children both create and react to situational events. Their own behaviors initiate and maintain reciprocal "give-and-take" interactions with adults. In turn, these reciprocal interactions, created by each child, become further opportunities for learning. Infants gradually learn that crying, cooing, smiling, body activity, and direct eye gaze make adults come to them in a regular manner. They begin to understand their own competence in shaping events in their world. It is

TABLE 3.1. Principles of Typical and Atypical Early Development

1. The child is an *active* participant in promoting development.
2. The child is increasingly *competent* in using adaptive abilities to change the environment.
3. Development is *interactive*; it depends on reciprocal exchanges between the child's neurodevelopmental functions and the social and physical aspects of the world.
4. The child's developmental course involves highly *organized* patterns of sensorimotor and cognitive–adaptive processes.
5. Development is *multidimensional*: it reflects the emergence of interrelated cognitive, sensorimotor, and social processes.
6. Development is characterized by the emergence of invariant and *sequential* stages or patterns of behavior.
7. Development proceeds according to *individual* rates.
8. Development consists of *variable* behavioral patterns of plateaus, regressions, and accelerations.
9. The child's behavior proceeds from undifferentiated toward highly *specialized* clusters of developmental skills.
10. Development, although involving "sensitive" growth phases, is *flexible*; alternative routes lead to the acquisition of the same basic adaptive skills.
11. Development and dysfunctions are caused by the interplay of multiple personal and environmental variables–*multicausal*.
12. The child's neurodevelopmental system is highly *sensitive* in responding to appropriately timed opportunities to practice and learn adaptive skills involving thinking, communicating, and socializing.

certainly true that environment and heredity are the raw materials for development, but the *interaction* of the child with the environment is the crucial factor.

Competent

Infants display a wide range of sensorimotor and adaptive skills at an early age. These abilities involve skills in such areas as visual–motor coordination, cognition, language use, and social attachment. As abilities in different processes become coordinated, children gain the capacity to exert greater control over their world. For example, with more refined coordination of visual and motor functions, infants can grasp and manipulate rattles and bells and learn that their movements make toys move and sound. This skill not only fosters a sense of mastery but also enhances attention, memory, and the capacity to form intentions to guide goal-directed behavior. Similarly, infant vocalizations and smiling also encourage social interactions with caretakers.

Interactive

Development and learning proceed because children, whether normal or handicapped, engage in reciprocal interactions with their world. The most basic adaptive act of the infant and young child is initiating and responding to changes in this environment. Thus, interactions with people and objects serve as continuous opportunities for the young child to activate and practice emerging abilities. Most major theories of child development stress the central role of the child's environmental exchanges in fostering growth and progress. Behavioral perspectives refer to these transactions as *stimulus–response opportunities* whereas Piagetian views talk of "co-occurrences."

Essentially, regular interactions with the environment enable the developing child to be continuously aware of a variety of events that involve such contiguous chains of behavior as the visual appearance of the mother and mother's vocal sound; moving the hand and touching a rattle that sounds; crying and the mother's approach to end crying. The child's ability to detect and remember such related events greatly influences the course of language, social, and cognitive development. Similarly, children with sensorimotor impairments have a reduced probability of experiencing connections between their own actions and the environmental changes that they can produce. Developmental intervention, in its most basic sense, must design natural but alternative experiences that increase opportunities or co-occurrences for the handicapped child.

Organized

The emergence and refinement of neurodevelopmental skills in children is a highly organized process. This process encompasses many areas of behavior (e.g., cognitive, language, affective, social, sensorimotor) that develop simultaneously and in a sequential fashion according to age and individual readiness. Transformations in developmental skills occur as children grow. These transformations take place when abilities merge, as seen in the influence of language on memory, reasoning, and self-regulation.

Multidimensional

Development consists of processes that have multiple functions that must be monitored separately. These processes involve multiple domains such as cognition, imitation, language comprehension and expression, gross motor skills, perceptual–fine motor abilities, social and emotional responses, self-care skills, self-regulation, and temperamental style. Such a breakdown is somewhat artificial but is a necessary basis for detecting developmental problems and planning individual learning experiences. Moreover, each of these general developmental processes consists of sequenced subskills that serve as the building blocks for acquiring more specialized competencies.

Sequential

Children do not pass through stages of development at the same age; however, most children attain the substages of cognitive, language, sensorimotor, and affective development in the same order. The acquisition of skills or abilities at earlier stages is a crucial prerequisite for the learning of more complex skills at later stages. In one sense, there is a "building block" character to skill development. Nevertheless, the process is gradual and relies on subtle quality changes in the individual child's perception of how behavior influences people and objects.

Individual

Despite the fixed order of growth in stages, each child develops specific skills at an individual rate. Furthermore, each child displays a unique temperamental style (e.g., content, difficult, hypersensitive, active, slow to adapt) that is partly innate and that influences the child's readiness to develop skills and to interact with people and objects. For example, the notion of individual rates and styles of development can be seen in the ages at which children typically acquire basic behavioral skills. By 8 months of age, 50% of children develop the ability to understand that an object still exists, even when it is hidden (object permanence). However, some children acquire that capacity as early as 6 months of age, still others as late as 15 months of age. Individual variations, whether involving normal differences or atypical deficiencies, must be considered in assessing and programming for young children.

Variable

A particular child does not always attain abilities in the areas of cognitive, language, motor, social, and self-help skills at the same time. Advances in one domain with slight lags in others are not uncommon. This pattern of variable rates of development is magnified in young children who experience sensorimotor and cognitive disabilities. For example, Martha is a 3-year-old child who shows average cognitive skills for her age but an immature style of playing with other children, adapting to strange situations, and separating from her mother. This behavior is more often typical of 2-year-old children. Similarly, some 3-year-old children with cerebral palsy may show nearly average learning abilities but severely impaired expressive language and upper-limb motor skills because of their neurological dysfunctions. Also, children with severe and profound mental retardation

develop cognitively according to the same invariant se~~
developing children but differ in terms of a slower an~~
of skill attainment. Children with Down's syndrome~~
variable rate of mastering such thinking skills as objec~~ _
relations, imitation, and causality.

Specialized

As children grow and develop, their behaviors become much more specialized in form and function. During the first 3 months of life, children's
behavior is characteristically imprecise and uncoordinated, owing to the
immaturity of the nervous system and the global and undifferentiated quality of sensory abilities (vision, hearing, touch) and motor functions (grasping and trunk control). However, with experience and maturation, children
learn to coordinate different behavioral functions so that their use becomes
much more specialized. Thus, the ability to track objects visually and to
focus enables the young infant to attend to rattles and rings placed in the
hand and to follow the movements of people and objects. Soon, the child's
sense of spatial relationships enables the coordination of vision with reaching and grasping to obtain toys that dangle out of reach. Thus, different
behaviors with separate functions are coordinated to form more specialized
behaviors, with unique functions.

Flexible

Hierarchical sequences of behaviors are characteristic of normal child
development. Nevertheless, research with groups of developmentally disabled children (blind, deaf, physically handicapped) indicates that the process of development and learning is *plastic* (i.e., it is possible to have alternative pathways and sequences for acquiring the same adaptive skills).
Despite the existence of "sensitive" growth periods when learning has its
greatest impact, alternative, adaptive developmental experiences can help
infants and young children acquire basic skills necessary for later learning.
Thus, blind children can acquire an understanding of the independent existence of hidden objects by learning to use their channels of hearing and
touch. Similarly, the child with cerebral palsy develops an understanding of
objects more through focused experiences in hearing and seeing rather than
through motor and tactile processes.

Multicausal

Current perspectives emphasize that multiple factors operate in shaping the
course of both normal and atypical development. Biological-genetic variables (prematurity, nutrition, family medical problems) and situational-

onmental variables (poverty, lack of appropriate learning experiences) eract to determine the child's future development and behavior.

Sensitive

Two interrelated concepts underlie the interactionist approach to developmental psychology: sensitive growth periods and "the problem of the match." The concept of *sensitive periods* refers to the belief that there are certain times when the child's neurobehavioral system is most receptive to stimulation and change. Thus, during these phases, appropriately timed learning experiences can have their greatest and most lasting impact. "We must hope to catch the child at exactly that time when environmental encounters will most effectively allow his or her hereditary potential to flourish" (Sprinthall & Sprinthall, 1981, p. 94).

Bound with the concept of sensitive periods is the strong belief that *stimulus variety* is essential for optimal development (i.e., providing diverse and frequent experiences that involve all sensory systems in encounters with people and objects). These opportunities are "peak" learning experiences that allow the child to understand how objects and events are related.

The crucial factor in effective learning during sensitive developmental phases is the "problem of the match." This concept, also called "goodness of fit," emphasizes that the type and amount of stimulation must be matched with each child's readiness to receive, integrate, and use it. Too much stimulation causes the child to be overwhelmed and frustrated, too little causes the child to become uninterested.

Learning experiences must take into account the child's behavioral style (e.g., quiet, content, active, irritable). The child's capacity to profit from different amounts of stimulation is influenced, for example, by poor attention, fear of loud noises, resistance to changes, and ability to understand new experiences. Between 5 and 8 months of age, an infant has the greatest readiness to learn about how objects are related. Simple informal games such as hiding toys under cloths, dropping objects into containers, and activating a jack-in-the-box toy are well suited to this stage. However, toys such as puzzles, telephones, and hammer–peg sets do not match the child's interests or developmental readiness at this time. A variety of well-timed learning opportunities and appropriate match with the child's needs and capabilities are the essential ingredients for developmental progress.

Three characteristics or principles regarding normal development are particularly applicable for understanding atypical development in young exceptional children: individual rates, multiple processes, and sensitive learning. In essence, each child's disabilities influence development in an individual manner. Similarly, because all areas of development are interdependent, functional disabilities in one area have an impact on the acquisition of skills in other areas. Nevertheless, my experience with young children has demonstrated that structured learning experiences provided during sensitive periods of growth can help each child to compensate for limitations and thus enhance developmental progress.

It is important to maintain the perspective that all developmental functions mature and emerge in an integrated fashion. It is not surprising that disabilities or dysfunctions in one area seriously influence the emergence of adaptive capabilities in other areas. The devastating impact of multiple disabilities on overall adaptive functioning is most evident, for example, in the areas of blind–deaf, cerebral palsy–developmental retardation. Table 3.2 presents information compiled from a variety of resources to illustrate the comparative impact of developmental disabilities on the timely emergence of cognitive–adaptive, and affective processes. The normal emergence of various capabilities is contrasted with the typical span of skill acquisition in children who are blind or have cerebral palsy. An analysis of such interrelated *dual* functions as reach–grasp and intentional actions, object constancy and separation anxiety, object constancy and reciprocal games, and smiling and approaching adults emphasizes the profound impact of physical and sensory impairments on cognitive and affective development.

Perspectives on assessing and educating young children with disabilities are intimately affected by these developmental principles. In particular, recent trends in special education emphasize a *functional* rather than a *categorical* approach to serving children with developmental disabilities. Rather than viewing them as occupying certain distinct categories (mentally retarded, neurologically impaired, emotionally disturbed), a functional perspective recognizes that children with different problems share dysfunctions across their behaviors and areas of developmental functioning. For example, Barry is mentally retarded and Martha has cerebral palsy, but both

TABLE 3.2. Developmental Disabilities and the Infant's Dual Cognitive–Adaptive and Affective Milestones

Process	Normal (months)	Blind (months)	Cerebral palsy (months)
Reach and grasp	3 to 5	10	14
Tactile–auditory patterns	4 to 6	9 to 12	15 to 20
Repeats purposeful acts	4 to 8	14	18
Extends arms to mother	3 to 5	8 to 12	18
Spontaneous smile	1 to 2	12	4
Object constancy	6 to 8	15 to 20	18
Separation anxiety	8 to 12	24 to 36	24
Word–object–person matches	12 to 14	20	18
Self-references (I, me)	30	36 to 54	42
Actual object representations	24 to 30	60	Incomplete
Reciprocal games (peek-a-boo)	6 to 8	14	12 to 14

may have severe deficits in their abilities to understand and use language. A functional description of the developmental skills that a particular child has or has not acquired in each behavioral area forms an accurate and practical basis for early intervention. Understanding normal developmental sequences in children, and how developmental disabilities inhibit and distort these sequences, enables early intervention specialists to serve infants and preschoolers with disabilities most effectively.

Research over the past decade has begun to detail the "typical" developmental progressions of children with multiple disabilities, but not enough is known. The following capsulized overview of developmental processes and disabilities in young children with disabilities is intended to provide substance to the "what" of developmental assessment and intervention and to highlight the complex interrelationships among emerging behavioral functions (Cohen & Gross, 1979).

NORMAL DEVELOPMENTAL PATTERNS

Cognitive Patterns

Definition

Cognitive developmental skills are a complex system of evolving problem-solving behaviors. These skills enable the developing child to understand complex interrelationships among people, objects, concepts, and events in the world—to comprehend, remember, compare, use, and master skills and experiences. One of the most important cognitive skills is the ability to integrate and apply clusters of related competencies in order to understand and solve problems in novel situations. This skill is the ability to transfer or generalize learning.

Perspective

Theories regarding cognitive skill development and learning come from Jean Piaget (1952) and Robert Gagne (1970). They add scope and substance to my view of emerging problem-solving abilities in young children. Piaget's cognitive developmental approach details the emergence and refinement of intellectual capabilities or styles of thinking in children; Gagne's focus on the learning process identifies the conditions under which behavior change and transformation in problem-solving occur.

Piaget advances the view that children learn by active sensory and motor play with objects and people in their world. Through this active, reciprocal partnership between the child and the environment, the child begins to form expectations about how objects and people behave. Each new experience adds to the child's perceptions of how behavior can influence events in the world (i.e., cause objects to move and people to come when the circumstances are right). In this evolving process, infants and young children modify their expectations about the world (*schemata*) and their ways of responding (*operations*) based on events happening as previously expected (*assimilation*) or requiring adjustments in typical behavior (*accommodation*). Discrepancies between old ways of behaving and the additional requirements of new situations cause uncertainty in the child (*disequilibrium*). This discrepancy serves as an incentive to promote a transformation leading to more effective ways of perceiving and responding. The four major stages, or phases of change, in the development of thinking skills according to Piaget are outlined with examples in Table 3.3. Two of these stages apply most readily to both typical infants and preschoolers and those with disabilities: the sensorimotor phase (0–24 months) and the intuitive or preoperational phase (24–48 months).

The salient feature of the *sensorimotor phase* is the child's exploration of the world through the combined use of the senses and fine and gross motor capabilities. The infant's activity is practical because it involves

TABLE 3.3. Characteristics and Achievements in Stages of Intellectual Development According to Piaget

Stage	Approximate age range (years)	Major characteristics and achievements
Sensorimotor period	0 to 2	Infant differentiates himself from other objects; seeks stimulation and prolongs interesting spectacles; attainment of object permanence; primitive understanding of causality, time, and space; means–end relationships; beginnings of imitation of absent, complex nonhuman stimuli; imaginative play and symbolic thought.
Preoperational period	2 to 6	Development of the symbolic function; symbolic use of language; intuitive problem solving; thinking characterized by irreversibility, centration, and egocentricity; beginnings of attainment of conservation of number and ability to think in classes and see relationships.
Period of concrete operations	6 or 7 through 11 or 12	Conservation of mass, length, weight, and volume; reversibility, decentration, ability to take role of others; logical thinking involving concrete operations of conservation of number and ability to think in classes and see relationships.
Period of formal operations	11 or 12 on	Flexibility, abstraction, mental hypotheses testing, and consideration of possible alternatives in complex reasoning and problem solving.

visual inspection, tactile manipulation, and responses to a variety of sounds. Reaching, grasping, mouthing, banging, and searching serve as the primary methods of beginning to understand objects and events. Each experience is novel and stands as an incentive and an experiential base for subsequent ones. Children in this phase gradually learn to coordinate sensory and motor functions to promote their continuing expansion of memories and knowledge about objects, people, and events. The results of learning in this phase include knowledge about how objects move and are obtained, and about their properties, the emerging separation of self and environment, and the beginnings of language and communication.

The *preoperational phase* signals a change in the child's style of learning (i.e., language processes gradually replace immediate sensorimotor experience as the primary method of thinking about the world). Children make rapid progress in the ability to label objects and communicate. Memory skills increase, and concept knowledge expands. Imitation, fantasy play, and an increasing understanding of the properties of objects are the hallmarks of this stage. The use of language for self-regulation is also a major achievement (Kopp, 1982).

Gagne's perspective, on the other hand, emphasizes the importance of identifying individual child characteristics (internal) as they match with environmental characteristics (external) to promote thinking and learning. External conditions for learning include the timing and mode of presenting developmental tasks to children. Similarly, internal child characteristics necessary for learning to occur include attention, motivation, and memory. *Learning* is a change in the child's behavior, or way of interacting with the world, that occurs because specific environmental conditions are present.

This match between child and conditions influences the quality of development. Pivotal to this view is the notion that structured stimulation (educational intervention) fosters effective learning. Similarly, the acquisition of more complex skills is dependent on prior learning of sequences of more rudimentary, prerequisite skills. Thus, a hierarchy of learning and developmental processes from basic to complex is fundamental. Table 3.3 illustrates the progression in this learning hierarchy. Basic skills in attending, object searching, and memory recall enable the child to perform behaviors that produce effects. These behaviors are used continuously because they are effective. Finally, such skills become useful in new circumstances that are different from the ones under which they were initially learned (generalization).

Normal Developmental Patterns

Throughout the early months, an infant's cognitive development is characterized by a variety of combined perceptual and sensorimotor strategies to explore the world rather than by the mental or symbolic strategies typical of later years. The young infant displays various motor patterns that demonstrate recognition and anticipation of selected people, objects, and events: "he behaves toward these objects and events with predictable, adaptive, and organized movements of his eyes, hands and mouth which suggest that he 'knows' certain things about them" (Cohen & Gross, 1979, p. 66). The phases of behavioral organization achieved within the first 24 months are increasingly sophisticated and enable the child to develop more effective strategies to understand and deal with the world. A gradual progression is observed from predominantly sensorimotor patterns in the first 24 months to verbally mediated behavior from 2 to 6 years of age (McCall, Hogarty, & Hurlburt, 1972).

During the first 4 months (0 to 4 months) infants display behavior that is largely reflexive and that undergoes refinement and integration. Through repeated use, such patterns as sucking, visual tracking, visual focusing, auditory responses, grasping, and head control are stabilized. These form the foundation for coordinated behavioral functions that are the prerequisites for cognitive development. Thus, visual and auditory functions become integrated as the infant achieves the ability to turn the head and eyes toward sound sources. Similarly, sucking and eye–hand coordination gradually emerge as the infant mouths objects, focuses on the hand and the object held, and then reaches for and grasps dangling objects. Nevertheless, some research demonstrates that the infant's ability to attend to and process auditory and visual information is relatively well developed early and is not wholly dependent on the refinement of reflexive motor patterns. For example, studies by Eimas (1975) with newborns in the first 3 weeks of life reveal that they can accurately discriminate between speech versus nonspeech sounds and show a preference for human vocalizations.

Finally, in this phase, the infant begins to develop a rudimentary sense of an ability to attain and move objects. Therefore, random contacts with objects, such as rattles that produce sounds and dangling mobiles that swing, become more frequent and goal directed as the infant attempts to repeat these interesting and pleasurable movements. This pattern of random to "intentional" contacts with toys is referred to as *primary and secondary circular reactions*, respectively.

In the following phase (4 to 8 months) previous patterns emerge under greater voluntary control. Children begin to behave toward toys in a manner that shows an understanding that objects are separate and constant (i.e., *object permanence*, see Table 3.4). Thus, reflexive responses are replaced by such goal-directed strategies as banging, throwing, and shaking as the child begins to explore individual objects in terms of their physical properties (texture, sound, color, movement) rather than solely the motor strategy available for such play. In addition, the infant will begin to reach and search for objects that are partially hidden by cloths and cups. The infant will anticipate the path of a moving ball that is screened in midroll.

TABLE 3.4. Stages in the Attainment of Object Permanence

Approximate ages	Search behavior
0 to 4 months	Nonvisual or manual searching
4 to 8 months	Searches for partially concealed objects
8 to 12 months	Searches for completely concealed objects
12 to 18 months	Searches after visible displacements of objects
18 months and older	Searches after hidden displacements of objects

Peek-a-boo games begin to generate interest at this stage. The infant grows in the ability to imitate motor and vocal patterns that already exist in the repertoire of skills.

At 8 to 12 months, the infant's behavior toward objects reveals a much greater goal-directed character. The infant is able to use new motor strategies to achieve desired results such as pulling a cloth to reach a doll resting on it, pulling an adult's hand to sustain an action, or reaching behind a plastic screen to retrieve a toy. In addition, the infant will now search for toys that are completely hidden and will imitate verbal and motor behaviors that are novel (e.g., tapping the head, wiggling the nose). The beginning ability to consistently apply sound labels to objects and people also advances thinking and concept development.

The 12- to 18-month phase stands as a transition point in which the infant depends less and less on sensorimotor means and begins to increasingly use perceptual thinking skills and language to deal with the world. Search behavior changes so that the child understands that if a toy is not under the first cup it must be hidden under the second. Although problem solving is still primarily trial-and-error in nature, the infant can begin to correct imitations that do not match an adult's.

At 18 to 24 months, the end of the predominantly sensorimotor phase is apparent as the infant begins to solve problems by "visualizing" solutions rather than by only using trial-and-error motor manipulation. The first 24 months of life are characterized as the *sensorimotor period* of cognitive development because of the necessity of immediate sensory input and motor manipulations for solving problems. The developmental phase from 2 to 6 years (24 to 72 months) is referred to as the *preoperational period* and represents a significant change in the child's thinking style and use of strategies. Specifically, language and conceptual knowledge allow the child to use symbols in place of actual objects or events in thinking and solving problems. The use of language to label, describe, explain, and indicate thoughts and wishes allows the child greater range in thinking style. Memory skills increase as the child is able to label objects and events to facilitate recall of them when they are absent. Perceptions of past, present, and future time also form. Because of the development of complex language abilities, children are capable of such intellectual strategies and symbolic operations as fantasizing through play, counting, sorting, sequencing, measuring, classifying, matching, recalling, explaining, and reasoning logically. However, much of the child's progress through this phase is a function of the nature of selective attention and the inability to view a problem from an alternative perspective.

Communication Patterns

Definition

"Language is a system of communication that allows two or more persons to exchange meaning" (Cohen & Gross, 1979, p. 1). This simple definition highlights the critical dimensions of the development of language capabilities. First, the development of language, thinking, and social skills is inextricably related. Meaningful use of language to express thoughts and feelings occurs only within a social context. Despite early prelanguage behaviors such as babbling, the use of language to convey *meaning* depends on the attainment of certain cognitive prerequisites (e.g., object permanence and imitation). Next, language is a complex symbol system involving elements of content and form. Thus, language consists of a child's expanding knowledge of objects, actions, descriptions, and concepts and their relationships to one another. Similarly, language has a form consisting of sounds, words, and grammatical structures used to expresses meaning—one's understanding of the essential concepts that underlie each word—and enable words to be related. The development of language is an amazingly complex process that has biological, cognitive, and social learning bases. Dysfunctions in any one system disrupt the course of functional communication skills in children.

Perspective

Research that describes, charts, and explains language development in children has greatly expanded in the past decade (Bloom & Lahey, 1978; Dale, 1979). The complex interrelationship between language, cognition, and self-regulation has been one of the most extensively studies areas (Meichenbaum & Goodman, 1971; Vygotsky, 1962).

Currently, the most influential theory regarding language acquisition centers on a field called *developmental psycholinguistics*. This area of study concentrates on the achievement of competence in language and communication. In the developmental psycholinguistic view, language competence is seen as the ability to understand, formulate, and use a symbolic communication system and is believed to be primarily a biologically determined process (Lenneberg, 1967). Although young children learn to use language for the purpose of social communication through pragmatic, learned interactions with others (McCormick & Scheifelbusch, 1984), the ability to understand and use language is presumed to have a neurological basis. At birth, children have the natural capacity to develop language as they interact with their world and gain information about how words are used, sentences formed, and meanings changed.

Within a psycholinguistic perspective, children are neurologically "programmed" to extract rules and regularities from the language that they hear spoken in order to form a *surface structure* of language. The surface structure consists of the orderly syntactic relations between classes of words. Similarly, children learn that words and sentences have a *deep structure* in which meanings change depending on the context in which they are used, for example, "a blind Venetian" and a "Venetian blind." Children develop a functional communication system both through an active process of making deductions about language from that which is heard and through modeling and being reinforced for the language used. Functional use of language can occur only within a social context.

Normal Developmental Patterns

The development of a system of communication entails three features of language: form, content, and use. According to the view of Bloom and Lahey (1978),

> Infants perceive and produce sounds (form); infants know about events in their immediate environments (content); at the same time, infants interact with other persons and objects in the context (use). . . . It appears that content, form, and use represent separate threads of development in the first year of infancy and begin to come together only in the second year as children learn words, sentences, and discourse. (pp. 69–70)

Most evidence to date indicates that language development is both biologically and environmentally determined. Certain language processes are linked closely with patterns of neuromotor development (see Table 3.5). However, children are active in processing language and making decisions about how words are used and sentences are formed.

Early language development consists of a variety of preverbal behaviors that involve both cognitive and social aspects. The formation of a meaningful communication system depends on the reciprocal relationship between mother and infant. The two most important dimensions of initiating early social communication are the transactional gaze patterns and smiling behavior. Consistent, maturationally determined patterns of crying (i.e., differentiated versus undifferentiated), pleasure-related cooing, and

TABLE 3.5. **Synchronized Motor and Language Patterns in Early Child Development**

At the completion of . . .	Motor development	Vocalization and language
12 weeks	Supports head when in prone position; weight is on elbows; hands mostly open; no grasp reflex.	Markedly less crying than at 8 weeks; when talked to and nodded at, smiles, followed by squealing-gurgling sounds usually called cooing, which is vowel-like in character and pitch-modulated; sustains cooing for 15–20 seconds.
16 weeks	Plays with a rattle placed in hands (by shaking it and staring at it), head self-supported; tonic neck reflex subsiding.	Responds to human sounds more definitely; turns head; eyes seem to search for speaker; occasionally some chuckling sounds.
20 weeks	Sits with props.	The vowel-like cooing sounds begin to be interspersed with more consonantal sounds; labial fricatives, spirants, and nasals are common; acoustically, all vocalizations are very different from the sounds of the mature language of the environment.
6 months	Sitting: bends forward and uses hands for support; can bear weight when put into standing position but cannot yet stand without holding on; reaching: unilateral; grasp: no thumb apposition yet; releases cube when given another.	Cooing changing into babbling resembling one-syllable utterances; neither vowels nor consonants have very fixed recurrences; most common utterances sound somewhat like "ms," "mu," "da," or "di."
8 months	Stands holding on; grasps with thumb apposition; picks up pellet with thumb and fingertips.	Reduplication (or more continuous repetitions) becomes frequent; intonation patterns become distinct; utterances can signal emphasis and emotions.
10 months	Creeps efficiently; takes sidesteps, holding on; pulls to standing position.	Vocalizations are mixed with sound-play such as gurgling or bubble-blowing; appears to wish to imitate sounds, but the imitations are never quite successful; beginning to differentiate between words heard by making differential adjustment.
12 months	Walks when held by one hand, walks on feet and hands, knees in air; mouthing of objects almost stopped; seats self on floor.	Identical sound sequences are replicated with higher relative frequency of occurrence, and words ("mamma" or "dada") are emerging; definite signs of understanding some words and simple commands ("show me your eyes").

(continued)

TABLE 3.5. (continued)

At the completion of . . .	Motor development	Vocalization and language
18 months	Grasp, prehension, and release fully developed; gait still propulsive and precipitated; sits on child's chair with only fair aim; creeps downstairs backward; has difficulty building tower of three cubes.	Has a definite repertoire of words–more than 3, but less than 50; still much babbling, but now of several syllables with intricate intonation pattern; no attempt at communicating information and no frustration at not being understood; words may include items such as "thank you" or "come here," but there is little ability to join any of the lexical items into spontaneous two-item phrases; understanding is progressing rapidly.
24 months	Runs, but falls in sudden turns; can quickly alternate between sitting and stance; walks stairs up or down, one foot forward only.	Vocabulary of more than 50 items (some children seem to be able to name everything in environment); begins spontaneously to join vocabulary items into two-word phrases; all phrases appear to be own creations; definite increase in communicative behavior and interest in language.
30 months	Jumps into air with both feet; stands on one foot for about 2 seconds; takes few steps on tiptoe; jumps from chair; good hand and finger coordination; can move digits independently; manipulation of objects much improved; builds tower of six cubes.	Fastest increase in vocabulary with many new additions every day; no babbling at all; utterances have communicative intent; frustrated if not understood by adults; utterances consist of at least two words, many have three or even five words; sentences and phrases have characteristic child grammar, that is, they are rarely verbatim repetitions of an adult utterance; intelligibility is not very good yet though there is great variation among children; seems to understand everything that is said to him or her.
3 years	Tiptoes 3 yards, runs smoothly with acceleration and deceleration; negotiates sharp and fast curves without difficulty; walks stairs by alternating feet; jumps 12 inches; can operate tricycle.	Vocabulary of some 1,000 words; about 80% of utterances are intelligible even to strangers; grammatical complexity of utterances is roughly that of colloquial adult language, although mistakes still occur.
4 years	Jumps over rope; hops on right foot; catches ball in arms; walks line.	Language is well established; deviations from the adult norm tend to be more in style than in grammar.

babbling (i.e., sound repetitions and intonations) predominate during the first 12 months of life. Patterns of jargon emerge as a form of transition in which the child plays with personal sound patterns and intonations that approximate adult speech.

At approximately 12 months of age, children begin to attach selected sounds to specific people and objects as the first words emerge. These sound–object matches focus on immediate wants (e.g., cup, ball, juice, mama). In addition, children tend to use the same sounds with different intonation contours to express several distinct wants or feelings, depending on the situation. They begin to use single words as if they were whole sentences (holophrases).

The *holophrase* marks a transition point in language development. Toward the end of the second year (18 to 24 months), true *syntactic* dimensions begin to appear in the child's language (i.e., the orderly pairing of two or more words to express thoughts). Comprehension of objects and pictures has increased rapidly. Thus, the content available for language use is magnified. At this point, children begin to understand regularities or rules regarding the relation of words in sentences. Two-word duos emerge that have a characteristic *pivot-open form* consisting of combinations of action, or indicator, words and nouns or adjectives. Early syntactic patterns combine form, content, and use in such constructions as "there book," "want milk," "hit ball," "baby fall," "where ball," and "give candy." Unique constructions such as "hands are messy" show that the child is actively processing the rules and meaning of language independent of direct imitation. Also, *telegraphic* patterns such as "where Daddy coat?" with omitted words and features represent the further extension of syntax.

Finally, from the third to the fifth years, expressive language expands greatly. Sentences increase in grammatic complexity, although one major idea dominates each sentence. Future tenses become widely used, and questions resemble adult forms. At 60 months of age, children have developed an adult linguistic form that can relate two or more ideas through relative clauses.

Parallel with syntactic development, children acquire an understanding of the *semantic* features of language. Semantic features are the meanings of individual words and surrounding words in sentences. Children initially comprehend that words are defined by their perceptual and functional features (i.e., the smell, look, feel, and sound of objects and what objects do). Children learn that a dog is shaggy, barks, has four legs, licks your face, and can run fast. Yet, as children learn specific features of specific objects, they begin to overgeneralize them to other objects. Thus, children initially begin to call all four-legged animals dogs. Gradually, they make more finely differentiated distinctions between objects and their features. The development of the understanding of meaning is intimately bound up with conceptual development as children begin to group objects into generic categories (e.g., things we ride, things that jump, things we eat) and begin to understand that certain words cannot be paired with other words because their meanings clash, for example, "bachelor's wife." Finally, children's understanding of meaning expands as they learn that meaning varies with the context in which words appear.

The language process of pragmatics emerges concurrently with syntactic and semantic processes. In fact, pragmatic and semantic skills are firmly related. Pragmatics refers to the evolving use of language for social communication. It is a reciprocal, two-person operation in which young children learn the functional meaning of words (semantics) as well as nonverbal behaviors (gestures) to express thoughts and intentions (McCormick & Scheifelbusch, 1984).

Affective–Social Patterns

Definition

The development of affective and social capabilities in children entails a complex cluster of interrelated dimensions including attachment, behavioral style, personal identity, self-regulation, and social and object play. Each of these behavioral processes plays a significant role in shaping the young child's sense of personal and interpersonal competence. Through early attachment bonds with caregivers, infants and young children develop a secure expectation about the regularity of people and events in their world. The loving and consistent nature of this affective bond allows children to model and develop a range of effective interpersonal behaviors. Yet, each child's unique behavioral or temperamental style, which has some hereditary basis, influences the course of social and emotional development (Thomas & Chess, 1977). Early play experiences with people and objects serve as the "proving ground" for children to model appropriate social interaction patterns, to test individual competencies, to learn compliance with rules and limits, and to develop skills for self-regulation.

Perspective

Several related viewpoints help to shape our knowledge about the substance and process of development in the affective and social area. One view is that of Bandura (1977), who maintains that much of our repertoire of interpersonal skills and personal competencies (e.g., self-efficacy) is developed through a process of social modeling. Simply stated, children imitate social behaviors that are valued and reinforced by adults; in addition, these behaviors (e.g., compliance, sharing) become self-perpetuating as they are effective in initiating and maintaining interactions with others. Nevertheless, cognitive and developmental readiness factors also exert a large influence.

Erikson (1959) offers a developmental perspective on psychosocial growth emphasizing that passage through successive stages in forming one's identity is influenced by the quality of parenting (see Table 3.6). in this process, it is assumed that children learn a basic sense of trust about the caring and constant nature of their world. Trust forms the basis for the child to successfully resolve other developmental tasks (e.g., conflicts) involving separating from parents, testing one's skills, and forming an individual sense of self.

Researchers believe that the process of *attachment* and *bonding* between caregiver and child, whether with or without disabilities, forms the solid base for future affective and social development (Ainsworth, 1973; Ludlow, 1982; Murdock, 1979). Attachment behavior, such as mutual smiling, touching, and talking, between parents and young children enables enduring interpersonal bonds to be established. Disruption or misinterpretation of these "signaling" behaviors, particularly with handicapped children, distorts growth in this area. Nevertheless, it is believed that each child's innate temperamental style (e.g., attention, mood, activity level, sensitivity) has an impact on parents' behaviors while they are providing care.

Much attention has been addressed to the issue of attachment and bonding with normal children, but little clinical research has focused on the attachment/bonding process with parents and children with disabilities (Blacher, 1998). A sensitive or "critical" period for the formation of the attachment bond between mother and child has been postulated, but some critics suggest that professionals have overemphasized the importance of this process and have, in the process, made parents feel anxious and guilty. Work with severely handicapped children suggests that their sensory, motor, cognitive, and affective disabilities make them incapable of supporting the emerging attachment bond with their parents that is so important.

TABLE 3.6. Erikson's Stages of Psychosocial Development

Life crisis	Favorable outcome	Unfavorable outcome
First year Trust–mistrust	Hope. Trust in the environment and the future.	Fear of the future; suspicion.
Second year Autonomy– shame, doubt	Will. Ability to exercise choice as well as self-restraint; a sense of self-control and self-esteem leading to goodwill and pride.	Sense of loss of self-control or sense of external overcontrol; the result is a propensity for shame and doubt about whether one willed what one did or did what one willed.
Third through fifth years Initiative–guilt	Purpose. Ability to initiate activities, to give them direction, and to enjoy accomplishment.	Fear of punishment, self-restriction or over-compensatory showing off.

Because of this, mothers often feel unusually stressed and discouraged by their seeming inability to engage their infants in interaction. This may contribute to the early "burnout" of parents as caretakers and teachers of their children. Child abuse can also be an outcome of such frustration. Nevertheless, research studies do show that even severely impaired infants have some adaptive responses that can be promoted in the development of the attachment bond (Blacher, 1984). Early intervention specialists must emphasize the teaching of certain skills to parents to help them to identify, anticipate, respond to, and elicit these subtle behavioral cues that can form the basis of the affective bond. Thus, such parent–child interactive therapy should be a major part of every program.

Finally, much recent research has focused on the emerging refinement of self-regulatory behaviors in children. These behaviors include the infant's attempts at self-consolation when crying and the young child's ability to modify behavior to meet the demands of new situations (Kopp, 1982).

Normal Developmental Patterns

The stable course of children's emotional and social development is firmly rooted in the nature of the caregiver–child relationship. Within this relationship, characteristics of the child and characteristics of the environment provided by adults intertwine to influence such early developmental processes as attachment, social play, separation and self-identity, emotional responses, and self-regulation (Anastasiow, 1981). Individual differences in child temperament and the ability to respond to the overtures of caregivers also are major factors in early affective development. In fact, children with diverse neurodevelopmental disorders tend to have an increased incidence of emotional behavior problems (Freidlander et al., 1982; Martin, 1982).

Table 3.6 presents one view regarding the general stages of socioemotional development during the birth to 6-year period (Erikson, 1959). The major achievements during these phases are early attachment to parents and the emerging capacity to separate oneself and become an individual. During the initial birth to 18-month period, children gradually gain a sense of trust regarding the parent's ability to nurture them and care for their needs. The process of attachment and bonding is central to this emerging sense. Cognitive, affective, and motivational aspects of an infant's behavior combine to influence the attachment process. Factors such as the infant's ability to recognize the major caregiver, to respond actively to caring behaviors, and to smile are essential in the formation of optimal bonds. Mutual patterns of touching, smiling, cooing, talking with varying intonations, rocking, face-to-face visual contact, and rhythmic starting and stopping of activity between caregiver and child encourage "learned" social interactions. Parental responses to smiling and crying that are dependent on the infant's state and needs allow infants to experience the impact of their own affective capabilities as well as typical adult responses to them. A secure attachment bond, then, serves as the child's base to begin gradual separation from the mother.

At 8 to 10 months of age, fear reactions to strangers and new situations emerge and also signal the discriminations required developmentally to begin the separation process. Each child begins to explore the environment by looking, reaching, and crawling away from the mother for short periods of practice. These periods increase with the ability to walk independently. In turn, the child's cognitive maturity allows the retention of a mental image of the mother and a sense that "she is still there," which emotionally "refuels" the child and enables continued exploration. This separation–individuation process is an extension of the child's attachment to the parents and signals the child's capacity to function with greater autonomy.

This phase of increased autonomy (18 to 36 months) marks the child's developing sense of self apart from others. Increases in cognitive, language, and motor skills enable children to function independently and to increasingly test their own capabilities to achieve self-mastery. During this phase, oppositional behavior, tantrums, and conflicts with parents regarding compliance with rules and limits are typical. Consistent limit setting with flexibility by parents is necessary to allow the child latitude in exploring and experiencing. The major achievement of this phase is the child's knowledge of competency to interact with and influence objects, people, and events with purpose and self-direction.

Finally, from 36 to 72 months of age, children further establish a sense of their own strengths and weaknesses, which includes modeling appropriate sex-role behaviors. Mastering basic self-care activities (e.g., toileting, dressing, grooming) and fantasy play regarding adult jobs and roles are typical of this period of testing and practicing. Firmer understandings of acceptable and unacceptable behaviors are also outcomes of this period.

Play

Another dimension of development that shapes socioemotional growth is *play behavior* in young children.

> For the child . . . [play] . . . makes it possible to relate to things that might otherwise be confusing, frightening, mysterious, strange, risky, or forbidden and to develop appropriate competencies and defenses. The active solution of developmental conflicts through play thus enables the young child to demonstrate and feel social competence. (Mindes, 1982, p. 40)

The process of play intricately involves the merger of cognitive, sensorimotor, affective, and social behaviors. Play is vital in facilitating the development of an understanding of social rules and limits, concepts regarding object relationships, personal preferences and competencies, and self-control. Patterns of cognitive play with objects proceed in the following order: (1) early exploratory schemes of mouthing, banging, and throwing; (2) fine motor manipulation; (3) constructive and creative play (e.g., drawing, measuring, building); (4) dramatic play (e.g., fantasy role-playing); and (5) games with rules. Early infant play involves solitary activities of manipulating objects, playing with vocalizations, and self-exploration. Gradually, young children begin patterns of parallel play with other children using toys similar to those used by others. Finally, group play patterns emerge from unorganized but associative playing to more organized styles of cooperation, sharing, and adhering to rules. All these styles and patterns of play serve as an indispensable vehicle for the child to develop important concepts: personal competence and self-regulation.

Self-Regulation

Self-regulation, the ability to monitor and control one's behavior in response to social expectations, is one of the most important features of affective development (Kopp, 1982). With increasing age, control evolves from primarily external sources (e.g., parental consequences) to internal child factors (e.g., personal verbal constraints, knowledge of social rules). Children learn appropriate social behaviors by modeling adult patterns that adhere to social rules. These patterns are reinforced in interactions with parents, teachers, and others. Gradually, these patterns, and the rules and expectations that underlie them, are internalized and form the basis for self-regulation. Kopp (1982) has synthesized much of the recent research on self-control capabilities in children in order to formulate a developmental progression scheme for the emergence of self-regulatory processes from birth onward (see Table 3.7). This progression devolves through five phases: neurophysiological modulation, sensorimotor modulation, control, self-control, and self-regulation.

The *neurophysiological modulation* phase (0 to 3 months) is characterized by the activation of various reflex operations to modulate states of arousal in the infant. Such behavior patterns as nonnutritive sucking for consolation, hand sucking to stop crying, withdrawing from intrusive stimuli (e.g., sounds, lights), and habituation are indications of the body's emerging neurophysiological capacity to maintain a steady state. As reflex patterns become organized, sleeping–awake states defined, and sensitivity to stimulation modulated, the basis for more voluntary regulation is established. Interactions with parents and caregivers further aid the infant in recognizing and adjusting to routines that support evolving internal control mechanisms.

TABLE 3.7. Developmental Phases in the Acquisition of Self-Regulatory Capabilities in Young Children

Phases	Approximate ages	Features	Cognitive requisites
Neurophysiological modulation	Birth to 2–3 months	Modulation of arousal, activation of organized patterns of behavior	
Sensorimotor modulation	3 to 9 months+	Change ongoing behavior in response to events and stimuli in environment.	
Control	12 to 18 months+	Awareness of social demands of a situation and initiate, maintain, cease physical acts, communication, etc. accordingly; compliance, self-initiated monitoring.	Intentionality, goal-directed behavior, conscious awareness of action, memory or existential self.
Self-control	24 months	As above; delay on request; behave according to social expectations in the absence of external monitors.	Representational thinking and recall memory, symbolic thinking, continuing sense of identity.
Self-regulation	36 months	As above; flexibility of control processes that meets changing situational demands	Strategy production, conscious introspection, etc.

The second phase is referred to as *sensorimotor modulation* (3 to 12 months) because the developing infant is able to generate voluntary motor functions such as reaching and grasping and to alter those patterns in response to events and stimuli in the world. These emerging abilities to coordinate sensory and motor functions help the infant to focus attention on objects; smile in response to caregiver approaches; reach for, search for, and obtain hidden objects; and engage in reciprocal games (e.g., peek-a-boo).

Parents and caregivers play an important role in encouraging infants to act on objects and to sustain those patterns by modulating their behaviors. Then, these patterns make the child more aware of the impact of these actions in changing the world. True "control" capabilities are dependent on the child's ability to distinguish his or her own actions from those of others.

The third phase is one of *control* (12 to 24 months). During this time, the child becomes aware of social or task demands established by adults and alters behavior accordingly. A wider range of behavior, such as initiating, sustaining, and ceasing activity, is now available for modulation. The major milestones involve the ability to comply with commands ("Don't run!") and the beginning capacity to monitor one's own actions. However, control is highly dependent on external cues about the appropriateness of behavior in specific situations. Moreover, this element of control is facilitated by the child's ability to engage in goal-directed, purposeful behavior and the awareness of the consequences of his or her actions.

The emergence of *self-control* and its refinement into *self-regulation* (24 to 36 months+) involves the capacity to comply with a command, to inhibit or delay behavior on request, and to behave according to rules and expectations. In particular, representational thinking and recall memory enable the child to relate his or her own behavior more firmly to specific consequences and adult dictates. Self-control is "self-initiated modification of behavior as a result of remembered information" (Kopp, 1982, p. 207).

Self-regulation differs in the quality of self-control capacities. Specifically, the child is more adaptable, more able to delay and wait in response to the requirements of situation (e.g., crossing the street). The child's emerging self-identity and more mature ability to reflect on and think about actions, as well as to remember and repeat back rules or alternative ways of behaving, serve as the cognitive underpinnings of self-regulation.

Sensorimotor Patterns

Definition

Sensorimotor development refers to the continually emerging interconnections between multiple sensory and perceptual systems (e.g., visual, auditory, tactile, kinesthetic, olfactory) and motor systems (e.g., reflex, fine and gross motor control). The complex interrelationship between sensory and motor systems is important to the development of basic cognitive processes and the skills requisite for learning.

Perspective

The progression of sensorimotor patterns follows the same course and developmental principles reflected in other functional processes, namely, sequential growth and progress from gross to finely differentiated states of functioning (Connor, Williamson, & Siepp, 1978; Cratty, 1979; Langley, 1980). Certain fundamental principles of sensorimotor growth assume that sensory input serves to both initiate and guide fine and gross motor patterns:

1. Interconnections between visual, auditory, kinesthetic, tactile, and motor systems provide feedback about the manner in which the body moves and enables the brain to alter movement patterns to explore the environment.

2. Development of sensorimotor patterns proceeds in a *cephalocaudal* (i.e., head to foot) and *proximal–distal* (i.e., trunk to extremities) direction. Control of the head and trunk are fundamental to balance, which is essential to independent walking. Fine motor precision occurs also with head–shoulder stability.

3. Basic movement patterns emerge through the differentiation and refinement of gross, prerequisite postural reflex mechanisms. While in the process of refining and mastering a particular motor skill, children practice elements of more complex skills that are next in developmental sequence.

4. As the neurological system matures, children become capable of dissociating movements in a selective manner. For example, infants gain more precise skills in grasping and manipulating objects as visual–motor coordination matures and more independent use of the fingers emerges.

In general, the ability to right one's position in space and to balance are automatic body responses that are critical to more refined fine and gross motor functioning. The total integration of sensory and motor dimensions is completed by 6 to 7 years of age.

Normal Developmental Patterns

The integration between visual, auditory, manipulative, and locomotor systems stands as the basis for subsequent learning and cognitive development (Cohen & Gross, 1979).

Research indicates that the auditory system is one of the most well developed at birth. Regularities in the behavioral responses of infants provide evidence of distinct developmental patterns in this area (see Table 3.8). The newborn infant demonstrates ability to perceive sound by a range of reflexive patterns consisting of eye blinks, brightening and widening of the eye, startle responses, and diffuse whole-body movements. At 3 to 4 months of age, the infant exhibits emerging abilities to localize sound sources by turning the head in their general direction. From this point, infants begin to localize sounds at various directions from the body in a more selective manner. It is evident that reflex and motor response patterns are the vehicles by which the infant displays perception of sound.

In a parallel fashion, the newborn infant demonstrates a capable, yet less mature *visual system*. At birth (0–2 months) visual acuity, visual

TABLE 3.8. Developmental Progression of Auditory Localization in Infants

Developmental age	Localization behavior
Newborn to 4 months	Arousal from sleep by sound signal.
3 to 4 months	Begins to make rudimentary head turn toward a sound.
4 to 7 months	Turns head directly toward side of a signal; cannot locate above or below.
7 to 9 months	Directly locates a sound source to the side and indirectly below.
9 to 13 months	Directly locates sound source to the side and directly below.
13 to 16 months	Directly localizes sound signals to the side and below; indirectly above.
16 to 21 months	Localizes sound signal on sides, below, and above.
21 to 24 months	Directly locates a sound signal at all angles.

accommodation, and ability of the eyes to move together to fixate on an object are all very immature functions. These visual limitations restrict the infant's attention to the most salient features of objects (e.g., size, pattern, movement, density). In this respect, infants prefer and appear "neurologically programmed" to respond visually to ordinary but complex patterns such as human faces. From 2 to 6 months, the infant's ability to fixate and attend to objects and people increases dramatically. New and unfamiliar objects seem to command the most attention; yet, the movement of objects begins to lose its exclusive control of attention as infants focus on the details of objects themselves. As infants are ready to reach and grasp, their visual system shows a preferential focus on the features of objects that facilitate motor manipulation.

The importance of vision as an impetus to functional *fine motor and gross motor development* cannot be overstated. Visual focusing and tracking serve to guide such precise motor functions as reaching, grasping, manipulating, and releasing. Head and trunk control develops in parallel fashion to eye–hand functions and establishes a stable basis for reaching and grasping. Full head control usually emerges at 6 months of age as the child gains the trunk stability to begin sitting independently. At this point, eyes and hands can coordinate functionally to locate and explore objects within reach at the midline of the body and grasping proceeds through the stages of (1) reflexive clutching of objects, (2) holding an object near the outer palm (ulnar palm), (3) holding an object near the palm between thumb and fingers (radial–digital), (4) a scissoring motion of the fingers, and (5) a precise use of the thumb and index finger to obtain small objects (precise pincer). With these skills in grasping and holding objects, the base is set for such precision skills as container play, block play, and drawing.

Similarly, gross motor patterns emerge and proceed toward independent locomotion. Such sequences as creeping, pulling to stand, standing supported, cruising along furniture, independent walking, stair climbing, running, jumping, and throwing generally characterize these patterns and will be fully discussed in Chapter 8.

ATYPICAL DEVELOPMENTAL PATTERNS

A variety of developmental disorders are responsible for the functional limitations that young children with disabilities experience. These diverse disorders can be observed in the categories that are traditionally used to classify children with developmental disabilities (e.g., Down syndrome, cerebral palsy, blindness, deafness, autism, language impairment. However, any dysfunction that involves the central nervous system and sensorimotor processes exerts a significant negative impact on the acquisition of neuro-developmental skills across all *interdependent* functions (e.g., cognition, language, play, social communication, sensorimotor exploration, self-care, and self-regulation) and transcends the narrow boundaries used in an attempt to characterize a particular disorder as unique and homogeneous. To illustrate this interdependent quality, a final discussion of atypical developmental patterns blends selected information about the early cognitive, affective, and sensorimotor deficits of young children with various developmental disabilities.

Sensory Disabilities

Children with visual, auditory, or multisensory (deaf and blind) impairments are at a profound disadvantage in their efforts to understand and respond to environmental stimuli. The lack of intergration between sensory and motor functions inhibits and distorts the full range of cognitive, affective, and communication processes in development.

Object Constancy

The coordination of visual and motor functions forms the basis for subsequent cognitive development in normally functioning children. Visual impairments highlight the need for dual auditory and tactile stimulation, whereas auditory deficits necessitate a focus on exaggerated visual cues. Multiple impairments point to the tactile mode as the alternate channel for information. The blind child reveals dysfunctions in visual attention, tracking, and discrimination of light sources, depending on the severity of the deficit. Thus, spontaneous search behavior for objects out of reach is precluded, as is the child's understanding of the permanent nature of contacts with people and objects. The child must be afforded experiences in which sounds can be used to direct reaching for toys that make noise or music. The child fails to search for a lost object because there are not natural cues to its position in space and little basis for believing that, once it is not felt or heard, it still exists. Moreover, the child fails to develop a sense of connection between self and actions, through reaching, finding, grasping, and losing objects.

Means–Ends

Without visual cues, the blind child fails to develop an understanding of the use of hands as functional tools for obtaining objects. Frequently, hands are held in an elevated, shoulder-high position, unprepared for contacts with or manipulation of toys. Self-stimulatory patterns of waving the hands over the eyes, rubbing the eyes to experience light sensations, and slapping the face become persistent if not interrupted and directed into purposeful tasks.

Causality

Visual impairments block children's understanding that their behavior causes objects to move or people to interact with them. Their inability to process and compare visual information impairs trial-and-error learning as well as intentional goal-directed behavior. Motivation is limited, and passivity and dependency are promoted by the fact that others must intrude to elicit behavior from the child. The establishment of auditorial directed reaching (i.e., the coordination of hand–arm extension to a sound source) is a prerequisite to independent creeping and motor movements in blind children.

Object Relations and Concepts

Not understanding the purpose for reaching and grasping limits the blind child's experience with objects. In turn, the ability to recognize different objects and understand their functional relationships (spoon, dish) is limited. Blind children develop a belief that objects materialize within their physical space by accident. According to Fraiberg (1977), visual functions serve to connect sound and touch in normal children before 4 months of age. Blind children display a 6- to 8-month lag in relating tactile and auditory attributes of objects. Therefore, without distinct concepts regarding the dimensions and attributes of whole, real-life objects, these children perceive large objects, such as chairs, as the isolated parts that they sometimes experience. Similarly, the severely physically impaired child's understanding of objects, attributes, functions, and names of functions are distorted, which influences the pace of linguistic and conceptual development.

Social Communication

The formation of enduring attachment bonds between the child with a severe disability, the parents, and other individuals is heavily influenced by the absence of visual responses and cues. Blind infants lack the capacity to extend their arms to reach for the mother to initiate a pattern of reciprocal interactions. Also, spontaneous and responsive affective behaviors, such as smiling, are often delayed until 12 months of age. In this context, caregivers tend to invest extraordinary energy in encouraging mutual responses but are faced with a frustrating and unrewarding style of detachment from the child, who cannot receive and respond to social cues (e.g., facial grimaces, gestures, smiles). Similarly, deaf children are often quiet and seemingly pre-occupied while signaling little need for adult attention. The lack of reaction to adult contacts, such as calling the child's name, may be personalized by the caregivers as "tuning out" or as oppositional behavior directed against them. Moreover, the associated absence of give-and-take verbalizations is detrimental to the emerging interaction between the adult and the deaf child.

Neuromotor Dysfunctions

The foundation for the development of cognitive-adaptive abilities is the integration and refinement of reflex motor patterns and their coordination with vision, touch, and hearing. "Thus, from the consolidation of early sensory and motor behaviors evolve the basic building blocks for subsequent learning" (Langley, 1980, p. 24). Whereas normal children create their own experiences to integrate these patterns, children with severe sensory and neuromotor impairments must have such opportunities created for them. The task experiences contained in developmental curricula provide specialized opportunities for sucking, grasping, visual–auditory attending, and movement to facilitate this learning for the child with cerebral palsy or other neurological impairments.

Object Constancy, Causal, and Means–Ends Relations

In the child with cerebral palsy abnormal tone and posture interfere with the integration of sensory and motor functions. The child demonstrates an inability to hold the head erect at the midline of the body as a result of the persistence of primitive reflex patterns that would have disappeared in normal children. This abnormal posture distorts visual attention and the localization of sound sources. In turn, problems with visual attention and auditory localization, coupled with dysfunctions in motor stability and equilibrium reactions, inhibit the child from reaching, grasping, and searching for toys. Moreover, absent or distorted experiences make the child unable to comprehend cause and effect relationships such as those involved in pushing a ball or repeating a motor response. The physical involvement of the arms and hands prevents the child from actively uncovering objects to discover and explore hidden toys. This inability precludes formation of a firsthand information base. Memory and knowledge of objects and their attributes is diminished, and the sense of personal competence in causing objects to move is limited.

Object Relations and Concepts

Severe physical impairment inhibits shifts of attention from object to object, movement toward sound sources, and tracking and locating objects out of view. Similarly, this lack of direct motor experience affects both a knowledge of the physical properties of objects and the child's awareness of his or her own body's position in space in relation to objects. The absence of control over arms, hands, and legs fosters a sense that these body parts are detached objects not under personal control. Poor motor control and distorted experiences with objects lead to a limited knowledge about the properties of objects (texture, dimension, shape, manipulation) and their uses, which in turn affects language and conceptual development.

Imitation and Social Communication

Severe neuromotor dysfunctions prevent the child from engaging in early reciprocal games such as peek-a-boo and pat-a-cake and matching and imitating adult gestures. Gestural and vocal imitation are blunted, which limits the child's sense of modeling such self-care behaviors as pulling off and putting on shoes and feeding with a spoon.

Abnormal body postures complicate the process of adequate bonding between caretaker and child. Cuddling produces body extensions and increased muscle tone, which the caregiver may interpret as rejection, irritability, or resistance. Moreover, hypertonicity and neurological difficulties prevent adequate respiration for sound production as well as preventing the ability to form fine mouth movements for vowel and consonant sounds. Absent is a sense of the communication value of sounds or fine motor gestures. Gross, whole-body movements and behavior problems become the child's mode of indicating wants or discomfort. Furthermore, a limited experiential base and poor sound–word–object correspondences impair language development.

Affective-Behavioral Disorders

Two aspects of the development of children with severe affective and behavioral disorders inhibit and disrupt the acquisition of adaptive capabilities: (1) neurological deficits that distort sensory input, and (2) a socially detached self-stimulatory style. Autism and the various forms of self-injurious behavior (e.g., Lesch–Nyhan syndrome) include these neuro-developmental deficits.

Object Constancy and Behavior–Object Relations

A child's understanding that objects exist independently depends on memory, visual representation, and visual attention. The autistic child's dysfunctions in regulating sensory (visual) input interfere with these processes. Poor attention, self-involvement, and frequent overreactions to sounds, sights, and textures inhibit the child from developing anticipatory behaviors and the ability to scan the environment to search for objects in an organized fashion. Perseverative behaviors, such as hand flapping, twirling, face slapping, touching, and smelling, prevent wider experiences in exploring the environment. Vision and hearing are used inappropriately and infrequently by autistic children as primary methods of exploring objects. Repetitive spinning and manipulation of tops and objects, such as cubes, offer increased sensory feedback but do not allow the child to attend to, remember, and discriminate the physical attributes and useful functions of objects. This style of behavior limits concept formation.

Social Communication

The autistic child's extreme lack of social responsiveness and failure to recognize and comprehend the value of the communication process are serious obstacles to the formation of attachment bonds. Such children show no desire for cuddling or interpersonal affection; instead, their bodies become tense and unresponding. The lack of eye contact, absence of crying when hurt, and failure to display a pleasant social awareness of others provide no reinforcement to caregivers. Moreover, the child's self-involvement and deficits in gestural communication, as well as idiosyncratic use of words and sounds, make social communication and concept formation a tenuous process. The most instrusive behavioral strategies are required to interrupt these detached patterns and to promote the acquisition of basic adaptive and social skills.

Developmental Retardation

Children with severe and profound retardedation develop cognitively according to the same invariant developmental sequence as children without a disability, but they differ in terms of a slower rate of overall skill acquisition. Although mental age matches the progressive attainment of sensorimotor abilities (language, grasping, manipulating) retarded children differ in the variable rate of attaining such parallel subskills as the recognition of object permanence, spatial orientation, imitation, and causation (Rogers, 1977). Children with Down syndrome also display this pattern.

Object Constancy and Causality

When the profoundly retarded child cannot attain an upright posture, visual and motor exploration of the environment and the ability to form concepts of body image and person–object relationships are limited. Moreover, research (e.g., Fantz, Fagan, & Miranda, 1973) demonstrates that children with Down syndrome show significant lags in their visual–perceptual development for the recognition of faces and novel stimuli. This may influence their ability to understand and complete a search for hidden objects and to respond to people socially.

Many severely retarded children show an inability to regulate responses to stimuli. Under- and overresponsiveness to various stimuli are common and prevent the formation of selective reactions to pleasant and unpleasant events. Thus, intentional motor acts may never develop and memories regarding the relationship between actions and consequences may never form.

Social Communication

Deficits in the child's ability to smile responsively and to maintain eye contact with the caregiver seriously impede the development of social communication. Responsive smiling is a subtle indicator of cognitive ability. Children with Down syndrome differ from typical children in the onset, frequency, and duration of smiling and eye contact with mothers. Therefore, the sustaining cues for social interaction are reduced. The child with brain damage and severe retardation lacks the cognitive capacity to interpret visual and gestural cues from the mother and, if multihandicapped, the motor ability to respond to and maintain the interaction. The capacity of such children to respond selectively and to show acceptance or rejection of people is seriously impaired.

SUMMARY AND IMPLICATIONS FOR PRACTICE

The use of a developmental perspective is indispensable for thoroughly understanding the behavioral progress of both children with and without disabilities. A developmental approach establishes expectancies for the emergence of a variety of abilities in children; it enables us to understand the complex interconnections among cognitive, language, social, sensorimotor, and affective processes; it reveals how disabilities distort the emergence of important adaptive skills in children. However, its most vital function is in establishing an operational base to blend assessment, intervention, and progress evaluation. With this effective mixture of philosophy, purpose, and practice, early developmental programs can be designed that will enhance the adaptive functioning and learning of young exceptional children.

Tables 3.9 and 3.10 provide a quick and easy-to-remember summary of the major principles of early development and their implications as guidepoints for "best practice" in early childhood measurement. Each of the 12 principles offers a rationale for why certain measurement practices are indicated because of their alignment with the processes of early development. The following section offers a summary list of essential guidepoints regarding relationships among these developmental principles and their implications for measurement in early childhood:

• Functional skills observed in everyday activities and routines are the only truly representative methods for measuring the capabilities of infants, toddlers, and preschoolers, since they are active agents in promoting their own development through interactions with their world; they are *active, interactive, and competent agents* in their own developmental progress.

• Early childhood measurement must sample children's skills comprehensively across interrelated and integrated developmental processes (e.g., cognitive–communication, cognitive–social, visual–motor, cognitive–motor, social–self-regulatory) and the sequential development of basic to

TABLE 3.9. Summary of Early Developmental Principles

1. Child's active participation in promoting own development
2. Competence using adaptive skills to change environment
3. Interactive exchanges with a stimulating social and physical environment—
   "developmental ecology"
4. Organized patterns of neurodevelopmental processes
5. Multidimensional interplay among developmental competencies and domains
6. Sequential stages of development
7. Individual rates of developmental progress
8. Variable developmental patterns
9. Specialized competencies from undifferentiated patterns
10. Flexible and "plastic" alternative routes to developmental competence
11. Multicausal factors for development and dysfunction
12. Sensitive periods for the timing and development of competencies

TABLE 3.10. Implications of Developmental Principles
for Measurement in Early Childhood

- Active: Functional tasks
- Competent: Natural problem solving
- Interactive: Everyday activities/routines
- Organized: Developmental processes
- Multidimensional: Full cross-domain sampling
- Sequential: Hierarchical stages
- Individual: Personal progress patterns
- Variable: Individual patterns of plateaus, regressions, gains
- Specialized: Sampling of simple to complex skills
- Flexible: Alternate response modes and paths to progress
- Multicausal: Sampling of ecological factors
- Sensitive: Precise measurement and intervention times

---

advanced competencies; developmental processes are, simultaneously, *organized, sequential,* and *multidimensional.*

- Each child (typical or atypical) shows *individual and variable rates and patterns* of acquiring developmental skills; moreover, developmental processes integrate simple early developmental skills (e.g., visual tracking) into complex and *specialized* competencies (e.g., eye–hand coordination in drawing). Thus, measurement in early childhood must emphasize intra-individual comparisons to showcase both these individual patterns and individual responses to instruction and intervention.

- Developmental trajectories in young children can be altered and enhanced through individually tailored interventions since developmental processes are *flexible and multicausal* and most amenable to enhancement during *sensitive periods* in development. Measurement in early childhood must serve as a support to uncovering alternate pathways through which young children with differences can learn; moreover, authentic assessment can make clear the interrelationships among individual pathways and the environmental supports that will strengthen their emergence and development as consistent and effective competencies in a child's life.

While this book is about measurement in early childhood, the principles detailed in this chapter also provide a practical rationale for both individual and group (systemic) interventions for children at developmental risk and with developmental disabilities.

Ramey and Ramey (1998) composed a seminal article that reviewed the seven essential dimensions of evidence-based early childhood intervention programs. These seven features, culled from 30 years of intervention research, show clear alignments with the principles of development regarding timing, sensitivity, authenticity, functionality, and scope. The principles are listed below:

1. Earlier and longer program participation results in greater early learning and school success.
2. Parent engagement in the program is critical for generalizing children's progress to real-life settings.
3. Direct child teaching and interventions and task engagement result in more enduring competencies than constructivist approaches.
4. Individualized care and teaching are important for all children.
5. High quality programs are critical for healthy development of all children.
6. Successful programs are characterized by comprehensive, interagency program supports in everyday settings and community-based leadership.
7. Preschool-to-school partnerships to continue supportive interventions into the early grades (K–6) are critical to promote generalization of learning and enduring success.

BEST-PRACTICE GUIDEPOINTS

♦ Understand and apply the 12 principles for typical and atypical development.

♦ Use a Piagetian framework to observe and understand developmental stages and progressions for all children.

♦ Analyze and use a comprehensive developmental curriculum to operationalize the stages of early development.

♦ Use a sequenced developmental curriculum to document observations about typical and atypical developmental progressions.

BEST-PRACTICE EVIDENCE

Ainsworth, M. S. (1973). The development of infant–mother attachment. In B. Caldwell & H. Ricciuti (Eds.), *Review of child development research* (Vol. 3, pp. 113–139). Chicago: University of Chicago Press.

Anastasiow, N. J. (1981). Socioemotional developmental: The state of the art. In N. J. Anastasiow (Ed.), *New directions for exceptional children: Socioemotional development* (Vol. 5, pp. 65–81). San Francisco: Jossey-Bass.

Bagnato, S. J. (1987). Normal and exceptional early development. In J. T. Neisworth & S. J. Bagnato (Eds.), *The young exceptional child: Early development and education* (pp. 64–100). New York: Macmillan.

Bandura, A. (1977). *Social learning theory.* Engelwood Cliffs, NJ: Prentice Hall.

Blacher, J. (1984). Attachment and severely handicapped children: Implications for intervention. *Journal of Developmental and Behavioral Pediatrics, 5*(4), 178–183.

Bloom, L., & Lahey, M. (1978). *Language development and language disorders* (pp. 69–70). New York: Wiley.

Capute, A. J., & Accardo, P. J. (1996). *Developmental disabilities in infancy and childhood* (2nd ed., Vols. 1 and 2). Baltimore: Brookes.

Cohen, M. A., & Gross, P. J. (1979). *The developmental sources: Behavioral sequences for assessment and program planning* (Vols. 1 and 2). New York: Grune & Stratton.

Connor, F. P., Williamson, G. G., & Siepp, J. M. (1978). *Program guide for infants and toddlers with neuromotor and other developmental disabilities*. New York: Teachers College Press.

Crain, W. (2000). *Theories of development: Concepts and applications*. New York: Prentice Hall.

Cratty, B. J. (1979). *Perceptual and motor developmental in infants and children* (2nd ed.). New York: Macmillan.

Dawson, G., & Fischer, K. W. (Eds.). (1996). *Human behavior and the developing brain*. New York: Guilford Press.

Erikson, E. H. (1952). *The origins of intelligence in children*. New York: International Universities Press.

Erikson, E. H. (1959). *Identity and the life cycle: Selected papers*. New York: International Universities Press.

Fantz, R. L., Fagan, J. F., & Miranda, S. B. (1973). Early visual selectivity. In L. R. Cohen & P. Salapatek (Eds.), *Infant perception: From sensation to cognition* (pp. 249–341). New York: Academic Press.

Fraiberg, S. (1977). *Insights from the blind*. New York: Basic Books.

Freidlander, S., Pothier, P., Morrison, P., & Herman, O. (1982). The role of neurological developmental delay in childhood psychopathology. *American Journal of Orthopsychiatry, 52*, 102–108.

Gagne, R. (1970). *Conditions of learning*. New York: Holt, Rhinehart and Winston.

Garwood, S. G. (1983). *Educating young handicapped children: A developmental approach* (2nd ed.). Rockville, MD: Aspen Systems.

Garwood, S. G., & Fewell, R. R. (1983). *Educating handicapped infants: Issues in development and intervention*. Rockville, MD: Aspen Systems.

Hanson, M. J. (1984). *A typical infant development*. Baltimore: University Park Press.

Kopp, C. B. (1982). Antecedents of self regulation: A developmental perspective. *Developmental Psychology, 18*(2), 199–214.

Langley, R (1980b). *The teachable moment and the handicapped infant*. Reston, VA: The Council for Exceptional Children.

Lennenberg, E. (1967). *Biological foundations of language*. New York:Wiley.

Lewis, V. (1987). *Development and handicap*. New York: Blackwell.

Ludlow, B. L. (1982). *Teaching the learning disabled*. Bloomington, IN: Phi Delta Kappa Educational.

Martin, H. P. (1982). Neurologic and medical factors affecting assessment. In G. Ulrey & S. J. Rogers (Ed.), *Psychological assessment of handicapped infants and young children* (p. 151). New York: Thieme Stratton, Inc.

McCall, R. R., Hogarty, P. S., & Hurlburt, N. (1972). Transitions in infant sensorimotor development and the prediction of childhood IQ. *American Psychologist, 27*(8), 728–748.

McCormick, L., & Scheifelbusch, R. L. (1984). *Early language intervention: An introduction*. Columbus, OH: Merrill.

Meichenbaum, P. R., & Goodman, J. (1971). Training impulsive children to talk to themselves: A means of developing self-control. *Journal of Abnormal Psychology,* 77(2), 115–126.

Mindes, G. (1982). Social and cognitive aspects of play in young handicapped children. *Topics in Early Childhood Special Education,* 2(3), 39–52.

Murdock, J. (1979). The separation–individuation process and developmental disabilities. *Exceptional Children,* 20(2), 176–184.

Piaget, J. (1952). *The origins of intelligence in children.* New York: International Universities Press.

Ramey, C. T., & Ramey, S. L. (1998). Early intervention and early experience. *American Psychologist,* 53(2), 109–120.

Rogers, S. (1977). Characteristics of the cognitive development of profoundly retarded children. *Child Development,* 48(3), 837–843.

Sprinthall, R. C., & Sprinthall, N. A. (1991). *Educational psychology: A developmental approach* (3rd ed., p. 94). Menlo Park, CA: Addison-Wesley.

Thomas, A., & Chess, S. (1977). *Temperament and development.* New York: Brunner/Mazel.

Vygotsky, L. S. (1962). *Thought and language.* Cambridge, MA: MIT Press.

CHAPTER 4

◆ ◆ ◆

What Are the Best Contexts
for Authentic Assessment?

◆

BEST-PRACTICE ISSUES

◆ Why are natural settings better than standardized situations for assessment of infants, toddlers, and preschoolers?

◆ How can analogue situations supplement authentic assessments in natural settings?

◆ Can the child's own toys and familiar situations be arranged to "occasion" desired behavior and still be considered authentic assessment?

◆ Is it appropriate to prompt and reward a preschooler's behavior during authentic assessment?

◆ Why is body position important when assessing the capabilities of children with disabilities?

◆ Can professionals work and play with children in "staged" situations and still be gathering authentic assessment information?

DEFINITION AND FEATURES

There are six important dimensions of authentic assessment that differ from testing practices. They are structured recordings; developmental observations; ongoing assessment; natural competencies; familiar people; and everyday routines.

Structured Recordings

Authentic assessment is not merely a process of passively observing children's behavior. Rather, it involves the use of standardized and field-validated schedules, protocols, or scales by professionals and parents to systematically record the extent to which developmental skills and various social behaviors are fully acquired, emerging, absent, or problematic in the child's repertoire. Various authentic curriculum-based instruments are available that enable individuals to structure and to systematically record observations to fulfill various early childhood intervention purposes (Bagnato, Neisworth, & Munson, 1997).

Developmental Observations

Observations for authentic assessment are based on age- or stage-referenced hierarchies of functional competencies that follow a developmental course; each early competency is a prerequisite for the next in a sequence of expected or desired behaviors. In many instances, these developmental competencies are mapped to the early learning standards in various states and, most often, they reflect teachable and applied skills that predict early school success (e.g., early literacy, social skills, self-control behaviors, basic concepts, pragmatic communication).

Ongoing Assessment

Authentic assessment for early childhood intervention is not a one-time event. Rather, it is ongoing or serial—occurring over various times of the day and different occasions. It is important that a full portrait of the child's skills contain representative samples of typical behavior from home, preschool, and community settings covering various activities and times of day—morning greeting, group circle time, lunch, snack, playground, computer work, bedtime, bathtime, parent–child activities.

Natural Competencies

One of the strengths of authentic assessment resides in the focus on children's typical behavior in a variety of everyday routines that are familiar to the child. Such naturally occurring behaviors reflect acquired or emerging competencies that arise in repeated home and preschool situations. These natural competencies reflect real-life problem-solving capabilities that promote future self-reliance and self-efficacy.

Familiar People

Rather than basing results upon the testing or observations of strangers (even though they may be credentialed professionals!), authentic assessment relies upon the ongoing observations of familiar and knowledgeable *caregivers*. Caregivers are defined as those individuals who know the child's typical or emerging competencies and idiosyncrasies, engage in repeated interactions with the child on a daily basis, and, of course, are familiar to the child; the child has some attachment to them. Such individuals can include child care providers, babysitters, grandparents, friends, teachers, therapists, and other team members in early intervention. Close knowledge and familiarity are crucial to reliable, valid, and representative assessments of all children, especially those with developmental delays and disabilities.

Everyday Routines

Observations are made of natural competencies that occur in typical settings, activities, and routines of the day both at home and in the preschool. These routines exert the influence of recurrent cues in the physical environment and interactions with adults and peers that promote or inhibit the expression of these natural competencies and ultimately affect early learning and future success at school, with others, and in the community.

THE IMPORTANCE OF DEVELOPMENTAL CONTEXT
FOR AUTHENTIC ASSESSMENT

Perhaps the central feature of authentic assessment is the environmental or developmental context that promotes or inhibits the child's early learning and progress. The natural environment of everyday routines is each child's *"developmental ecology."* This ecology identifies the total nurturing environment for the child, including parents, teachers, peers, and various other caregivers as well as the diverse physical and social environments where interactions with these figures occur. Thus, for all children, assessment in and of this ecology or context is critical for accurate, valid, and representative appraisal of strengths and needs.

In Chapter 2, I discussed the authentic assessment alternative to conventional testing in early childhood intervention. One of the features of this description was the continuum of measurement contexts. In this chapter, I focus on the most authentic contexts or developmental ecologies in the continuum for assessment of young children—natural and analogue. Figure 4.1 illustrates the continuum of major contexts for measurement that are used by professionals. The continuum proceeds from the most authentic contexts, on the left (i.e., natural and analogue), to the least authentic and most contrived (i.e., simulated and clinical), on the right. Again, the use of natural or analogue contexts for authentic assessment is best practice with preschoolers, not contrived testing circumstances and procedures.

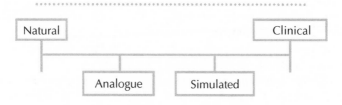

FIGURE 4.1. Continuum of measurement contexts.

Natural Contexts

Authentic assessment is based on the underlying concept that children express their typical behavior and performance best in familiar environments that contain reinforcing physical and social cues for early learning and progress. This describes *natural contexts*. To be sure, many children are raised and cared for in natural environments that are not reinforcing or nurturing and may even be detrimental. Nevertheless, the child's typical behavior and interactions in everyday routines foster the best understanding of current capabilities and predictors for future progress. Also, appraisal of the physical and social environment enables professionals to detect features of the environment that both promote and inhibit performance and to plan modifications that will promote gains.

Assessment in natural environments is required by the Individuals with Disabilities Education Improvement Act (IDEIA) and the Office of Special Education Programs. Recommended professional standards such as these of the Division of Early Childhood (DEC) and the National Association for the Education of Young Children (NAEYC) also require teachers and other professionals in collaboration with parents to use natural and unobtrusive tactics, methods, and instruments that capture real-life functioning in real-life settings. Authentic assessment in natural environments is not merely an arbitrary or contrary personal decision. Rather, authentic assessment in the child's own developmental ecology is required by law, promoted by professional standards for credentialing, aligned with strong developmental and behavioral theories and practices, and supported by an emerging research evidence base.

Natural contexts for infants, toddlers, and preschoolers encompass physical environments, routines, activities, materials, peers, and adults. An exhaustive catalogue of these contextual features is unnecessary, but I list here some for illustration to help set the stage for authentic assessment. Natural contexts for assessment include home, preschool, and community settings. Within the home, children's behavior is influenced by many factors including parenting behaviors, availability of multisensory toys, use of the television and computer, daily schedule, and siblings. Observational assessment by both parents and professionals can record such naturally occurring functional competencies as finding a remembered toy at the bottom of the toy box, opening and closing doors, unlocking locks, turning the television on and off, using remote controls, pretend play with favorite toys, sharing or fighting with brothers and sisters, turn-taking in games, using a chair to climb to a cupboard to get the cereal box, following mother's directions to "bring me the salt shaker," following steps in making a pizza together, indicating wants and needs by crying and gestures, and describing a favorite videotape.

Within the preschool, children show their competencies in such activities as playing in the sandbox, counting toy animals, lining up and sorting types of toy animals, retelling the details of a story read aloud the day before, sharing Play-Doh with a peer, making a sculpture from clay, identifying common signs and words, using the bathroom, understanding basic concepts in daily activities such as "big box," "little fish," "on the windowsill," and "behind the door." Each of these situations couples a functional competency with an activity within a setting with materials. Children demonstrate their competencies clearly in many ways and situations during a day. Professionals need merely to have technically adequate recording tools that enable them to observe, capture, and score these natural competencies in order to summarize skills and needs. Using natural settings, professionals are not straitjacketed by scripted and restricted materials and situations and expected responses for assessment. Children who do not show cause–effect, object permanence, or other problem-solving behaviors using the unmotivating and contrived toys and tasks in most test kits will most often show their "true" competencies in natural settings or with familiar adults in such daily activities as flipping the light switch, finding a ball that has rolled under the couch, and steering a shopping cart around a display in the grocery store. Natural contexts enable children to display their spontaneous competencies in any way possible; observers can note the reinforcing or inhibiting features of the environment that affect the display of the behavior, and thus the child's current skills and performance levels, as well as make suggestions for improving care, instruction, and learning.

The early developmentalists got it right: natural observation in natural settings offers the richest picture of children's capabilities. In the modern era, our charge is to select, use, and even develop tools and technologies that allow us the flexibility to unobtrusively capture and document real-life performance in real-life settings rather than depending on contrived, laboratory-like situations and tasks.

Analogue Contexts

Analogue contexts are a beneficial complement and, sometimes, alternative to full natural contexts. *Analogue contexts* refer to natural contexts in which the activities, materials, toys, and even people are arranged, managed, and selected so as to "occasion" or prompt behaviors that may not be readily observed or that are inconsistent in the child's repertoire. In analogue contexts, teachers, parents, and other professionals can choose toys and circumstances that will likely stimulate the child to act. For example, if one is concerned about a child's ability to share, take turns, and follow game rules in preschool because the child shies away from peers and group activities, the situation can be arranged and managed to increase the likelihood that the child will show the desired behavior. A familiar peer can be chosen to play with the child in a quiet section of the classroom with the teacher guiding the play in a fun game that requires turn taking. The teacher can set the rules and encourage the children to play; first, one can observe the children's natural play tendencies. If spontaneous sharing, rule following, and turn taking are not observed, the teacher can model such behavior and then praise the child for showing expected behavior following the model or prompt. In this case, the child's performance would indicate an "emerging" skill—one that is available in the child's skill repertoire, but not yet consistent. In analogue contexts, selection of multisensory and response-contingent toys and devices (i.e., microswitch on a drumming bear, touch-activated communication devices) is critical to appraisal of the full range of functional capabilities for a child and the environmental conditions that prompt those capabilities.

Analogue contexts are useful most often with children who have developmental delays and disabilities or challenging social behaviors. For children with special needs, it is common that their behaviors are inconsistent, and their skill sets are meager. Also, latencies or lags in behavioral response times occur because of neurophysiological dysfunctions. For children with cerebral palsy, acquired brain injuries, autism spectrum disorders, and significant developmental retardation, analogue contexts can provide strong supporting information about possible higher-level and emerging capabilities that are not observed spontaneously, but rather require environmental stimulation and organization for display.

CONSIDERATIONS IN STAGING
AUTHENTIC ASSESSMENTS FOR PRESCHOOL CHILDREN
IN ANALOGUE CONTEXTS

Traditional styles of evaluation require children to sit at a table, respond on demand, and perform without rewards, and require testers to impassively follow standardized procedures. Teachers, psychologists, and others who work with preschoolers sense that they must use different arrangements and styles of interaction when assessing preschool children. We must recognize the emotional needs and behavioral styles of toddlers and preschoolers and adjust interactions accordingly or our efforts will fail. The aims and methods for assessing preschoolers are quite different from those for school-age children. Professionals require keen observational skills, creative flexibility in procedures, and, most of all, sensitivity to detect and respond to the young child's interests, moods, and needs. These attributes are magnified in importance and "put to the test" when assessing young children with developmental disabilities. For authentic assessment in analogue situations, teachers, psychologists, and other caregivers must be both good playmates and good managers of behavior. Simply, professionals must be skilled in staging a preschool assessment.

Staging refers to arranging the physical and social environment, selecting toys and materials, and adjusting one's language and style of interaction to sustain the preschooler's attention and social interactions in order to ensure *optimal* child performance during the observational assessment.

Behavioral Styles of Typical Preschoolers

Often, behavior that we consider of concern in school-age children is developmentally appropriate for the preschool child. For example, inattention, distractibility, impulsiveness, overactivity, noncompliance, and some degree of aggressiveness are worrisome when observed in a fourth-grade child. However, these behaviors are expected with preschool children. No wonder that it is so difficult to diagnose attention disorder and hyperactivity during the preschool years! Often, the diagnosis is a reflection more of the adult's lack of tolerance rather than the child's intrinsic problem. There are four behavior patterns that are developmentally appropriate for typically functioning preschoolers and necessitate general strategies for reducing their impact on performance in the analogue setting.

Fear of New Situations

Typically, preschool children may be fearful or wary of new situations. This can include difficulties separating from the parent, fear of unfamiliar people, and reactions to failure on new activities. For this reason, a quick systematic desensitization procedure is usually effective. This involves a positive, gradual, low-demand approach to allow the young child time to adjust to the new situation. Have the parent present, initially, in the classroom or analogue situation to reassure the preschooler that you, your toys, and the situation are safe. Talk to the parent first while allowing the child to explore the room freely to allow time for this reassurance to occur naturally. Novel toys placed selectively about the room encourage the child's discovery and provides you with the opportunity to make contact in a nonthreatening way and to set the stage for a rewarding play interaction that will encourage the child to play apart from the parent.

Encourage the child to play with the toys and materials in a more structured place and manner. Select toys appropriate for a wide age or ability range. As you begin, be certain to choose toys and materials that will maintain the child's interest and task orientation. It is crucial to intersperse easy and difficult tasks—particularly with young children who have motor, behavior, language, and social interaction problems. The child will give up on tasks easily if they are viewed as too hard and failure is possible. For example, gross motor tasks and verbal reasoning tasks must be interspersed and alternated to maintain interest. If the child is unable to complete a task after two to three attempts, switch to an activity he or she has completed successfully before and allow the child to gain some success at something familiar. Completion of a task is often more reinforcing than social praise alone.

Overactivity and Distractibility

Professionals must remember that only a few preschoolers have learned a "set" for paying attention, answering questions, and doing activities on demand. For these reasons, reintroducing tasks at a later time after modeling and observing spontaneous play behavior are necessary to discover if the child really has acquired a particular skill or concept. Attention span may be fine for familiar tasks, but may vary markedly with other demands, including the use of two-step directions, increases in item difficulty, directions to look, listen, and draw at the same time, and an emphasis on the child's least well-developed skill area. Be vigilant to reduce competing stimuli, choose naturally exciting tasks, give frequent praise, and separate the steps for doing auditory, visual, and verbal tasks.

Negativism and Oppositional Behavior

Preschoolers have little experience in staying with an activity just because someone says so. Moreover, their natural push toward independence and autonomy is a recipe for conflict if one fails to understand these dual factors of lack of experience and natural noncompliance. In analogue assessment situations for which time is limited, professionals should rather establish an atmosphere of cooperative turn taking—"working and playing together." Start with games or active toys that permit turn taking. This models the behaviors appropriate for preschoolers and also allows them the opportunity to be rewarded for (unwitting) compliance! Once again, it is important to intersperse structured, perhaps tabletop tasks, with more free play opportunities as a reward. For example, formal puzzle tasks can be followed by drawing activities or picture identification tasks, followed by free play with puppets. More than one and often several observational assessments in different situations are necessary to move beyond situational opposition and noncompliance to achieve an optimal survey of the pre-schooler's competencies.

Perseveration

Repetition of behavior is a common occurrence with preschoolers. Young children may perseverate because they are rewarded for it or, for example, because they know only one way of playing with a toy. Professionals can reduce perseveration by teaching new responses (e.g., cause–effect play versus banging) through modeling, and then reinforcing these different, new behaviors through praise. Similarly, they can praise "hard work" and guessing or trying on unfamiliar and difficult tasks rather than only success. Using the preferred perseverative task to reward work on the more difficult, less desirable one is often effective.

Analogue Contexts for Preschoolers at Risk and with Mild Delays

Several considerations are important when organizing analogue situations for young children with suspected or mild developmental difficulties, including those at high risk for learning disabilities, attention disorders and hyperactivity, communication disorders, and possible mental retardation. These considerations have been arranged below into five major clusters: physical environment; body positioning; attitude and interactive style; routines and transitions; and motivation and management.

Physical Environment

The condition of a classroom or analogue situation greatly affects the behavior and adjustment of young children. Such factors as room lighting, temperature, noise, and even arrangement of furnishings can ruin the best staged setting. Psychologists should strive to reduce distractions by any convenient means, such as room dividers or carrels if possible or, more likely, by positioning chairs and tables away from distracting noises and movement and toward corners.

Planning of *room layout* is critical for many children. This means placing and arranging chairs, tables, and toys strategically about a room so that the child has easy access to the materials and distance is maintained from doors and windows. In fact, the familiar environment of the preschool setting or home should be considered the best context in which to evaluate the child's skills. Here the child knows the materials, understands what is expected behavior, feels comfortable, and will more likely be less wary of strangers.

Body Positioning

One of the most crucial and generally neglected considerations is body positioning for the child. Professionals must recognize that young children do not have the same skill in trunk control and equilibrium that older children do. Therefore, the *importance of proper choice of child-sized tables and chairs* cannot be overstated when working and playing at tables. The child should be seated at a chair that is padded, allows feet to bear weight slightly on the floor, and, preferably, has arm rests or sides to contain and stabilize the young child. Similarly, the table surface should be approximately waist high and allow the child proper position, height, and leverage for such tasks as drawing, assembling, and block building. Some children with neuromotor immaturities are affected quite negatively by improper body positions, presumably because they must concentrate on maintaining balance and position. Thus, they fail to attend and persist on tasks because they are tense and preoccupied. Moreover, the young child should spend no more than 15 minutes at the chair and table at any one time, and should be given the opportunity to work and play in other positions.

Attitude and Interactive Style of the Professional

The professional arranging an analogue situation for observation must be flexible in maintaining a structured play atmosphere that motivates the child to do his or her best. The professional cannot be afraid of "acting like a fool" to keep the child attentive, aroused, and task oriented. This requires one to respond to the child's interests and preferences to some degree while also imposing structure.

Preschool children respond best when adults identify their behavioral and temperamental needs beforehand and react accordingly to signs of anxiousness, fear, or loss of interest. Many children work best with a *side-by-side seating arrangement* on the floor or at the table. This may involve seating the child in a chair and at a table tailored to size. Instead of sitting across from the child, the adult should sit beside the child (ata 60- to 90-degree angle) with an arm placed lightly about the child's shoulder. This serves to gently contain the child and cue him or her about the expected behavior of sitting and working at a table for certain tasks. During a play-based assessment analogue situation, toys and activities should be presented from the child's side in a *calm, gradual approach* with fluid changes from activity to activity. This also conveys the message that "we are working and playing, together." Often, using a *soft, quiet voice* models slow, deliberate habits for the child. This also requires him or her to listen more carefully for directions and to attend better. Using this soothing manner, the adult can also shape the child's behavioral style by a combination of physical prompts and verbal cues as needed, such as "Remember, we look before we point"; "Let's use our little voice"; "Show me quiet hands" (accompanied by a manual prompt). This style illustrates clearly that effective assessment behaviors are the same as effective teaching behaviors.

Routines and Transitions

Routines and transitions between routines are very important for any preschooler, especially those with language, learning, and behavior problems.

Preparation for transitions will greatly reduce disruptive, off-task behavior. Preschoolers must be told beforehand what changes are coming and what they will be doing so that they know what to expect. This attention to preparatory routines will ease the transition and reduce the possibility of resistance, fear, and tantrums. Similarly, *frequent breaks* must be taken between activities and situations to extend the child's endurance and to maintain attention and task performance.

In addition, other contextual factors encourage optimal performances. The *presence of parents and peers* in the analogue situation is often important for young preschoolers who need reassurance. In addition, parents share a complementary base of information with the professional, who can refer to and explain the meaning of a child's behavior more clearly. However, the analogue situation should be viewed more broadly as a time to appraise the child's capacity to practice separating from parents and peers and adjusting to new circumstances. *Cooperative games and high-interest toys* such as arcade video games and movable, sound-producing cars and trains with microswitches frequently allow the adult and young child to become comfortable with each other.

Motivation and Management

The combination of *balanced work and play* with structure and management increases motivation and fosters optimal performance.

The *use of rewards* is vital with preschoolers. Preschool specialists should regularly use stickers, tokens, social praise, and task-embedded reinforcers such as novel activities to establish and maintain motivation through incentives. A developmental hierarchy of reinforcers can be used that is based on an initial scrutiny of the child's level of development and social competence. Similarly, professionals must also view their job as evaluating the child's ability to change behavior through positive management and limit setting. Preschoolers should be given choices as a way of encouraging cooperation while emphasizing that compliance is required ("You can play with either the train or the bear; which do you want?").

Young children need *models for behavior*. Preschoolers feel more secure and are more compliant when they know what will happen, how they are expected to behave, and how adults will respond to their behavior.

Thus, the analogue assessment session is inevitably a controlled situation for observing the young child's competence in adjusting to more structured routines and learning important prerequisite behaviors. Answering questions, completing puzzles, and drawing designs at a table is a strange, new experience for many preschoolers, who have been unaccustomed to following directions and staying seated. We must analyze how quickly they can learn prerequisite skills. Modeling and demonstration of expected behaviors are important as well as rewards for effort and compliance. However, it is just as important to evaluate children's *reactions to limit setting*. Professionals should feel that not only is it okay to discipline preschoolers, but that it is required and necessary. Planned ignoring of inappropriate behavior and social praise for desired behavior are basic strategies. Also effective are combined verbal and physical prompts to direct eyes to pictures, to encourage pointing at pictures instead of hitting cards, and for reducing impulsive grabbing of materials. These management strategies must be used to shape appropriate looking, listening, waiting, and sharing. In extreme circumstances, time out in a chair at a corner for tantrum behavior may be required; similarly, we must not be afraid to show an angry face with an angry or displeased voice tone when disciplining a child in order to heighten the cues that distinguish appropriate from inappropriate behavior for the young inexperienced preschooler. A "wimpy" or impassive approach may not provide the contrast needed to stop ongoing inappropriate behavior. Of course, many children may need only a slight sign of displeasure from the adult. The required level of reprimand must be detected by the alert and sensitive professional.

Finally, *word choice and phrasing* are important, especially given the limited memory skills of the young child with a language disorder for long and multiple directions and and his or her limited understanding of only the basic words and concepts. Preschool teachers and specialists must recognize the necessity of using *active, concrete directions* with young children. "Look with your eyes" is superior to "pay attention." "Listen with your ears" can be accompanied by a manual cue such as holding your ears out. When first entering the room for the analogue situation, the adult can prepare the child sufficiently by simply saying, "I have some new toys to show you in my room; we can work and play together with them." Other examples may include "Put your finger on the car" instead of "Show me the car." With some children, it may be necessary to use short telegraphic statements (when there is a severe lack of language) such as "Kermit—sit," "roll ball," or "ball under chair."

In summary, a combination of novel, active, multisensory toys, behavior management strategies, varied room arrangements, and judicious word choices can combine to allow young children who are at risk or have mild delays to display capabilities in the analogue situation that approximate performance in the "real world," and show their best selves.

Analogue Contexts for Children with Low-Incidence Disabilities

Professionals are challenged and often frustrated when called upon to observe and profile the capabilities of young children with severe functional limitations. Aside from temperamental and behavioral considerations, accommodations must also be made for the child's sensory, neuromotor, cognitive/linguistic, and affective/behavioral limitations. Special arrangements are necessary in these circumstances to circumvent disabilities and to maximize performance by using both environmental and, often, prosthetic adaptations to the usual assessment context. Young children with prominent disabilities include those with visual impairments, hearing impairments, severe developmental retardation, neuromotor impairments (e.g., cerebral palsy), and affective/behavioral disorders (e.g., autism spectrum disorder). The following sections pose key guidelines in staging an analogue authentic assessment for each disability group.

Sensory Impairments

VISUAL IMPAIRMENT

One of the most important staging considerations for children with visual impairment is allowing sufficient time for the child to orient and *adjust to the unfamiliar environment*. The use of a team approach using a *vision specialist* during the observational sessions represents best practice. These children must have time to explore toys gradually and to orient to the room arrangement through the combined use of hearing, smell, taste, and touch. The professionals must be as sure of the child's *residual vision* as possible since children are rarely totally blind; similarly, children often resist using their prescription lenses or parents forget to bring the child's glasses. Removing distractions, providing one toy or task at a time, and prompting touching of different toys and textures broaden the child's experience and gradually foster awareness of surroundings.

It is vital that the child be provided with a *distraction-free, well-defined work area* with accessible boundaries such as a defined play area or a table tray with higher sides. Next, choosing *multisensory toys* is in order. Carefully choose toys that seem to match the child's stage of play skills gauged by your observation and parental report. In general, toys must be movable, sound producing, air producing, oversized, and textured, have high-contrast colors and illumination, be easily manipulated, and have raised and single line features.

Preschool specialists must be skilled in using instructional strategies and knowledgeable about developmental expectancies for young blind children. Verbal directions must be more concrete and active than usual; a combination of *verbal descriptions and manual prompts* must be used in providing access to toys, materials, and tasks. Preparatory descriptions of the toys and tasks being presented and what the child will be doing with them are helpful procedures. Children must also be told when to start and stop an activity to orient them in time. For example, "Sara, this is a fuzzy rabbit. He has big, long ears with bells on them that make noise. We can feel the ears with our hands and hear the bells with our ears. They are big and long! Hear the sound [verbal and manual guidance]? This toy over here is a big box. Let's feel how big and deep it is. You can almost go inside it." (Manually guide the child's hand into the box.) "Now, feel the rabbit on the floor beside you with your hands (assessor rings bells). Hear the bells? Get him! Now, put him in the big box." The specialist must use auditory and tactile cues in working with the child to assess the ability to search for an object out of reach (object permanence) and to follow a direction regarding location. The reward is success in the task, hugging, and social praise. *Exaggerated up-and-down voice intonations* should be used to help the child distinguish between different feeling states, for example, happiness and excitement for task completion, surprise for a new event (jack-in-the-box pops up), and firmness for stopping inappropriate behavior (e.g., eye poking). Gradually present and remove activities for the child to smooth transitions and to increase readiness for the next activity with little upset.

Know *developmental expectancies* for blind preschoolers. They show some general though prominent functional deficits that must be considered during assessment. Blind children may not use their well developed gross motor skills until they have learned to move out in space toward a sound cue; thus, sounds must first have reinforcement value for them. They show delays in social communication and initiation, such as smiling and reaching out to touch a familiar adult's face. Also, these children typically show gaps in knowledge of concepts. They may know the name for something but be unable to describe it accurately because of their lack of experience.

Finally, it is often necessary to deal with the child's self-stimulatory behaviors such as hand flapping, eye poking, and twirling or spinning. These "blindisms" can be managed by using combinations of various behavior techniques including sensory extinction, interruption, and alternate sensory activities.

HEARING IMPAIRMENT

A screening for *residual hearing* is an essential first step in any authentic assessment that includes establishing an analogue situation. The use of hearing aids and body pack amplifiers must be determined beforehand. Assessment of hearing impaired children requires very specialized skills. Ideally, the teacher and other team members should have previous experience with deaf and hearing impaired preschoolers and must be trained in the use of a *total communication approach* including signing and gestures.

However, this is rarely the case; thus, consultation with a communication disorders specialist and/or *hearing specialist* during the assessment is a key to accurate assessment; in short, a team approach is essential!

The room environment for the child should be as free as possible of visual *distractions* and ambient noise and vibrations. Consider the *room arrangement* beforehand, especially lighting and direct seating across from the child so that full facial attention is obtained. Again, *multisensory toys* and tasks must be carefully selected. Visual and motor or tactile characteristics are most important; thus, toys should be movable, vibrating, colorful, textured, and highly arousing (e.g., pop-up toys, visual computer displays).

Once again, *instructional strategies* are important. Physically prompt the child's eyes and face to the task; reward with smiles, touching, facial expressions, and clapping. Use demonstrations, pantomime, and manual guidance to teach trial tasks beforehand to prepare the child. Make gestures very demonstrative and exaggerate facial expressions to convey direction and meaning. At times, allow the child to feel your throat vibrations for help in distinguishing words and sounds.

The use of *nonverbal and/or universally designed assessment content and deaf norms* is absolutely critical. Developmentally, young children with hearing impairments generally show serious delays in speech and language production. Behavior problems with shyness, wariness, and social withdrawal are not uncommon and must be considered in establishing rapport. With older preschoolers, puppet play and interactive computer games can help foster trust, interest, and cooperation. In language assessment with such toddlers, it is often helpful to demonstrate comprehension through the paired use of concrete and pictured objects. For example, a toy rabbit can be matched with a picture of a rabbit.

Developmental Retardation

For infants and preschoolers with severe cognitive deficits, combinations of the strategies for other disabilities are necessary. Team members must *consider atypical patterns of development and behavior* when assessing preschoolers with severe cognitive and functional limitations. These characteristics include variable attention and arousal, high and low muscle tone, changeable moods, fleeting social communication, little or no initiation of interactions, self-stimulatory patterns, seizures, and nonpurposeful and infantile play patterns (e.g., mouthing, banging, shaking, throwing).

Body position and choice of toys are two important staging dimensions. It is important to conduct the assessment with other team members, preferably the teacher or an occupational or physical therapist who understands the crucial importance of body position on optimal performance. Such children can be positioned in feeder or car seats so that upright positioning and head control are promoted. Another technique is to seat the child in the therapist's lap to support the child upright. The use of visually stimulating, response-contingent, colorful, movable, sound-producing toys will in itself prompt and shape adaptive responses better than toys with single indistinct features. Nevertheless, manual prompts are necessary to allow the child to initiate behavior; then, the psychologist can redo a task and observe whether the adaptive behavior is repeated independently without prompts. *Emphasize social interaction* heavily in the assessment. Face-to-face vocal play for children with limitations can be conducted using peek-a-boo games, gently blowing air on the child's face to stimulate smiling, matching vocalizations, and employing other emotional responses. Another simple game consists of placing the child on his or her back while the teacher or other caregiver uses high-pitched, up-and-down vocalizations (like a slide whistle) and moves his or her face near and then away from the child. Using this game, you can assess sustained attention, social communication, arousal, and evidence that the child wants the game to continue (secondary circular reactions). Often, a Piagetian framework for cognitive developmental assessment is very useful to suggest tasks and procedures for eliciting cause–effect, means–end, imitative, and object search behaviors from preschoolers with severe developmental retardation.

Neuromotor Impairments

Consistent with the cognitive deficits frequently accompanying neurological impairments, children with cerebral palsy are not able to discover and explore their worlds through motor exploration. In addition, they often learn to be helpless since their motor deficits prevent them from gaining toys that they want; this establishes a cycle in which parents and others dominate interactions and do things for them. They then become dependent and passive while never having the experience of testing their own capabilities—the key to developing a sense of personal competence or self-efficacy.

The aim of the analogue authentic assessment is to *circumvent the neuromotor deficits* as much as possible to isolate evidence of intact conceptual, problem solving, and social communication skills—a tall, but not impossible order.

As an inviolable principle, professionals, especially psychologists, should never assess children with neuromotor impairments unless they pair with a physical or occupational therapist or teacher skilled in proper positioning techniques. *Proper positioning* for each child all too frequently makes the difference between an accurate appraisal and one that, while seemingly true,, dramatically underestimates the child's concepts and competencies. The child with cerebral palsy or acquired brain injuries, for example, should be observed over several situations and times, and by several people so that the child's typical methods of communication can be determined. *Consultation with the therapist or teacher* will provide direction on the most effective positioning arrangement according to the child's level of muscle tone, arm and hand use, and trunk and head support. Often, young children with physical impairments interact and perform best when seated in their *adaptive wheelchair with a table tray*. The chair offers the advantage of structure, confinement at a table, foot support for leverage, and trunk support by an H-strap over the chest and shoulder wedges that position the arms forward for better hand use at the midline of the body. At a table surface, it is usually helpful to use a sticky or nonslip surface, which can be attained with removable Dycem products that prevent toys from sliding. Another arrangement may involve seating at a corner chair with a high back and wedges and blocks for trunk support. For children with more severe limitations, the use of a beanbag chair is recommended to mold body positions; also, working with the child in a side-lying position (on the side) that offers best hand use is important. Systems such as *Every Move Counts* (EMC; 1989) have been field validated for children functioning below the 18-month stage. EMC forms the basis for an effective combination of sensory and communication assessment strategies involving observation, analogue methods, and prompting attuned to the purpose of creating an individualized plan for instruction and therapy. Proper positioning alters muscle tone, reduces the negative effects of persistent primitive reflexes, and aligns the head and body for optimal facial orientation, reaching and grasping, and manipulating. While using testing procedures, *Developmental Potential of Preschool Children* by Haeussermann (1958) is still the best detailed resource on assessing young children with cerebral palsy since it was prescient in advocating the movement toward functional assessment, modifications to detect optimal capabilities, and assessment–intervention linkages.

Assessing the child's most *reliable response mode* is another key step in staging. The team must explore alternative modes such as eye localization to pictures and objects, changes in facial (emotional) expressions, eye blinks, global gestures for the child with athetoid cerebral palsy, and yes–no head shakes. The use of microswitches on action toys for cause–effect play and alternate computer-based communication systems must be explored and used as part of the assessment.

In summary, authentic and analogue assessment of young children with neuromotor impairments dictates using adaptive equipment, determining the best response mode, properly positioning the child, and allowing sufficient time for the child to try a task before offering verbal or manual guidance.

Affective/Behavior Disorders

Staging an analogue assessment for a child with autism spectrum disorder is one of the most challenging and frequently exhausting experiences for both parents and professionals. A *team approach* is necessary with such children; the use of an *authentic assessment protocol for natural observation* is essential to greatly reduce ambiguity and to appraise comprehensively the child's capabilities and intensity of service needs. The protocol should be a multisource, multidimensional survey that synthesizes information from parent interview, observation of parent–child interaction, ratings of atypical and functional characteristics, and appraisal of verbal and, especially, nonverbal concept development and problem solving. Authentic curriculum-based measures such as the Autism Diagnostic Inventory (ADI-R; 1994) and the Adaptive Behavior Assessment System (Harrison & Oakland, 2003) are extremely useful since they allow all team members to contribute to the assessment and help to determine the severity of the disorder and range of functional competencies in order to direct intervention.

Two aspects of autism seriously disrupt developmental progress: a presumably neurogenetic basis that distorts sensory input and often results in self-stimulatory behavior; and serious deficits in social interaction and communication. These same qualities make staging a formal assessment extremely difficult. A combination of table and free play activities should be arranged in the analogue setup that alternates *verbal, nonverbal, and reciprocal tasks.* For structured activities, it is often best to use a chair and table to contain the child and/or an assistant to *interrupt inappropriate behaviors.* Often, these children show an unusual attachment to certain toys, such as a Gumby doll or horse or, typically, toys that spin and move. These can be used as activity reinforcers for completing various assessment tasks. Interspersing verbal and nonverbal tasks is crucial, for example, object/picture identification followed by assembling a disjointed cat puzzle. Of critical importance in analogue situations is observation of the interaction between the child and his or her parents, stressing expression and acceptance of affection, rhythmic habit patterns, symbolic play with toys, ability to cope with changes, and, above all, eye contact and initiation of social interaction. These observational sessions should be designed to elicit the child's typical responses to environmental stimulation, including negative reactions such as screaming, self-involvement, tantrums when routines are disrupted, and catastrophic reactions to transitions.

BEST-PRACTICE GUIDEPOINTS

Analogue Contexts for Typical Preschoolers

♦ Desensitize fears.
♦ Expect inattention.
♦ Reduce distractions.
♦ Give simple, active directions.
♦ Use real toys.
♦ Use child-sized furniture.

♦ Work and play together.
♦ Alternate easy and difficult tasks.
♦ Ensure multiple sessions and times.
♦ Model, prompt, and reward new behaviors.

Analogue Contexts for Preschoolers at Risk and with Mild Delays

♦ Rearrange natural home and preschool settings.
♦ Provide extra structure with toys and activities.
♦ Emphasize optimal positioning.
♦ Play but be in charge.
♦ Acquaint child with peers and adults first.
♦ Include parents and favorite toys and games.
♦ Maintain a reassuring and positive manner.
♦ Allow breaks.
♦ Reward through praise and favorite activities.
♦ Alternate work and play.
♦ Use active, concrete directions..
♦ Model prerequisite behaviors.
♦ Set limits as needed.

Analogue Contexts for Preschoolers with Moderate and Severe Disabilities

SENSORY IMPAIRMENTS

♦ Appraise vision and hearing.
♦ Consult with specialists.
♦ Use multisensory materials and methods.
♦ Exaggerate gestures, expressions, and voice.
♦ Use universally designed content and disability-specific norms.

DEVELOPMENTAL RETARDATION

♦ Limit stereotypical behaviors.
♦ Use response-contingent toys.
♦ Emphasize social interactions.

NEUROMOTOR IMPAIRMENTS

♦ Team with physical therapist/occupational therapist, teacher, and parent.
♦ Stress individual positioning.
♦ Use adaptive equipment and accommodations.
♦ Discover best response modes.

AFFECTIVE/BEHAVIOR DISORDERS

♦ Use a formal observational protocol.

♦ Limit self-stimulatory behaviors.

♦ Emphasize nonverbal and reciprocal tasks.

♦ Appraise parent–child and child–peer social interactions.

BEST-PRACTICE EVIDENCE

Bagnato, S. J., & Campbell, T. F. (1993). Comprehensive neurodevelopmental evaluation of children with brain insults. In G. Miller & J. Ramer (Eds.), *Static encephalopathies of infancy and childhood* (pp. 27–44). New York: Raven Press.

Bagnato, S. J., & Neisworth, J. T. (1985). Assessing young handicapped children: Clinical judgment versus developmental performance scales. *International Journal of Partial Hospitalization, 3*(1), 13–21.

Bagnato, S. J., Neisworth, J. T., & Munson, S. M. (1997). *LINKing assessment and early intervention: An authentic curriculum-based approach* (3rd ed.). Baltimore: Brookes.

Bronson, M. B. (2000). *Self-regulation in early childhood.* New York: Guilford Press.

Haeussermann, E. (1958). *Developmental potential of preschool children.* New York: Grune & Stratton.

Harrison, P., & Oakland, T. (2003). *Adaptive behavior assessment system* (2nd ed.). San Antonio, TX: The Psychological Corporation.

Korsten, J. E., Dunn, D. K., Foss, T. V., & Francke, M. K. (1989). *Every move counts: Sensory-based communication techniques.* San Antonio, TX: The Psychological Corporation.

Lewis, V. (1987). *Development and handicap.* New York: Blackwell.

Lord, C., Rutter, M., & Le Couteur, A. (1994). *The Autism Diagnostic Interview, Revised.* California: Western Psychological Services.

Lynch, E. M., & Struewing, N. A. (2005). Children in context: Portfolio assessment in the inclusive early childhood classroom. *Young Exceptional Children, 5*(1), 2–10.

Robeck, M. C. (1987). *Infants and young children: Their development and learning.* New York: McGraw-Hill.

◆ ◆ ◆

CHAPTER 5

Can Professionals "Test without Tests" for Authentic Assessment?

◆

with RICHARD LeVAN

BEST-PRACTICE ISSUES

◆ Can natural observations be used to assess intelligent behavior?

◆ How does typical child behavior in daily routines reveal "true" developmental competence?

◆ Can natural observations be used to conduct valid assessments?

◆ How can assessment competencies in measures be reorganized around daily routines to structure "shopping for skills"?

Preschool children naturally display patterns of development and behavior that frequently limit the use of formal and standardized evaluation procedures. Disabling conditions including sensory impairments, motoric involvement, and speech–language disorders further compromise the utility of such measures. Based on direct experience, an alternative strategy for the assessment of young children with disabilities is necessary.

Richard LeVan, PhD (deceased), was affiliated with the Sara Reed Children's Center at Gannon University in Erie, Pennsylvania.

Brief clinical sampling can be used as the basis for making structured judgments regarding development. In the context of skill hierarchies, this information is useful in designing programs for intervention. This chapter describes principles and techniques of brief clinical sampling. Examples of the applications of brief clinical sampling with young children with disabilities are given.

ADVENTURES IN ASSESSMENT

To say that Clarence was an active child would have certainly understated the case. This 3½-year-old was clearly hyperactive, impulsive, and constantly on the go. Gross motor skills were good. Those who knew Clarence were fully aware of his agility. Observed expressive language was limited. Clarence communicated using an intricate blend of noises and gestures. No limitations of vision or hearing had been reported. Development of instructional programs for Clarence had been difficult. He also presented management problems both at home and in his preschool classroom. Behavioral and medical interventions had not been successful in producing any notable gain in self-regulation.

The assignment was to conduct further assessment with Clarence and obtain information that would be useful in promoting his overall development. As far as testing Clarence, others had tried before. They came away exhausted with no more than a qualified IQ somewhere in the range of 35 to 50. The assignment was accepted with determination. Instruments were selected and the assessment, which was conducted at home, began. A few short minutes later it was over. Even with the best attempts to structure the setting, the tiny toys of the test were of little value in drawing and holding attention. Once neatly organized in small boxes, they were left in disarray. Beads and blocks had become projectiles and were scattered about the floor. Because of the "less than optimal" level of cooperation, testing was discontinued.

This assessment had given Clarence a chance to work up an appetite. His mother placed him in his high chair, strapped him in, and securely snapped on the tray. Lunch was served. When the phone rang, Mother left the kitchen to take the call. In a matter of seconds, Clarence unbuckled his strap and quickly released the latches to his tray. He pushed his chair to the edge of the counter, climbed up, opened a cabinet, and removed two large rings of keys. Fast thinking about what action should be taken to manage Clarence in his mother's absence was not fast enough. He unhooked both the top and bottom latches of the back door, selected the proper key to open the lock, and exited to the backyard. He darted into the garage, where he unlocked the car, inserted the key in the ignition, and was preparing to take himself for a ride. At that point, Mother interrupted his travel plans and escorted Clarence back to the kitchen to finish his lunch. Evidencing no surprise, she calmly announced, "He does it all the time."

In this brief scenario, Clarence displayed several important developmental skills. Intentionality was clearly present as Clarence executed the steps of his escape in a purposeful and well directed manner. Observed skills included basic problem solving, perceptual discrimination, an understanding of objects by use, and an awareness of cause–effect relationships. This story of Clarence illustrates a theme known all too well to the veterans of assessment with young children. Skills that are not demonstrated in more formal testing may be elicited and observed later in other less structured and less formal settings.

PRESCHOOLERS AND TESTS

It is fortunate that not all preschool children are as active or as difficult to manage as Clarence. However, those working with young children do understand that they typically are quite active and their ability to maintain attention on tasks is limited. Young children like to be on the go rather than sitting still. They are highly inquisitive and enjoy exploration of their surroundings. The unique characteristics of the preschool child have been noted (Paget & Nagle, 1986).

From a Piagetian perspective, preschoolers show patterns of cognitive development that are qualitatively different from those of older children and adults (Piaget, 1952). Their preoperational thought is idiosyncratic and highly intuitive. Concept development is limited. Young children assimilate new experiences into existing patterns of thinking much more readily than they can accommodate or change these patterns to meet external demands. For this reason, they do much better in imaginative play than they do in conforming to structure or rules.

Reviewing the characteristics of preschool children in this context initially appears to be an unnecessary exercise. Who does not understand that very young children have patterns of development and adjustment that are qualitatively different from older children and adults? Perhaps because of its simplicity, this concept is typically overlooked in the design and construction of tests for preschool children.

Within the tradition of psychometric measurement, tests have been developed to appraise developmental skills. Standardized procedures are used to present selected tasks. The child's performance is judged according to set criteria and then translated into a score that provides an indication of standing in some normative group. Hopefully, this information will then be used to answer original assessment questions.

In testing, emphasis is placed on control of the child and on compliance to standard procedures. Test materials are supplied. These materials may or may not be of interest to the child. To ensure uniformity, the manner and sequence of eliciting responses is fixed. Verbal instructions may be quite formal and the complexity of such instructions may often exceed the concept development of the child at risk, let alone the child with a disability.

The value of such standard procedures in preserving reliability and validity in normative measurement is certainly supported. However, procedures that emphasize control, uniformity, and direction are incompatible with the identifying characteristics of young children. Preschool children are not too content working in one spot for very long and their curiosity is not well satisfied by most of the "fun" materials in test kits.

While completing a formal test with any young child is a challenge, the task becomes even more difficult when conditions that may adversely affect the child's ability to receive information and make responses are encountered. Limitations of vision or hearing, language problems, and impaired motor skills all may significantly limit performance. Problems with compliance associated with shyness, separation difficulties, or oppositional features, which are frequently seen in young children, may also compromise the demonstration of skills.

The adverse effects of these difficulties on performance are even greater when standardized procedures associated with testing place additional limits on the presentation of tasks and the evaluation of performance. Under such conditions, it is very difficult to make appropriate adaptations in materials, manner of presentation, or evaluation criteria to accommodate special needs.

SAMPLING DEVELOPMENTAL SKILLS

In the assessment of young, handicapped children, adherence to procedures that permit the quantification of performance may actually thwart efforts to obtain richer, more valuable information about what the child does and does not do in several domains of functioning. This information is essential in designing and implementing appropriate programming for the child. The value of identification of skills and the establishment of a "linkage" between assessment and intervention has been discussed (Bagnato, Neisworth, & Munson, 1989).

With a recognition of the limitations of more formal or test-based evaluation procedures, alternative strategies for obtaining valuable information regarding emergent and established skills are available. A creative strategy in the assessment of young children with disabilities involves the use of structured "clinical judgment" in appraising development and functioning in several domains (Bagnato & Neisworth, 1985; Simeonsson, 1986). The use of clinical judgment in assessment represents an effort to overcome the limitations of more traditional psychometric approaches and provide information that is more directly useful in guiding appropriate instruction for the child.

In applying judgment-based assessment strategies, it is extremely important to discover what the child does do. Assessment will always be based on identification of emergent and established skills within several developmental areas. This information could be obtained from parent or teacher report, observation, or direct interaction with the child. While reports are of value, observation and direct interaction with the child often provide more useful information. A critical limitation of observation is that the observer will see only behaviors that are elicited by natural demands of the situation. More information may be obtained through direct interaction with the child as the observer then has the opportunity to elicit or "draw out" specific skills that may not be readily identified through observation alone.

The use of observation and direct interaction with a child to obtain a sampling of skill development is certainly not an innovative assessment technique. *The innovative component is the attempt to free such observation and interaction from the constraints of standardized procedure and to place the focus properly on the child's natural skills.* The objective is to make the assessment strategy conform to the characteristics of the young child with a disability rather than to force compliance to specific standardized procedures.

In sampling, the emphasis shifts from controlling the child to providing the child with multiple opportunities to express developmental skills. The objective of sampling developmental skills is to describe the child's capabilities. Efforts are directed at obtaining the very best sample of behavior that documents skill development. Sampling of skills provides a basis for formulating clinical judgments and designing appropriate programming.

SHOPPING FOR SKILLS: AN ASSESSMENT ANALOGUE

Have you done your grocery shopping this week? A trip to the supermarket is hardly an adequate analogy for conducting developmental assessment with young children. Those who study the complex neurological bases of cognitive development would certainly shudder at such a simplistic comparison. However, there are points of similarity worth exploring. In the market, goods are shelved in a somewhat orderly fashion based upon group or use. Although the precise arrangement may vary from market to market, there is a general pattern of organization that is recognized by most shoppers. To promote efficiency, the shopper prepares a list to guide the pursuit. Knowing the layout of the market may be helpful in preparation of the list and in procuring the goods. Of course, the list does not map out an exact route. You can start at any point, pick up items as you go, and come back to get what you missed. Bargains can be selected from special displays in any aisle and at any time.

Much like the shopper in search of supplies, the evaluator is searching for *samples of behavior*. The child's repertoire of developmental skills may be seen as following some logical groupings. Although the precise arrangement will vary from child to child, there are generally recognized patterns of organization. Like the efficient shopper, the evaluator prepares a *shopping list to guide the sampling of child behavior*. Knowing the patterns of child development is helpful in preparing the list and in obtaining samples of skills. The list does not map out an exact route for eliciting and observing specific developmental skills. You can start at any point, pick up additional skills as you go, and always go back to find those skills that may have been missed. A bargain or unexpected demonstration of skills can be picked up at any time. The shopping list provides the evaluator with clear indication of essential skills that should be sampled to assess development. With the list, assessment time is used in the most efficient manner. Emphasis is on procuring the skills rather than on the order or techniques of procurement.

Commercially available developmental inventories often are based on detailed analyses of skills. Under ideal circumstances with competent and cooperative preschoolers, such refinement may promote precision. Under the more typical conditions of assessment, highly detailed skill analysis may not be possible. The detailed list can be a distraction and the user may become overly involved in procedures for defining and eliciting responses. As a result, the focus on the child's response and capacities becomes blurred and much valuable information may be lost.

An example of a fairly simple shopping list to guide sampling of developmental skills in the communications area is provided in Table 5.1. A shopping list for basic cognitive skills is presented in Table 5.2. These lists are based, in part, upon skills noted in common developmental inventories. They are not comprehensive lists but rather offer suggestions for sampling representative behaviors in several skill areas. Similar listings covering these and other skills in the fine/gross motor, self-help, and personal–social areas could be easily developed. The idea is to follow basic developmental sequences and age/stage expectancies and create a list to meet your own shopping needs.

TABLE 5.1. Shopping List for Communication Skills

Developmental areas	Skills to be sampled
	Prespeech
Orienting	Orients to sound
	Orients to voice
Responding	Responds selectively to voice
	Responds to name
Gesturing	Gives greetings
	Indicates needs
Vocalizing	Makes cooing, babbling sounds
	Imitates sounds
	Receptive language
Identifying	Identifies body parts
	Identifies common objects
	Identifies colors
Following directions	Follows one-step direction
	Follows two-step direction
	Follows complex directions
Developmental areas	Skills samples
	Expressive language
Naming	Names people
	Names body parts
	Names common objects
	Names less common objects
Stating needs	States need to eat, drink
Describing action	Describes own actions
	Describes action of others
Speaking socially	Responds to questions
	Initiates discussion

SAMPLING STRATEGIES

In sampling, the focus remains on the child. The setting and materials used serve only to facilitate the demonstration of developmental skills. The objective is to elicit and describe developmental skills in a functional manner. Techniques involved in sampling are directed toward eliciting the child's best performance.

Setting

Sampling of developmental skills can be accomplished in any setting. However, young children can more readily express skills in familiar surround-

TABLE 5.2. Shopping List for Basic Cognitive Skills

Developmental areas	Skills to be sampled
	Association
Matching	Matches objects one to one
	Matches by color, shape, size
	Matches by two dimensions
Sorting	Sorts on one dimension
	Sorts on two dimensions
	Organization
Classifying	Assigns to class by use
	Assigns to class by category
Ordering	Orders by size
	Orders by quantity
	Comprehension
Displaying awareness	Attends to persons
	Attends to objects
Exploring relations	Effects circular reactions
	Effects cause–effect patterns
	Shows intentionality
	Follows complex directions
Understanding	Shows use of common objects
	Shows use of uncommon objects
	Shows action sequences
	Shows action for situation
	Recognizes absurdities
	Memory
Attending	Tracks visually
	Pursues objects
	Listens in sustained manner
Retention and recall	Matches visually by memory
	Matches auditorily by memory
	Identifies single object by recall
	Identifies multiple objects by recall
	Repeats digits or sentences
	Concepts
Identifying direction	Demonstrates up, down
	Identifies object's position
Quantifying	Identifies big, little
	Tells "how many"
	Counts
Identifying time	Shows temporal sequences

ings where they can be given some latitude to freely engage in exploratory activities. The child's home or preschool classroom are often good settings. In cases where children must be seen in an office, clinic, or hospital setting, it is important to provide space and materials that will allow simulation of a more comfortable setting. The assessment can move from place to place and, in each new setting, the child and evaluator may identify opportunities for demonstrating skills.

The child's parents and teachers can often be very helpful in obtaining a good sampling of the child's capabilities. They can be enlisted to assist in all phases of the assessment. Attention can be given to how parents and teachers can be most helpful rather than to the plotting of schemes for "separating" the child from them. Only in those cases where the presence of others is clearly detrimental to the child should separation be considered.

Materials

Materials that come with many commercially produced tests or developmental inventories are often unfamiliar, too small, and not particularly attractive to the child. Young children respond notably better to three dimensional, larger, more colorful materials. In most cases, appropriate materials are available in the child's home, school, or play setting. Young children will frequently demonstrate a specific developmental skill with such materials that they did not demonstrate with unfamiliar, less attractive materials.

Sampling does not require any specialized materials. With appropriate consideration to age, just about anything that can be used by a child to demonstrate a skill can and should be used in sampling. Objects in the room (e.g., chairs, tables, doors, phone, toys) can be materials for sampling both receptive and expressive vocabulary skills. Anything of which there is more than one (e.g., shoes, cups, bananas, gloves) is a suitable material for matching activities. Things that come in sets (e.g., toy blocks, plates, toy cars) or things that represent a category (e.g., fruits, tools, clothing) can be used in sorting tasks ranging from simple to complex. Objects that have specific uses (e.g., telephone, can opener, paint brush) are suitable for sampling basic comprehension skills. Collections of objects or toy representations of such objects that are often used together (e.g., can, can opener, pan, stove, plate) provide an opportunity to elicit complex sequences of behavior that reflect sophisticated understanding. Any objects that provide sensory feedback when acted upon (e.g., bells, light switches, remote control carts) present opportunities for demonstrating awareness of cause–effect relationships. Objects of varying sizes (e.g., large teddy bear, small teddy bear) can be used to demonstrate concept development. Other than concerns for safety, there are no limits to the possible uses of available materials in the sampling of skills.

Procedures

Using the shopping list of skills as a general guide, the assessment can proceed in a sequence that is most convenient. It is often helpful to work within general skill areas or domains (e.g., language, basic problem solving, basic concepts). Within the identified area, assessment moves from more basic to more complex skills. Attempts may be made to elicit responses in areas that correspond to the child's interests. Following the child's natural exploratory activity and eliciting skills associated with such activities may be useful in engaging children. Adaptations for children with disabling conditions can be made as needed. Simultaneous expression of skills in several domains is frequently noted and increases the efficiency of the assessment strategy. Skills and capabilities are noted and recorded as they are demonstrated.

Helpful Hints

1. Begin with a relaxed approach focusing on establishing and maintaining rapport with the child. Sampling is a "child-centered" approach and retaining this orientation is of critical importance. Pace and scope of the assessment are adjusted to accommodate the needs of the child.

2. Enlist the help of parents, teachers, therapists, and others who are familiar with the child. They can often be very helpful by identifying routines, activities, or settings in which the child may commonly demonstrate the skill or skills you are attempting to elicit.

3. Incorporate familiar toys, games, and play activities. They offer multiple opportunities to elicit skills in a comfortable manner. Ask for help in identifying the games and activities that are familiar for this child.

4. Do not hesitate to try out new ways of eliciting responses n a creative manner. Adapt presentation and response modes to accommodate children with sensory, motor, or speech–language impairments.

5. As children may be encountering many different toys and materials, care must be taken to protect the safety of children.

6. Take time to enjoy your work. Assessing young children is fun. This is particularly true when the assessment strategies conform to the characteristics of the children.

CLARENCE: THE ADVENTURE CONTINUES

Back in the kitchen, under close surveillance, Clarence was finishing lunch. It would soon be time for another try. Efforts would be directed at obtaining a brief clinical sampling of emergent and established developmental skills using a shopping list to guide the assessment.

Identification, Directions, and Concepts

Observation established good orientation to sounds and voices. He was clearly responsive to his name. Clarence was invited to play the "show me" game. Moving from room to room, Clarence pointed out objects as they were named. Fairly common and easy items (e.g., ball, television, doggie) were introduced first. More difficult items were requested as the assessment progressed. Items were interspersed to maintain a successful response pattern and avoid frustration. Receptive skills were much stronger than suggested by previous performance on receptive vocabulary tests. Finding real objects in the context of a game was far more productive than pointing to black and white line-drawn pictures in a static and structured setting.

Building on this success, it was relatively easy to involve Clarence in other receptive language activities. In formal assessment, he had little interest in pointing to body parts on himself or in pictures. In play, he readily pointed out body parts as named on a large teddy bear in the corner of the play room. When asked to "put this hat on Teddy's head" or "put this shoe on Teddy's foot," he quickly complied. Other one-step directions involving play with Teddy were readily followed.

It was a good time to produce a few directional concepts. Clarence placed Teddy in, under, and on top of a box as directed. He liked the idea of another "bear" joining the activities and identified "big bear" and "little bear." He also took the bears "up the steps" and "down the steps" with good compliance.

Attempts were made to elicit more advanced skills. Clarence did not correctly identify objects that were less common and he was not successful in identifying colors. He did not complete directions involving more than one element. With consideration to age, these skills may be included as objectives in programming for Clarence.

Exploration and Understanding

Clarence was an active explorer of his environment. He had already discovered many cause–effect relationships. Turning on lights, ringing the doorbell, operating water faucets, and changing the channel with the remote control were all comfortably in his repertoire.

It was time for a different version of the "show me" game. The objective was to find objects by described use. He evidenced good understanding of common uses. In response to "show me what we cook on," he identified his sister's play stove. This attracted his interest. With the toy pots and pans, he cooked a meal. Steps in the process were performed in the correct order with proper use of food and utensils. Even the finer details of proper seasoning were not neglected.

Toy dishes and cups were used to set the table. When Clarence was busy in the kitchen, one of the cups was turned upside down. When Clarence came to pour the coffee, he quickly noted the incorrectly placed cup and turned it right side up. He also smiled curiously when he noticed the shoe placed on the plate. Clarence was quick in identifying this odd entree and the other contrived absurdities.

Matching, Memory, and Classification

Two shoes, two apples, and two cups were placed on the floor. The two shoes were held up, the match was noted, and they were placed together. The cup was then held up and Clarence was invited to find the "match." He matched the cup and the apples, and performed well with other paired objects.

Once ability to match was documented, it was quite easy to assess visual memory. One set of objects (shoe, orange, cup) was kept in clear view on the floor while the "mates" to these items were placed out of sight behind the sofa. When Clarence was not looking, one of the objects was covered with a box and Clarence was asked to go behind the sofa to find the mate to the hidden object. Short-term memory for one object was good.

On the toy farm, there were many animals and people. There were also cars, trucks, and tractors. Efforts were made to assess more sophisticated classification skills by moving people to one pile and animals to another pile. Clarence was asked to place toy animals and people in the appropriate piles. He was not successful with this task.

As in the other areas assessed, it is possible to document specific skills evidencing association, organization, and memory. With an understanding of developmental hierarchies, appropriate objectives can be established and strategies for promoting skill acquisition designed.

Naming and Expressing Needs

Throughout the assessment, Clarence did not produce any discernible words. Sounds were used for naming with "wroom" for car and "woof" for doggie. He did well in gestural expression. When given toy musical instruments (e.g., guitar, horn), he did well in demonstrating their appropriate use. Needs to drink, eat, use the bathroom, and go for a ride were all clearly expressed in gesture. Attempts to elicit some easy sounds (e.g., "ball," "mom") were not successful.

ACTIVITY-BASED ASSESSMENT
IN EARLY CHILDHOOD INTERVENTION:
OPERATIONALIZING SHOPPING FOR SKILLS

Early childhood intervention researchers have observed that teachers and other professionals value authentic assessment but often find it difficult to implement. The purpose of authentic assessment is to create a "map" or alignment among children's competencies, appropriate interventions, and everyday activities, routines, and settings.

Rather than contrived tabletop testing procedures, authentic assessment relies on structured, yet natural observations of children's daily behavior in natural contexts. Many professionals find it difficult to implement authentic assessment because most commonly used authentic curriculum-based and play-based scales organize competencies by developmental domains (i.e., cognitive, language, motor) instead of by daily routines (i.e., greeting, bath, group circle, playground, stories), both at home and preschool. Thus, the scales themselves may hinder the "natural" process of observation for many people

In the last decade, researchers have developed some field-validated procedures through federal grants that enable teachers and others to reorganize and map functional competencies to daily routines. These procedures operationalize the "shopping for skills" process. Various approaches share the same strategy of mapping observable functional competencies to everyday routines: Activity-Based Assessment (Bricker, 1998; Grisham-Brown & Hemmeter, 1998); Ecological Congruence Assessment (Wolery, Brashers, & Neitzel, 2002); Embedded Assessment (Cook, 2004); and Routines-Based Assessment (McWilliam, 2003).

Steps to Implement Activity-Based Assessments

Cook (2004) presents a simple and useful step-by-step model for activity-based assessment, which includes five steps:

1. *Regroup assessment competencies within an authentic measure.* Using an authentic, curriculum-based assessment measure such as the Assessment Log and Developmental Progress Chart from the *Carolina Curriculum for Preschoolers with Special Needs* (Johnson-Martin, Hacker, & Attermeier, 2004), reorganize the expected competencies of children in order of chronological age under broad categories—all attention and memory items grouped irrespective of domain, such as cognitive or language (e.g., attention and memory) to create a hierarchical sequence of simple to complex functional competencies (see Table 5.3). Then, examine the competencies and determine those that are easily grouped into specific categories so as to make them easier to observe—for example, all singing and rhyming items grouped together (attention and memory: rhymes/songs).

2. *Map regrouped competencies to daily routines.* An easy guide for authentic assessment is created by analyzing and choosing those competencies that can be readily observed in one daily setting versus another. Some of these common preschool classroom routines typically include arrival,

TABLE 5.3. Reorganized Assessment Items

Broad categories—items developmentally listed	Specific categories—items grouped
1. Attention and memory	**1. Attention and memory: Rhymes/songs**
h. Says or sings at least two nursery rhymes or songs in a group or with an adult (2.5–3 years).	h. Says or sings at least two nursery rhymes or songs in a group or with an adult (2.5–3 years).
i. Identifies from four or more pictures one seen briefly (3–3.5 years).	q. Sings songs or says rhymes of at least 30 words (4–4.5 years).
j. Names one of several objects or pictures shown, named, and then hidden (3–3.5 years).	**2. Attention and memory: Stories**
k. Repeats a sequence of three digits or words (3–3.5 years).	o. Recalls one or two elements from a story just read (3.5–4 years).
l. Repeats four-word sentences with adjectives (3–3.5 years).	r. Recalls three to four elements from a story without prompts (4–4.5 years).
m. Remembers and names which of three objects has been hidden (3.5–4 years).	**3. Attention and memory: Digits/words**
n. Describes familiar objects without seeing them (3.5–4 years).	k. Repeats a sequence of three digits or words (3–3.5 years).
o. Recalls one or two elements from a story just read (3.5–4 years).	l. Repeats four-word sentences with adjectives (3–3.5 years).
p. Matches both color and shape of an object or picture seen only briefly (3.5–4 years).	**4. Attention and memory: Objects seen briefly**
q. Sings songs or says rhymes of at least 30 words (4–4.5 years).	i. Identifies from four or more pictures one seen briefly (3–3.5 years).
r. Recalls three to four elements from a story without prompts (4–4.5 years).	j. Names one of several objects or pictures shown, named, and then hidden (3–3.5 years).
	m. Remembers and names which of three objects has been hidden (3.5–4 years).
	p. Matches both color and shape of an object or picture seen only briefly (3.5–4 years).
	5. Attention and memory: Objects unseen
	n. Describes familiar objects without seeing them (3.5–4 years).

Note. From Cook (2004). Copyright 2004 by the Division for Early Childhood. Reprinted by permission.

large-group activity, snack, story time, and transitions. This alignment of observable competencies by observational settings establishes a systematic approach for authentic assessment (see Table 5.4).

3. *Create developmentally appropriate activities to prompt and probe elusive competencies.* Professionals can use common toys and materials in the preschool and pairing of peers to "set the occasion" for children to display some behaviors that may not be readily observed, such as following prepositional directions and counting.

TABLE 5.4. Types of Assessment Items Embedded into Daily Routines

Arrival

- *Adaptive/undressing:* taking off coat, hat, mittens, and boots; unbuttoning, unzipping, and unsnapping
- *Gross motor:* walking up stairs
- *Social:* responding to a greeting

Departure

- *Adaptive/dressing:* putting on hat, mittens, and boots; buttoning, zipping, and snapping
- *Gross motor:* walking down stairs
- *Social:* responding to parting remarks

Large-group activity

- *Cognition:* Calendar/weather, time, patterns, numbers, counting, same/ different, size, shape, color, opposites, rhyming, classifying, sequencing, prepositions
- *Language:* grammar, verbal, expression, questions, listening
- *Social:* attending, performing for others, responsibility (jobs), participation
- *Adaptive:* solving problems, making rules

Center time

- *Social:* Level of social and cognitive play, responsibility, selecting materials, cleaning up, following rules and procedures, sharing
- *Fine motor:* stringing beads, putting together puzzles, imitating/copying block and peg designs, manipulating clay, drawing, printing, painting, lacing
- *Cognition:* size, shape, color, counting, opposites, rhyming, classifying, sequencing, prepositions

Snack

- *Adaptive/feeding:* using a spoon, fork and knife, pouring, requesting food, using manners (please/thank you), cleaning up
- *Language:* pragmatics/conversational turn taking, staying on topic

Bathroom

- *Adaptive/toileting:* bowel/bladder control
- *Adaptive/grooming:* washing/drying hands
- *Adaptive/dressing:* buckling/unbuckling
- *Language:* indicating toileting needs

Story time

- *Cognition:* memory of story content, concepts delineated in the story, colors, same/different, opposites, rhyming words, numbers, counting, size, length
- *Language:* listening, answering questions about the story, completing a partial story
- *Social:* attending, participation

Music

- *Cognition:* memory of rhymes and songs, imitating actions and words
- *Language:* listening to and following directions
- *Social:* attending, participation
- *Gross motor:* walking on a line, hopping, jumping, skipping, running, marching

Transitions

- *Gross motor:* standing on one foot, walking on a balance beam, hopping, jumping, skipping
- *Cognition:* concepts/shapes and colors, memory of rhymes and songs
- *Language:* following directions, listening

Outside play

- *Gross motor:* running, running around obstacles, walking on a line/balance beam, walking backwards, throwing, catching and kicking a ball, jumping, climbing, hopping
- *Language:* following directions, listening

Note. From Cook (2004). Copyright 2004 by the Division for Early Childhood. Reprinted by permission.

4. *Design an authentic observation form.* Next, professionals can create an observational form that integrates observed competencies with observational settings across children. This efficient process allows teachers, for example, to observe and compare the competencies of several children simultaneously (see Figure 5.1).

5. *Complete the authentic assessment.* Once observational performance data are collected for each child, the information from the authentic observation form can be rerecorded and scored on the original assessment protocol form—in this case, the Carolina Curriculum's Assessment Log and Developmental Progress Chart.

A similar format is illustrated by Grisham-Brown and Hemmeter (1998), in which functional categories such as making choices, reaching and grasping, initiating social interactions, and cause–effect tool use are operationalized by specific behavioral competencies that exemplify each category and can be observed in specific settings (i.e., center time, small group—art, going to park with parents) (see Figure 5.2).

For authentic assessments, the advent of Palm Pilot and Tablet PC technologies has made this assessment process much more unobtrusive, efficient, and easy to accomplish.

BEST-PRACTICE GUIDEPOINTS

♦ Recognize that exemplars of intelligent behavior or problem solving (e.g., finding the correct toy at the bottom of the toy box, steering a shopping cart around obstacles, getting objects out of reach) can be readily observed and recorded in natural daily routines instead of on contrived test tasks.

♦ Use commercially available authentic curriculum-based assessment measures to structure natural observations in everyday routines.

♦ Be sensible in grouping competencies that can be observed in certain settings to increase ease and efficiency.

♦ Engage parents in the gathering of authentic performance information on their children in daily routines at home.

♦ Establish analogue, but natural situations within the home or classroom using typical toys and objects and peer pairings in which hard-to-observe and inconsistent behaviors can be prompted or occasioned.

Assessment Planning Guide		Ben	Juan	Tira	Reem
Music		*Date*	*Date*	*Date*	*Date*
Attention and memory: ***Rhymes/songs***	*Criterion*				
h. Says or sings at least two nursery rhymes or songs in a group or with an adult (2.5–3 years).	Most words correct				
q. Sings songs or says rhymes of at least 30 words (4–4.5 years).	Words may be repeated				
Story time					
Attention and memory: Stories	*Criterion*				
o. Recalls one or two elements from a story just read (3.5–4 years).	Without question prompts				
r. Recalls three to four elements from a story without prompts (4–4.5 years).	Without question prompts				
Teacher-directed activities					
Attention and memory: ***Digits/words***	*Criterion*				
k. Repeats a sequence of three digits or words (3–3.5 years).	Two different sequences				
l. Repeats four-word sentences with adjectives (3–3.5 years).	Five different sentences				
Attention and memory: ***Digits/words***	*Criterion*				
i. Identifies from four or more pictures one seen briefly (3–3.5 years).	Several different occasions				
j. Names one of several objects or pictures shown, named, and then hidden (3–3.5 years).	Five occasions				
m. Remembers and names which of three objects has been hidden (3.5–4 years).	Three or more occasions; errors rare				
p. Matches both color and shape of an object or picture seen only briefly (3.5–4 years).	Five times; no errors				
Attention and memory: ***Digits/words***	*Criterion*				
n. Describes familiar objects without seeing them (3.5–4 years).	Uses three accurate descriptive terms (questions allowed)				

FIGURE 5.1. Systematic observation form excerpt. From Cook (2004). Copyright 2004 by the Division for Early Childhood. Reprinted by permission.

Daily Schedule of Activities	Goals			
	Making choices	Reach and grasp	Initiate social	Cause–effect (tool use)
Center time	Choice between playing in the block center or housekeeping	Reach and grasp blocks to build a tower	Greet other children by vocalizing or making eye contact upon coming to center	Use switch to turn on dump truck at "building site"
Classroom chores	Choice between watering plants or feeding fish	Reach and grasp attendance slip—reach to place on desk in office	Initiate contact with school secretary to get her attention upon entering office to drop off attendance slips	Use switch to greet other teachers and children in the hall while doing her chore
Snack/ cooking activity	Choice between making pudding or milkshakes	Reach and grasp cooking utensils to stir and cook	Make eye contact with peers to let them know it's their turn to stir	Use switch to activate blender or mixer
Small group—art	Choice between art materials (paint or modeling clay)	Reach and grasp built-up paintbrush handle	Initiate interaction with adult to ask for assistance with painting	Use switch to request color of paint
Going to park with parents	Choice between slide or swing	Reach and grasp to hold on to swing or sides of slide	Make eye contact or vocalize to let parent know she wants to be pushed in the swing	Use switch to play music while she is on the playground

FIGURE 5.2. Activity matrix. From Grisham-Brown and Hemmeter (1998). Copyright 1998 by the Division for Early Childhood. Reprinted by permission.

BEST-PRACTICE EVIDENCE

Bagnato, S. J., & Neisworth, J. T. (1985). Assessing young handicapped children: Clinical judgment versus development performance scales. *International Journal of Partial Hospitalization, 3*(1), 13–21.

Bagnato, S. J., Neisworth, J. T., & Munson, S. M. (1989). *Linking developmental assessment and early intervention: Curriculum-based prescriptions* (2nd ed.). Rockville, MD: Aspen.

Bricker, D. (1998). *An activity-based approach to early intervention.* Baltimore: Brookes.

Cohen, M. A., & Gross, P. J. (1979). *The developmental resource: Behavioral sequences for assessment and program planning* (Vols. 1 & 2). New York: Grune & Stratton.

Cook, R. J. (2004). Embedding assessment of young children into routines of inclusive settings: A systematic planning approach. *Young Exceptional Children, 7*(3), 2–11.

Grisham-Brown, J., & Hemmeter, M. L. (1998). Writing IEP goals and objectives:

Reflecting an activity-based approach to instruction for young children with disabilities. *Young Exceptional Children, 1*(3), 2–10.

Johnson-Martin, N. M., Hacker, B. J., & Attermeier, S. M. (2004). *The Carolina Curriculum for Preschoolers with Special Needs—Assessment Log and Developmental Progress Chart.* Baltimore: Brookes.

Linder, T. (2002). *Transdisciplinary play-based assessment: A functional approach to working with young children.* Baltimore: Brookes.

McWilliam, R. A. (2003). *The routines-based assessment report form (RBA).* Unpublished measure.

Paget, K. D., & Nagle, R. J. (1986). A conceptual model of preschool assessment. *School Psychology Review, 15*(2), 154–165.

Piaget, J. (1952). *The origins of intelligence in children.* New York: International Universities Press.

Simeonsson, R. J. (1986). *Psychological and developmental assessment of special children.* Boston: Allyn & Bacon.

Wolery, M., Brashers, M., & Neitzel, J. C. (2002). Ecological congruence assessment for classroom activities and routines: Identifying goals and intervention practices in childcare. *Topics in Early Childhood Special Education, 22*(3), 131–142.

CHAPTER 6

◆ ◆ ◆

How Does Authentic Curriculum-Based Assessment Work?

◆

BEST-PRACTICE ISSUES

◆ Is "teaching to the test" justifiable and acceptable?

◆ Why is curriculum-based assessment (CBA) the optimal method for team assessment?

◆ Why are psychometric test items poor CBA tasks?

◆ What is "treatment utility" in assessment?

◆ Why are serial assessments critical in early childhood intervention and CBA?

Many professionals rely upon conventional norm-referenced testing in their work with children. It is true that instruments with adequate technical qualities enable us to determine the status of a child with respect to a referent group. Such testing seems, thus, useful for diagnostic purposes (i.e., determining the clinical category closest to the child's performance and attributes). However, diagnostic testing (i.e., finding the appropriate disability category) with preschoolers is not particularly useful with respect to either the mission of early childhood intervention or the professional practice standards in early childhood. Comprehensive assessment in early childhood must have immediate and continuous benefits for the child in terms of planning programs and interventions that work. Conventional tests and testing practices, however, fail to be useful for early childhood intervention for two core reasons: they require situations and behaviors that are divorced from the child's natural developmental ecology; and they fail to accomplish the most important reason for assessment in early childhood—to plan beneficial goals and programs for children. Bronfenbrenner (1977) succinctly summarized the contrivances and limitations of traditional practices best:

> Much of developmental psychology [early childhood assessment] as it now exists is the science of the strange behavior of children with strange adults in strange settings for the briefest possible periods of time. (p. 513)

Educators and therapists are much more concerned about what children can do or not do than what they are or are not (i.e., retarded, "disturbed," "learning disabled"). Thus, for years educators have complained about the low "treatment utility" of psychometric, trait-based assessment. Intelligence quotients, personality profiles, and other measures of global ("g" factors) or alleged characteristics offer little guidance to the teacher or parent who must decide what to teach and what materials and strategies would be most effective. Further, diagnosis of infants and young children is especially difficult and fraught with pitfalls. Very young children may be most uncooperative during formal testing. Infants, toddlers, and preschoolers are difficult to assess, change rapidly, and often require adaptations in assessment that may violate the standardization procedures required for norm-based assessment.

In addition to the usual problems associated with accurate and reliable testing of youngsters, various functional disabilities impose stimulus and response limitations that further complicate normative testing, making it questionable at best. Given the treacherous nature and low treatment utility of even well calculated diagnostic testing, it is no wonder that teachers and therapists have demanded assessment that is more relevant, practical, and directly linked to intervention. Indeed, federal law requires assessment that is *noncategorical* and yields a profile of the child's *specific* functional strengths and weaknesses across multiple developmental areas. The Individuals with Disabilities Act (IDEA) (1997, 2004) requires that "children's eligibility for early intervention shall be determined through a functional assessment conducted in the 'natural environment.' "

Authentic curriculum-based assessment is widely accepted by both early childhood special educators and early childhood educators as the best means for supplying the specificity and relevance needed for preschool program planning. Note, again, that it is the *purpose* of the assessment that must be considered when selecting best practices and measures. It is essential for psychologists to be skilled in developmental curriculum-based assessment (CBA) to increase their credibility and value to other early intervention professionals.

DEFINITION OF AUTHENTIC
CURRICULUM-BASED ASSESSMENT

Authentic CBA is a form of criterion-referenced measurement wherein curricular objectives act as the criteria for the identification of instructional targets and for the assessment of status and progress, conducted in natural environments by parents and professionals working together.

Criterion-referenced assessment has been employed for some time in therapy and applied behavior analysis. The major purpose of such assessment is to evaluate attainment of preset standards. Behaviorally based instruction and therapy often involve a changing criterion design wherein the requirement for reinforcement is progressively raised. Similarly, programmed instruction and precision teaching involve measurement of behavior to check for mastery of objectives. CBA is clearly an application of criterion-referencing or goal-attainment scaling for educational purposes. Even more specifically, *developmental* CBA uses developmental landmarks, expectancies, or hierarchical functional content as potential instructional goals and objectives.

PURPOSES OF CURRICULUM-BASED ASSESSMENT

Expert use of CBA is central to quality early childhood intervention. Developmental CBA is the optimal approach for accomplishing four important tasks: identifying program entry points, program planning, progress monitoring, and program evaluation. Each of these functions of CBA is discussed and illustrated later in this chapter.

CBA provides the needed closeup of child developmental or functional status. It not only identifies where the child is within an array of objectives but also permits monitoring of progress. It detects what the child can do and cannot do, giving clear entry points within the program's curriculum. The monitoring function of CBA is particularly useful: it tracks child progress (formative assessment), demonstrates accumulated progress (summative assessment), and offers continual information on the effectiveness of instruction (corrective feedback); in fact, for 20 years in early childhood special education, response to intervention (RTI) has been accomplished through CBA. Clearly, CBA is a most direct means for identifying the entry points within an instructional program and for pacing and altering instruction.

Besides providing entry points and tracking progress, it is important to note a third distinct advantage of authentic CBA: it can invite and evaluate interdisciplinary team collaboration. Developmental curricula and corresponding assessment usually include several areas of development (i.e., motor, language, cognitive, social, and adaptive). Teaching, therapy, and tracking of curricular progress in each developmental domain can be done by parents and professionals working together. The child's progress within and across developmental domains can be charted, reflecting the contributions of specialists and detecting special areas of difficulty. CBA can "pull together" a team involving a physical therapist, psychologist, speech–language therapist, early childhood or special education teacher, parent, and even pediatrician. CBA has been used and field validated in several types of settings: private early childhood centers, Early Head Start and Head Start, family child care, home-based early intervention, inclusive early intervention classrooms, and hospital clinic and pediatric rehabilitation programs. Each member can contribute to and assess relevant developmental objectives. No other form of assessment encourages and structures interdisciplinary collaboration as specifically as CBA.

Finally, there is yet another advantage of *developmental* CBA: it provides a form of norm-referenced assessment. Normal developmental curricula are based on developmental landmarks (i.e., skills manifested by most children at various ages) that have been validated over years of clinical experience. Using two-word sentences is generally characteristic of 2-year-olds. This capability is a norm (developmental landmark) and a curricular objective. When curricular objectives are based on child development norms, child achievement can be judged relative to other same-age children. The 3-year-old who learns to walk shows mastery of the curricular objective but also a serious delay relative to the 12- to 15-month norm for walking. Good developmental CBA, then, also yields a normative picture of the child's development. Research in early intervention has shown that certain authentic, developmental CBA measures equal and even surpass conventional, norm-referenced tests in the early identification of children eligible for early intervention.

The curriculum-based scale within the developmental curriculum lays the foundation for profiling specific child strengths and weaknesses and for mapping and evaluating the course of intervention. Clearly, then, the choice of an appropriate developmental curriculum is crucial and fundamental.

BENEFITS OF A DEVELOPMENTAL CURRICULUM

Most curricula include objectives across several major developmental domains. Because of its specificity, curriculum-based developmental assessment provides direct guidance for writing learning objectives—a kind of blueprint for care, instruction, and intervention. Using a map metaphor, we may view CBA as a way to find specific directions for starting on a "developmental journey." The curriculum is the map that includes crucial landmarks, many potential destinations, and clear routes toward the destinations. The curriculum "map" should be detailed enough to permit progress checks (how far we have gone), accommodations for various handicaps (alternative routes), and comprehensive and balanced objectives (covers a large territory). Without a curriculum, IEP objectives must be generated piecemeal, perhaps without a broader or longer view of where the child is going or should go. Without a curriculum, it is difficult, confusing, and hazardous to specify entry objectives, to individualize program planning, monitor progress, and evaluate program impact. Since getting the right map for a trip is important, the necessity of selecting the right curriculum cannot be overestimated. An early childhood program without a curriculum will benefit from using one that is program appropriate (i.e., that fits the children's needs, staff philosophy, and capabilities). If a program does not employ a specific curriculum, professionals can use a generic curriculum that includes developmental goals and objectives that span the early learning domains for most children and is feasible for staff use.

DEVELOPMENTAL CURRICULA

The *developmental milestones* recognized in child development are organized into curricula that comprise *developmental objectives* for teaching children who experience developmental delays or dysfunctions. A developmental curriculum, then, is composed of developmental objectives (i.e., critical capabilities that are targets for instruction and therapy). A given milestone (e.g., uses two-word sentences) obviously has dozens of precursive or prerequisite skills. Since much of development is incremental and involves a "building" process of increasing differentiation and integration of competencies, hierarchies of developmental objectives can be described. Through task analysis, observation, and logic, curricula incorporate *sequenced developmental hierarchies* that become "ladders" or sequences for instruction. Figure 6.1 illustrates a developmental task analysis or hierarchy of skills for the area of attention/task completion from the *Help for Special Preschoolers* (Furuno et al., 1984) curriculum. Note the increasing complexity and independence in skills required with increasing age and the graduated scoring by functional level (2 = mastery, 1 = emerging, 0 = absent). Such scoring aids in curriculum entry determinations, progress evaluations, and goal planning.

Determining where a child is within a curriculum yields a profile of current capabilities (i.e., curriculum-based appraisal of developmental status). Identifying subsequent developmental objectives for instruction and therapy becomes *prescriptive* developmental assessment. It should be noted that developmental objectives are not—and should not be—psychometric test items. Only *functional* developmental objectives should be emphasized

Curriculum-based Developmental Assessment

D.A.	Developmental Task Analysis: ATTENTION/TASK COMPLETION	Functional Level
30-36 mo.	Starts task only with reminders and prompts	2
36-48 mo.	Completes 10% of task with little sustained attention	2
42-48 mo.	Attends to task for 5 minutes with no distractions	2
42-48 mo.	Remains on-task for 5 minutes with distractions	1
48-60 mo.	Starts task with no reminders or prompts	1
46-50 mo.	Completes 25-50% of task with some prompts	1
48-60 mo.	Attends to task for 10 minutes with no supervision	0
48-60 mo.	Remains on task for 10 minutes with distractions	0
60-66 mo.	Completes 50-75% of task with some prompts	0

FIGURE 6.1. Developmental task analysis: Attention/task completion. Items from the H.E.L.P. Hawaii Early Learning Profile Furuno et al. (1984).

since they contribute to the child's increasing mastery of the social and physical world (e.g., initiates social interactions with adults; operates mechanical toys; attends to a talk for 3 minutes with distractions). When assessment instruments designed for diagnosis are normed and subjected to psychometric refinements, the items that survive the process are included in a test because they differentiate statistically between age or diagnostic groups; these items and content are not worthy of teaching. Standing on one foot and stacking three blocks, for example, are familiar items on norm-based developmental assessment devices. It is dubious that such skills in isolation should actually be instructional objectives.

Domains and Subdomains

Curricular content is usually grouped into useful developmental categories or *domains*. Typically, developmental curricula include the domains of cognitive, language, social–emotional, and motor development. Other domains are often variations or combinations of these basic four categories. Self-help, sensorimotor, psychomotor, social competence, communication, problem solving, and affective development are some of the terms that will be encountered when examining the numerous available curricula.

Domains are usually broken into two or more *subdomains* (i.e., dimensions of developmentally related but different capabilities). Language development, for example, can be analyzed into such subdomains as expressive, receptive, pragmatic, gestural, and imitation. These subcategories are useful for organizing and planning instruction, even though the assignment of a skill to one category or another may sometimes be arbitrary.

Subdomains are composed of developmentally related objectives arranged in hierarchies—easier to harder or primitive to advanced development. These objectives can readily be tailored to the child and written into lesson plans and IEPs. A few new curricula are organized within *strands*; these are interrelated skills that cut across domains and that can be taught or practiced concurrently. Using a telephone, for example, includes language, social, cognitive, and motor objectives: strands or cross-referencing are practical ways to avoid teaching fragments and to optimize balanced progress. One practical approach to implementing interrelated developmental objectives is to weave them into the existing program's schedule of activities. Some teachers design a matrix with the several scheduled activities as rows and a child's (or group's) several domain objectives as columns (Figure 6.2). Lessons centered around an activity such as snack time can include specific language, social, motor, and cognitive objectives. These same objectives can continue to be taught, generalized, and maintained in other routines and activities. Indeed, most day care or preschool scheduled activities provide opportunities for the building of interrelated and collateral developmental competencies.

Lessons

In the narrow sense, a curriculum refers to just the organization and content of developmental objectives; increasingly, however, published curricula include several other components.

Lessons or suggested activities are also usually included. Indeed, some curricula feature recipe-type lesson cards that many teachers and aides are more than happy to use.

Child's Name <u>Roxann</u>

Date <u>9/90</u>

Current Program Titles (abbreviated):

<u>Language 1—vocalizing three-word sentences; Language 2—g, h, k initial sounds;</u>
<u>Social 1—vocalizing peer names; Social 2—initiating interaction using play organizers;</u>
<u>Cognitive 1—identifying letters; Personal care 1—street crossing; Personal care 2—</u>
<u>coat (dressing); Gross motor 1—tricycle riding; Fine motor 1—name writing</u>

ACTIVITY	CURRICULAR DOMAIN					
	Language	Social	Cognitive	Personal care	Gross motor	Fine motor
Greeting	$1^a x^b$ 2x	1xxxxx		1x*		1x
Play		2xxxxx*			1xxxxx	
Circle	1x 2x	1xxxxx*				
Centers	1x 2x		1xxxxx*			1xxxxx*
Story	1x 2x					
Break/rest	1x 2x					
Art/music	1x 2x					1x
Game (gross motor)				2x		
Lunch	1xxxxx* 2xxxxx					
Break/rest						
Play		2xxxxx			1xxxxx*	
Departure	1x 2x	1xxxxx		1x 2x*		

ᵃnumerals correspond with IEP objectives.
ᵇrefers to number of trials.
*denotes when skill is to be measured.

FIGURE 6.2. Activity-by-objectives matrix.

Lessons are sometimes described, along with suggested materials, in a booklet or three-ringed binder. Some curricula provide discussions of selected teaching strategies and learning principles. Behavioral and Piagetian principles and related methods are the most frequently cited.

Many early childhood educators are eager to use "canned" lessons, activities, materials, and room arrangements. The day is busy enough without the burden of inventing lessons for small groups and individuals. On the other hand, many teachers resent too much "scripting" of lessons, preferring suggested activities that can be tailored to their situations. Staff preferences in this regard should be determined before curricula are purchased.

Curriculum Placement Estimates

A number of curricula include a form or procedure for rapid placement of the child in the curriculum. An estimate of capabilities is done through testing, observing, or interviewing to discover roughly where the child may be functioning in each domain (and sometimes subdomain). Entry behaviors are then identified as starting points for instruction.

Parent Materials

Parent materials and home-based activities are highly desirable components of some new curricula. With the increasing emphasis on family involvement, and indeed, new infant legislation that requires a family focus, parent–child activities are a welcome component. Furthermore, older, more widely used curricula are now being published with supplemental materials to be used at home to accommodate families.

It should be noted that "parent involvement" can mean several things. Sometimes materials and activities supplied to parents assist them in teaching toward the same objectives as in the preschool program (parents-as-teachers approach). Increasingly, parent materials and activities are becoming focused on helping *parents as parents*, emphasizing parent–child reciprocity, constructive interaction, and "joint action routines." This approach broadens the scope of curricular objectives and attempts to enhance the quality of family–child development.

Progress Charts and Forms

Finally, most good curricula have some means for tracking child progress and displaying developmental status. Some use a simple check-off sheet or form for noting date of mastery; others provide some useful profile chart or actual progress "tracks." These curriculum-based assessments can, and should, be shared with parents. Usually, graphic displays of child *change* are appreciated most by parents. Quarterly and annual curriculum progress summaries are valuable when summative assessment or program evaluation is attempted.

In summary, then, published curricula contain hierarchies of developmental objectives organized into domains and subareas or strands, and often include quick entry appraisals, continual and periodic progress monitoring, parent materials, and suggested lesson plans.

SELECTING DEVELOPMENTAL OR FUNCTIONAL CURRICULA

Since the selection of a curriculum and its assessment components is a most important program decision, it must be done with deliberation. The topics included in this selection should help in the selection process (Figure 6.3). The three major dimensions to consider are child, setting, and curriculum characteristics.

Child Characteristics

Obviously, the nature of the children enrolled in a program is the preeminent consideration. Developmental age and disability are the two major aspects of importance with regard to child characteristics.

Developmental Age

Programs for youngsters are usually organized around age levels. The most frequent groupings are infant (0–2), toddler (2–3), preschool (3–5), and kindergarten or readiness (5–6) programs. Infant and transition/readiness programs are increasingly seen as important services beyond the usual preschool age group. Armed with fairly convincing evidence and professional support, infant advocates have successfully lobbied for federal policy and public law.

Kindergarten transition and school readiness programs are proliferating to smooth the transition between preschool/child development–type programs and education/school-based programs. Transition programs are especially important where the differences between early childhood and elementary programs are greater and when children need structured programs to shape school readiness.

Note that the *developmental* age (not chronological age) is the major information usually needed. The comprehensive services of many toddler/ preschool programs can usually accommodate children of chronological ages and developmenal ages 2–5.

CONCERNS IN SELECTING A DEVELOPMENTAL CURRICULUM

Curriculum _____ Publisher _____

Address _____

Phone _____

1. What is the population?
   Developmental Age ____   Handicap Specific/Adaptable
   Program Type: ____ Home ____ Center   ____ Clinic
                              ____ Individual   ____ Small Group

2. What areas are covered?
   ____ Gross Motor   ____ Fine Motor   ____ Own Care
   ____ Language   ____ Cognitive/Problem Solving
   ____ Social/Emotional   ____ Other

3. Are these areas covered in a balanced manner? _____

4. Are the areas presented in a sequential manner? _____

5. Does the organization provide or permit cross-referencing or strands? _____

6. Does the material lend itself to normalization and integration? _____

7. Type of family involvement:
   ____ Parent Centered   ____ Notes/Information Sheets ____ Sibling Activities

8. What training is needed?
   ____ Study of the Manual ____ Workshop   ____ Consultation

9. How are lesson plans formatted?
   ____ Clear   ____ Require extra preparation time
   ____ Easy to use   ____ Adaptable to handicapping conditions

10. Is curriculum-based assessment facilitated?
    ____ Formative (day-to-day)____ Summative (long-range)
    ____ Clear   ____ Easy to use

11. Is data support available?
    Field Tested _____ Teacher Recommended _____
    Number of Children _____ Type of Programs _____

12. How durable are the materials
    Sturdy constructed materials _____ Amount needed _____
    Consumables _____ Extra materials _____
    Special features _____

13. What is the cost?
    Basic curriculum _____ Extra manuals _____
    Consumables _____ Other supplies _____

FIGURE 6.3. Checklist for evaluating and selecting developmental curricula. From Bagnato and Neisworth (1991). Copyright 1991 by The Guilford Press. Reprinted by permission.

A complication may arise with certain developmental disabilities when one area of a child's development (e.g., motor) is at an infant level when other areas are well within the preschool developmental age. In such cases, it might be necessary to use two curricula. Again, some curricula do include infant through readiness content. These age-comprehensive curricula are most useful when children evidence uneven development.

Disability/Severity

The more specific and severe a disability, the more likely a specialized (dedicated) curriculum will be the optimal choice. Children with relatively severe vision, hearing, neuromotor, or behavioral/emotional difficulties often require specialized techniques and materials. Further, clinical technique and teaching methods must be adapted to meet sensory/response limitations. Curricula dedicated to a specific disability will usually be the best choice when teaching groups with the same disability (e.g., deafness) or severe disorder (e.g., autism).

Many newer curricula do provide general suggestions and sometimes specifics for accommodating various (usually mild to moderate) disabilities. Hopefully, the "adapted-to-disability" feature will become part of most new curricula.

Setting Characteristics

Most early childhood curricula have been developed for use in preschool centers; other settings that provide programs to many special needs youngsters are best served by a setting-appropriate curriculum. Setting-specific curricula are available for use in home, hospital, and day care situations. Home based curricula are certainly not new, but are now even more important when infant education and family involvement are considered.

Sometimes home-based curricula are used in conjunction with part-time center-based programs. Additionally, a few curricula focus on parenting skills, which are especially important for new parents of infants who are born prematurely or have specific physical and neuromotor limitations.

Hospital and clinic settings deserve special curriculum content. The staff and techniques involved with the intensive care unit, child-life program, or neonatal intensive care unit require objectives and activities tailored to the situation. These restrictive settings are temporary, but child development activities are crucial to offset early developmental problems and delays if not the negative effects of treatment itself.

Curriculum Characteristics

I have already discussed the benefits and components of a good curriculum. Here, I refer to *qualities* to look for after child and setting characteristics are satisfied. These eight qualities are summarized below and are included on the curriculum evaluation form at the end of this chapter (Figure 6.3).

Full Age and Domain Coverage

Full age and domain coverage may be important to a program. Obviously, a mixed-category, inclusive program would require a curriculum capable of accommodating a wide age range. Important also is coverage of all major areas of development. Children's weak areas must not be addressed at the expense of progress and even regression in other developmental domains. Parallel, balanced progress is feasible with a curriculum that covers all major dimensions of child development. Inclusiveness also refers to comprehensiveness of objectives within each domain. Some curricula include many more objectives per domain than others. Generally, a greater number and more detailed objectives are desirable when working with more severe and specific disabilities.

Family/Parent Involvement

Active support for and involvement of parents in the child's early education is crucial and yields greater benefits. Parent–professional collaboration may greatly enhance child learning, generalization across settings, and maintenance of progress. Further, there may be benefits to siblings, relatives, neighbors, or others who come in contact with better parenting and teaching. Some curricula offer specific suggestions and even plans for home based activities, teacher–parent discussions, and parent skill training. Often, teachers will be able to involve a parent in the center as well as at home. In any event, the family is increasingly seen as the focus for concern, rather than the child isolated from the home context. Curricula that include family participation have distinct advantages: they are in the spirit of the new laws and policies that emphasize family collaboration and they greatly assist in maintenance and generalization of center-based learning.

Inclusion

With the proliferation of inclusive early childhood programs, curricula that promote involvement with typical peers become especially needed. Objectives should move the child with a disability progressively to more typical, age-appropriate capabilities. Likewise, the management and instructional methods suggested must, when feasible, become more "normal" and compensatory (i.e., less contrived and prosthetic). Social integration can be encouraged through activities that include cross-age tasks in which children at differing developmental levels can participate. Through integration activities, cross-age tutoring, and other suggested projects and unit plans, some curricula especially offer opportunities for normalization and integration; these integration qualities are usually emphasized in the promotional material for the curriculum.

Progress Monitoring

Authentic curriculum-based developmental assessment presumes a developmental curriculum that includes developmental hierarchies within the several domains. Much has already been said about how progress tracking and program evaluation can easily be accomplished when a good curriculum is in use. As discussed, most newer curricula offer a mastery check-off sheet or some other way to keep track of what objectives have and have not been achieved.

Criteria for mastery are often recommended, although the teacher may want to use other standards. The often seen "90% of the time" may not make as much sense as "three consecutive times correctly," or "four days in a row." Teachers will usually want to construct criteria that not only are suitable for use within a daily lesson but also reflect a recognition of maintenance and generalization.

Effort/Benefit Ratio

To be effective, a curriculum must be properly implemented. Some curricula seem excellent until put into practice. The needed time and effort may not be tolerated, even though the later payoff may be great. Sometimes well-designed, thorough curricula take longer to put in place; a consultant or model program can be quite instructive and save much trial and error.

An admonition about the cost of curricula may be helpful: excellent curricula are commercially available for $50–$75; do not pay much more. Those curricula in the $100+ range often include materials (e.g., puppets, blocks) that are easily found elsewhere. A few curricula are worth more if they are age inclusive (0–8), disability specific or sensitive, and include a tracking system to facilitate formative and summative evaluation.

Information Base

One of the best ways to select a curriculum is to examine research literature, brochures, or curriculum manuals for information regarding the efficacy and utility of the curriculum during field-based research.

Unlike psychometric tests, technical adequacy data focus on treatment validity. Outcome-related information regarding child progress in terms of numbers of curriculum objectives achieved with and without prompts, the efficacy of curricular links and instructional strategies, time needed to train staff, and staff satisfaction reports are most useful. When available, technical reports are a valuable resource for selecting a curriculum; when no information is available, the consumer should beware.

TWO TYPES OF AUTHENTIC CURRICULUM-BASED ASSESSMENT

Curriculum-referenced and curriculum-embedded assessment are both forms of CBA, each with its own strengths and weaknesses according to the purpose for assessment. CBA has become the preeminent form of measurement within early care and education and early intervention programs. (For a complete review of the features and use of exemplary CBA systems, refer to Bagnato, Neisworth, and Munson (1997).

Curriculum-Referenced Assessment

Developmental or functional scales whose specific item content can be readily cross-referenced or "linked" to similarly based curricula are termed *curriculum-referenced*. A number of "generic" curricular scales exist that can be described as composites of specific curricula and are therefore compatible with commonly used curricula. Most of these authentic scales have been nationally standardized; they are considered norm/curricular hybrids since they retain features of both types of measures. Instruments such as the Brigance Diagnostic Inventory of Early Development (BDIED-R; Brigance, 1991), the Battelle Developmental Inventory (BDI; Newborg et al., 2005), the Adaptive Behavior Assessment System II (ABAS II; Harrison & Oakland, 2003), and the Basic School Skills Inventory—3 (BSSI–3; Hammill et al., 1998) provide a means for assessing specific skills common to most curricula that contain developmental task analyses. Professionals who are skilled in the use of curriculum-referenced scales are able to profile the child's specific strengths and weaknesses and make recommendations that are cast in terms of a program's specific curriculum. Thus, results on the BDI, for example, may be used to recommend entry objectives and IEP objectives based on the Hawaii Early Learning Profile (Parks, 1992) or other similar curricula. Curriculum-referenced scales provide a bridge or common base applicable across program-specific curricula.

Curriculum-Embedded Assessment

If the curriculum itself is used as the source for both testing and teaching, the instructional and assessment items are, of course, identical. Curriculum-embedded assessment refers to use of the specific program curriculum content and objectives for assessment purposes. Many curriculum-embedded scales have been field validated for use with children who have specific disabilities. As the content of the CBA scale departs from the actual curricular items, the assessment results may require some extrapolation or interpretation. Using this approach, assessment can take much time. If the teacher is conducting the assessment, the curriculum-embedded method is most feasible. Once this is done, progress monitoring is relatively easy and becomes a part of typical instructional work routines.

Tables 6.1 and 6.2 profile and summarize information on exemplary curriculum-referenced and curriculum-embedded assessment measures.

TABLE 6.1. Curriculum-Referenced Measures

Scale	Publisher	Age/Grade	Domains
Adaptive Behavior Assessment System (ABAS; Harrison & Oakland, 2003)	Psychological Corporation	0–89	Communication, Community use, School/home living, Functional preacademics, Health and safety, Leisure, Self-care, Self-direction, Social, Motor
Ages and Stages Questionnaire (ASQ; Bricker & Squires, 1999)	Paul H. Brookes	4 months to 5 years	Communication, Gross motor, Fine motor, Problem solving, Personal–social
Basic School Skills Inventory (BSSI; Hammill & Leigh, 1998)	PRO-ED	48–107 months	Spoken language, Reading, Writing, Math, Classroom behavior, Daily living
Battelle Developmental Inventory (Newborg, 2005)	Riverside Publishing	0–7 years, 11 months	Adaptive, Personal–social, Communication, Motor, Cognitive
Communication and Symbolic Behavior Scales (CSBS; Wetherby & Prizant, 2002)	Paul H. Brookes	CA: 6–72 months, DA: 6–24 months	Communication, Symbolic behavior
Developmental Observation Checklist System (Hresko, Miguel, Sherbenou, & Burton, 1994)	PRO-ED	0–71 months	Motor, Social, Language, Cognition
Pediatric Evaluation of Disability Inventory (PEDI; Haley, Coster, Ludlow, Haltiwanger, & Andrellos, 1992)	PEDI Research Group	6 months–7.5 years	Self-care, Mobility, Social function
School Function Assessment (SFA) (Coster, Deeney, Haley, & Haltiwanger, 1998)	Harcourt Brace	Kindergarten–Grade 6	Participation, Task supports, Activity performance: physical, cognitive/behavioral tasks

TABLE 6.2. Curriculum-Embedded Measures

Scale	Publisher	Age	Domains
Assessment, Evaluation, and Programming System for Infants and Children (AEPS; Bricker, 2002)	Paul H. Brookes	0–6 years	Fine motor, Gross motor, Adaptive, Cognitive, Social, Social communication
The Carolina Curriculum for Preschoolers with Special Needs (Johnson-Martin, Attermeier, & Hacker, 1990)	Paul H. Brookes	0–60 months	Cognition, Communication/Language, Social skills adaptation, Self-help, Fine motor, Gross motor
Every Move Counts (Korsten, Dunn, Foss, & Francke, 1993)	Psychological Corporation	0–18 months	Sensory response, Communication
Hawaii Early Learning Profile: (HELP; Parks, 1992)	Vort	0–60 months	Cognitive, Language, Gross motor, Fine motor, Social–emotional, Self-help, Regulatory/Sensory

AUTHENTIC ASSESSMENT FOR INTERVENTION USING CURRICULUM-EMBEDDED SCALES

Curriculum-based developmental assessment is the primary technique used to plan instructional and therapeutic programs for infants, toddlers, and preschoolers who are at developmental risk and who have developmental delays and/or disabilities. Among all other forms of assessment, CBA is unique: assessment items are also curricular objectives based on developmental norms for functional sequences. This offers a way to pinpoint specific strengths and weaknesses, track child progress, synchronize team efforts, and estimate developmental status. With the emerging national outcome benchmarks from the Office of Special Education of the U.S. Department of Education as well as state early learning standards, early childhood intervention programs will find such scales essential for charting child attainments and progress during participation in the program.

Early intervention programs include finely graded CBA developmental skill sequences to identify appropriate goals for all children, even those with the most severe limitations. Perhaps the most critical assessment feature of CBA is serial or repeated evaluations over time to document progress in learning and the effectiveness of instruction. Clearly, CBA is an exemplary "best practice" in psychology and education. In the future, more ecological methods of CBA are anticipated. This means that curricula and assessment strategies will be devised to identify the characteristics of the child's environment, including parents, family circumstances, stressors, classroom arrangements, and adult–peer interactions. The objective is to identify and respond to not only the child's individual skill needs but also dimensions of the physical and social environment. Creative advancements in authentic curriculum-based developmental assessment technology are clearly in the works, including Palm Pilot observational assessments, Web-based computer interfaces, and automatic progress monitoring.

Curriculum-based developmental assessment is a natural partner of developmental instruction and is used before, during, and after programming; a close-up of these three assessment phases follows.

Before Instruction

The "before" measure is certainly important; it tells the teacher where to begin with instruction. Children who have developmental differences cannot be presumed to possess all the skills of same-age "typical children." By using a hierarchy of developmental landmarks and competencies, the professional can identify what skills a given child displays, which ones are missing or delayed, which ones would be reasonable IEP goals, and which skills should be taught next. The assessment information can be collected by diverse means: observation, interview, and elicited performance. The "before" assessment provides valuable *program-entry* information that matches initial instructional objectives with a child's current capabilities; this makes sense from both behavioral and cognitive-developmental perspectives.

Most good programs use comprehensive developmental curricula—organized lists of sequential and hierarchically arranged skills in the several areas of development. Great precision for entry into the curriculum is possible, of course, when the child is assessed on the actual objectives within the program's specific curriculum. CBA includes a graduated scoring system that can detect small increments of learning (0, 1, 2, 3 or +, -, +). Extended observation, probes, and assessments are needed to check the child's mastery of actual, detailed, program-specific curriculum objectives. Sometimes an abbreviated procedure is used for program-entry assessment. A program may use an assessment device that *samples* the developmental objectives contained in its specific curriculum. Using such assessment devices provides at least rough estimates of where a child is in a specific developmental curriculum. This method is much faster but, as indicated, does not provide the exact position of the child in all areas of a specific curriculum.

During Instruction

Assessment of the child's progress *during* program participation might also be estimated through an instrument that samples the curriculum. Many teachers, however, prefer to use the program's curricular objectives them-selves as a kind of checklist. In this fashion, the teacher can continually track the child's (intra-individual) own progress within the program curric-ulum. This information is useful, of course, in guiding instruction and for planning the next objectives. This feedback function is a crucial strength of CBA and is central to direct instructional technique.

Parents are especially interested in their child's progress, and CBA is most valuable in this regard. Some commercially available preschool curric-ula actually include a chart or form that permits a graphic display of child progress.

After Instruction

Finally, summative assessment after program involvement (end of year, transition to new program) may also be accomplished by using the curricu-lum itself or an assessment device that samples the content of typical pre-school curricula (i.e., a curriculum-referenced instrument). Professionals often encourage the use of a standardized authentic curriculum-referenced assessment device as well as the curriculum itself for summative assessment. When properly chosen, both will sample the same or similar objectives as in those a given program. Further, since the authentic scale is not based on any single curriculum, it roughly relates to many curricula and thus acts as a comparative concurrent measure to check accuracy. When a child moves from one program to another, it is cumbersome to compare child status in curriculum A with curriculum B. The curriculum-referenced device can act as the information bridge between developmental programs.

SEQUENCE OF STEPS
FOR CURRICULUM-BASED ASSESSMENT

Repeated appraisals during instruction can document change and deter-mine whether modifications may be needed in instructional strategies. This assessment–prescription–evaluation model has been referred to as a "test–teach–test" approach, or developmental assessment/curriculum linkage (Bagnato, Neisworth, & Munson, 1997). Evidence of the child's progress is not based on comparative evaluations with other similar children, but rather on the child's previous performance levels as a reference point and higher-level goals as criteria to be mastered. In practical terms, an initial comprehensive appraisal of skills within several developmental domains and subdomains provides a baseline assessment of current skills and defi-cits. Early childhood intervention specialists can then determine individual-ized goals along the developmental or instructional sequence that become the focus of teaching and therapy. Finally, with these goals as benchmarks, the child is reevaluated at some predetermined time to detect evidence of progress. With progress, more challenging clusters of related skills are then established to amplify the child's individualized plan. The following five-step sequence forms the basis for developmental curriculum-based assessment:

1. Appraise the status of developmental skills within the major functional domains.
2. Determine functional ranges in each developmental domain.
3. Identify "transitional points" of skill acquisition in each domain.
4. Select related objectives that match the child's current level of skill acquisition in each domain within the developmental sequence and teach to mastery.
5. Reevaluate to monitor developmental change and generalization of learning across persons, situations, and materials.

Step 1: Appraise Developmental Status

Certain authentic curriculum-based developmental scales such as the Developmental Observation Checklist System (DOCS; Hresko, Miguel, Sherbenou, & Burton, 1994) can function as curriculum-referenced measures since they are "curriculum compatible." They are hybrid norm-based scales that contain similar but more global developmental sequences compared to the curriculum-based scales. However, unlike school-age curricula and intelligence tests, the parallel content of norm-based developmental skill measures and preschool curriculum-based measures generates some valid "assessment/curriculum linkages" (Bagnato, Neisworth, & Munson, 1997).

The skills and developmental domains surveyed in both types of instruments are similar. Thus, a diagnostic specialist such as the developmental school psychologist or the early childhood special educator can use authentic norm-based scales to appraise landmark developmental skills, then calculate developmental ages (DA) and developmental quotients (DQ) that describe a particular child's level in each developmental domain and subdomain, including cognitive, language, perceptual/fine motor, social–emotional, gross motor, and self-care.

Curriculum-embedded scales, however, may be used more directly to appraise developmental levels. Both curriculum-referenced and curriculum-embedded scales can be used to establish developmental levels and thus enter a child into an appropriate level within the curriculum, such as skill sequences appropriate for the 24- to 36-month level.

Step 2: Determine Functional Ranges

Once the child has been entered into appropriate curriculum levels for each developmental domain, an analysis of each item or task within the sequence at that developmental level must be made to determine the extent to which the infant or preschooler has acquired that skill and its behavioral components. The procedure involves an appraisal of which skills are fully acquired (+), absent (–), or emerging (±) within all major developmental areas. Thus, a *range* of functioning can be ascertained within each developmental domain.

Step 3: Identify "Transitional Skills"

The next step in the sequence involves isolating those specific skills that are only partially acquired or emerging (±). Examples include an infant's beginning coordination of eyes and hands in reaching for a brightly colored mobile or a preschooler's beginning discrimination of 12 different forms in a shape-matching task. In both instances, the child may have acquired components of the final skill but be unable or inconsistently able to complete the task as expected. Intervention is now directed toward full skill acquisition on these tasks in the developmental sequence. Transitional skills are ideal instructional objectives since they are usually at the optimal challenge level for the youngster—not too hard, not too easy. These transitional competencies are curriculum entry points, or *linkages*, for individualized curriculum planning and progress evaluation purposes.

Step 4: Link Curriculum Goals to Transitional Skills and Teach to Mastery

With identification of the child's transitional skills, individualized goal planning is accomplished by designing lessons that involve these transitional skills in various *purposeful* and natural activities such as when drawing and writing, matching shapes in group circle time activities, and labeling pictures during storytelling and prereading groups, and during lunch and toileting routines. Instruction is most effective when clusters of related skills are taught together across people and settings and also across curriculum areas so that uneven development is prevented. This also prevents teaching to isolated tasks, which produces the learning of nonpurposeful splinter skills. Most commercially available developmental curricula include field-tested strategies for grouping transitional skills for individual and group instruction and for matching appropriate instructional techniques (such as shaping and prompting) for teaching certain tasks. Mastery criteria are established by the program and each teacher; however, criteria typically involve 80–90% completion of a task without prompting over a number of trials or when the skill occurs under several conditions. Most intervention specialists believe that mastery and generalization of trained skills occur when that skill is repeatedly displayed with different people, in different settings, with different materials, and under circumstances distinct from the training conditions.

Step 5: Reassess Developmental Skills and Profile Gains

Frequent formative evaluations are needed to provide evidence of developmental changes in the transition skills that have been the focus of instruction. Such evaluations typically occur on a monthly, weekly, or even a per session basis depending upon program resources. Most often, progress assessments occur every September, January, and May. The curriculum-embedded scale is used once again to assess gains within several curricular areas. Again, the emphasis is not upon rote, isolated completion of splinter skills, but rather on the functional or purposeful use of such skills in play, social, and/or self-care routines. Frequent reevaluations enable the program staff to determine areas of change and to also detect domains in which no progress is apparent. These clinical evaluations allow the team to reconsider the effectiveness of their teaching and therapy methods. Once this reevaluation is completed, the process is repeated by determining the next range of fully acquired, emerging, and absent skills so that a child's individualized goal plan can be revised. This reciprocity between curriculum-based assessment and developmental instruction is the sine qua non of contemporary early intervention.

BEST-PRACTICE GUIDEPOINTS

♦ Recognize CBA's prominent historical use in early childhood intervention.

♦ Use developmental CBA to plan program prescriptions.

♦ Monitor goal mastery and progress with CBA.

♦ Structure parent–professional collaboration with CBA.

♦ Map a child's individual program with a developmental curriculum.

♦ Focus on *functional goals* within multiple developmental domains.

♦ Evaluate the developmental sequences and functional skill hierarchies.

♦ Select appropriate curricula and scales by developmental age; severity of disability; program characteristics; age and domain coverage; parent involvement; focus on inclusion; progress evaluation elements; and field-derived evidence base.

♦ Choose curriculum-referenced scales for linkage to many curriculum types.

♦ Use curriculum-embedded scales and accompanying curricula to meet group and idiosyncratic child needs.

♦ Emphasize a "test–teach–test" approach with CBA.

♦ Appraise preintervention baseline competencies.

♦ Determine ranges of acquired, emerging, and absent skills.

♦ Link transitional skills and curricular goals/expected competencies.

♦ Teach skills to mastery.

♦ Monitor skills acquisition regularly during intervention.

♦ Evaluate overall progress in multiple domains by comparing beginning-of-year and end-of-year levels of attainment.

BEST-PRACTICE EVIDENCE

Bagnato, S. J. (2005). The authentic alternative for assessment in early intervention: An emerging evidence-based practice. *Journal of Early Intervention, 28*(1), 17–22.

Bagnato, S. J., & Mayes, S. D. (1986). Patterns of developmental and behavioral progress for young brain-injured children during interdisciplinary intervention. *Developmental Neuropsychology, 2*(3), 213–244.

Bagnato, S. J., Mayes, S. M., Nichter, C., Dorriota, V., Hamann, L., Kuner, S., et al. (1988). An interdisciplinary neurodevelopmental assessment model for brain-injured infants and preschool children. *Journal of Head Trauma Rehabilitation, 3*(2), 75–86.

Bagnato, S. J., & Neisworth, J. T. (1985). Efficacy of interdisciplinary assessment and treatment for infants and preschoolers with congenital and acquired brain injury. *Analysis and Intervention in Developmental Disabilities, 5*(1–2), 107–128.

Bagnato, S. J., & Neisworth, J. T. (1991). *Assessment for early intervention: Best practices for professionals.* New York: Guilford Press.

Bagnato, S. J., & Neisworth, J. T. (1995). A national study of the social and treatment "invalidity" of intelligence testing for early intervention. *School Psychology Quarterly, 9*(2), 81–102.

Bagnato, S. J., & Neisworth, J. T. (1999). Collaboration and teamwork in assessment for early intervention. *Child and Adolescent Psychiatry Clinics of North America, 8*(2), 1–17.

Bagnato, S. J., Neisworth, J. T., & Munson, S. M. (1997). *LINKing assessment and early intervention: An authentic curriculum-based approach* (3rd ed.) Baltimore: Brookes.

Bagnato, S. J., Suen, H., Brantley, D., Smith-Jones, J., & Dettore, E. (2002). Child developmental impact of Pittsburgh's Early Childhood Initiative (ECI) in high-risk communities: First-phase authentic evaluation research. *Early Childhood Research Quarterly, 17*(4), 559–580.

Bagnato, S. J., & Yeh-Ho, H. (2006). High-stakes testing of preschool children: Violation of standards for professional and evidence-based practice. *International Journal of Korean Educational Policy, 3*(1), 23–34.

Bricker, D. (2002). *Assessment, Evaluation, and Programming System for Infants and Children* (2nd ed.). Baltimore: Brookes.

Bricker, D., & Squires, J. (1999). *Ages and Stages Questionnaires (ASQ): A parent completed, child-monitoring system*. Baltimore: Brookes.

Brigance, A. H. (1991). *Brigance diagnostic: Inventory of early development, revised edition*. Billerica, MA: Curriculum Associates.

Bronfrenbrenner, U. (1977). Toward an experimental ecology of human development. *American Psychologist, 32*(7), 513–531.

Coster, W. J., Deeney, T., Haley, S. T., & Haltiwanger, J. T. (1998). *School function assessment*. San Antonio, TX: Harcourt Brace.

Furuno, S., O'Reilly, K. A., Hosaka, C. M., Inatsuka, T. T., Allman, T. L., & Zeisloft, B. (1984). *Hawaii Early Learning Profile and Activity Guide*. Palo Alto, CA: VORT Corporation.

Hammill, D. D., Leigh, J. E., Pearson, N. A., & Maddox, T. (1998). *Basic School Skills Inventory (BBSI)* (3rd ed.). Austin, TX: PRO-ED.

Haley, S. M., Coster, W. J., Ludlow, L. H., Haltiwanger, J. T., & Andrellos, P. J. (1992, October). *Pediatric Evaluation of Disability Inventory (PEDI)* (Version 1.0). Boston: PEDI Research Group.

Harrison, P. L., & Oakland, T. (2003). *ABAS II: Adaptive Behavior Assessment System* (2nd ed.). San Antonio, TX: Psychological Corporation.

Hresko, W. P., Miguel, S. A., Sherbenou, R. J., & Burton, S. D. (1994). *Developmental Observation Checklist System*. Austin, TX: PRO-ED.

Individuals with Disabilities Education Act, 20 U.S.C. § 1432(5), 1435(a)(1) (1997).

Individuals with Disabilities Education Improvement Act, 20 U.S.C. § 1414(b) (6) (50a) (2004).

Johnson-Martin, N. M., Attermeier, S. M., & Hacker, B. (1990). *The Carolina Curriculum for Preschoolers with Special Needs*. Baltimore: Brookes.

Korsten, J. E., Dunn, D. K., Foss, T. V., & Francke, M. K. (1993). *Every Move Counts*. San Antonio, TX: Psychological Corporation.

Macy, M. G., Bricker, D. D., & Squires, J. K. (2005). Validity and reliability of a curriculum-based assessment approach to determine eligibility for Part C services. *Journal of Early Intervention, 28*(1), 1–16.

Neisworth, J. T., & Bagnato, S. J. (1991). Curriculum-based assessment (CBA) in early childhood education. In J. Salvia & C. Hughes (Eds.), *Curriculum-based assessment: Testing what is taught* (pp. 255–269). New York: Macmillan.

Neisworth, J. T., & Bagnato, S. J. (1992). The case against intelligence testing in early intervention. *Topics in Early Childhood Special Education, 12*(1), 1–20.

Neisworth, J. T., & Bagnato, S. J. (1996). Assessment for early intervention: Emerging themes and practices. In S. L. Odom & M. E. McLean (Eds.), *Early intervention for infants and young children with disabilities and their families: Recommended practice* (pp. 23–57). Austin, TX: PRO-ED.

Neisworth, J. T., & Bagnato, S. J. (2004). The mismeasure of young children: The authentic assessment alternative. *Infants and Young Children, 17*(3), 198–212.

Newborg, J. (2005). *Battelle Developmental Inventory* (2nd ed.). Itasca, IL: Riverside.

Parks, S. (1992). *Inside HELP: Hawaii Early Learning Profile (HELP): Administration and Scoring Manual.* Palo Alto, CA: VORT.

Sparrow, S. S., Cicchetti, D. V., & Balla, D. A. (2005). *Vineland-II Adaptive Behavior Scales.* Circle Pines, MN: AGS Publishing.

Squires, J., Potter, L., & Bricker, D. (1999). *Ages and Stages Questionnaire (ASQ)* (2nd ed.). Baltimore: Brookes.

Wetherby, A. M., & Prizant, B. M. (2002). *Communication and Symbolic Behavior Scales* (1st normed ed.). Baltimore: Brookes.

CHAPTER 7

◆ ◆ ◆

Can Clinical Judgments Guide Parent–Professional Team Decision Making for Early Intervention?

◆

with EILEEN McKEATING-ESTERLE

BEST-PRACTICE ISSUES

◆ Does clinical judgment have a valid role in assessment of infants and preschoolers for early intervention eligibility?

◆ Why is it important to match the model of teamwork with child and family needs?

◆ Why are multidisciplinary teams not recommended in early childhood intervention?

◆ Is there an evidence base for use of clinical judgment or informed opinion for early intervention?

◆ Can professionals and parents reach consensus decisions about the needs of young children with special needs?

◆ Is there a way to quantify collaborative team decision making about early intervention services?

Despite the interest in and policy mandate for clinical judgment or "informed clinical opinion" in the early intervention field, no clear defini-

Eileen McKeating-Esterle, MS, is a Research Assistant in the Early Childhood Partnerships program at the Children's Hospital of Pittsburgh.

tion has been posed to describe what it is. Moreover, only a few research studies exist to document the best methods, technical adequacy, and results of clinical judgment. Perhaps the most widely cited source in the early intervention field on clinical judgment or informed clinical opinion is Shackelford (2002) and its earlier versions (Biro, Daulton, & Szanton, 1991) distributed by the National Early Childhood Technical Assistance Center (NECTAS). Despite the informative value of this document, the authors offered no definition on the construct of "informed clinical opinion" itself. The definition that was posed focused instead on the methods ("qualitative and quantitative information"), content ("difficult-to-measure aspects of developmental status"), and purpose (to determine status and need for early intervention) for clinical judgment. As reported by Hayes (1990), one of the better definitions of clinical judgment is attributed to Goodnow (1988), referring to assessments by parents and other lay individuals: "Clinical judgment, defined as inference or evaluation derived from intuition and/or personal experience, is the basis of many daily routine assessments by parents and professionals" (p. 2).

The definition and evidence base for clinical judgment with infants, toddlers, and preschool children is, at best, undefined. Nevertheless, early interventionists and policy makers advocate the importance of informed clinical opinion for two major reasons: (1) state and federal regulations for Part C of the Individuals with Disabilities Education Act (IDEA) promote the flexible use of informed clinical opinion with difficult-to-evaluate infants and toddlers who may have developmental difficulties; and (2) parents and team members can integrate broader, qualitative information (without formal tests) to answer difficult questions about the status and service needs of young children. Part C regulations mandate informed clinical opinion as one of several techniques "to determine the existence of a condition that has a high probability of resulting in developmental delay" (p. 7). Clinical judgment is regarded widely as an important adjunct when other more formal measures fail to be appropriate or useful. Moreover, informed clinical opinion offers the necessary flexibility to integrate data from interviews, observations of natural play behaviors, and data from multiple lay caregivers and records to guide the determination of probable delay or disability and to establish the basis for early intervention services.

Clinical judgment or informed opinion is useful, unavoidable, and widely practiced in early childhood intervention, particularly for eligibility determination and team decision making about services in Part C. This chapter presents applied strategies that will enable teams of parents and interdisciplinary professionals to use clinical judgments to guide authentic assessment and decision making and fulfill early intervention purposes. The utility of clinical judgment is illustrated in five sections that cover (1) operational definition and background; (2) the evidence base supporting essential practice characteristics; (3) models of teamwork; (4) exemplary clinical judgment systems for authentic assessment and team decision making; and (5) an example of the System to Plan Early Childhood Services (SPECS) team decision-making model.

CLINICAL JUDGMENT:
OPERATIONAL DEFINITION AND HISTORICAL CONTEXT

Clinical judgment, or informed clinical opinion, refers to the knowledgeable perceptions of caregivers and professionals about the elusive and subtle capabilities and contexts of children that must be defined and quantified such that individuals or teams are able to reach accurate decisions about eligibility for early intervention. Clinical judgment or informed clinical opinion becomes particularly important when standardized measures are inappropriate or unavailable (IDEA, 1997; IDEIA, 2004) and is most effective when it goes beyond measurement to involve collaborative decision-making strategies that integrate information from various aspects of children's lives." (Bagnato, Smith-Jones, Matesa, & Fevola, 2005, p. 1)

Since the 1950s clinical judgment has been a widely studied concept or phenomenon, especially in psychology and medicine. Meehl's (1954) seminal review comparing clinical and statistical prediction encouraged a flurry of studies of the phenomenon. However, the majority of the research was conducted in university-based laboratory settings and had very few implications for practical applications. A recent meta-analysis by Grove and colleagues (2000) examined studies that compared clinical versus mechanical (statistical and actuarial) prediction techniques in the psychological and medical literature. Recent research has demonstrated the greater accuracy of actuarial methods compared to clinical judgment methods (Dawes, Faust, & Meehl, 1989). While not directly germane to early intervention, the meta-analysis may have some application to alternative early detection strategies such as presumptive eligibility.

Nevertheless, clinical judgment has intuitive appeal and persists as an evaluation methodology in many health and human service fields. The nursing literature details the rationale for, teaching of, and application of clinical judgment in nurse-midwifery (Greener, 1988) and decision making about life-threatening conditions (Benner & Tanner, 1987). The field of communication disorders has produced research and position statements on the use of clinical judgments in a comprehensive decision-making process about the presence and type of speech–language disorder exhibited by individuals (Records & Weiss, 1990). In pediatric medicine, Glascoe and Dworkin (1993) have published research and position statements on the factors, or "judgment heuristics," that influence physicians' abilities to discriminate typical from atypical child development.

Within special education and school psychology, researchers hold differing positions on the role, usefulness, and technical adequacy of clinical judgment in a broad assessment-based decision-making process. Gresham and colleagues (Gresham, Reschly, & Carey, 1987) conducted research on the accuracy of teacher judgments in distinguishing between students with learning disabilities and those without learning difficulties. The results demonstrated that teachers' judgments were as accurate as decisions based on the use of standardized tests of intelligence and achievement. Functional classification systems based on the use of clinical judgment in team decision-making processes have been proposed and examined, although only descriptively (Iscoe & Payne, 1972). Arguably, the most thorough study of research on assessment and decision making in special education has been conducted by Ysseldyke and colleagues (1983) through the University of Minnesota Learning Disabilities Research Institute. Specific to clinical judgment, the researchers determined that school psychologists and special education teachers were able to differentiate between students who were low-achieving and learning disabled with only 50% accuracy whereas introductory psychology students evidenced a 75% accuracy rate. Moreover, their research indicated that team decision-making processes about special education eligibility were flawed and based more often on nonperformance data such as socioeconomic status, family issues, and physical attractiveness.

There have been few publications on clinical judgment and its associated variants, such as informed clinical opinion and judgment-based evaluation, and still fewer high-quality research studies specific to early intervention. Two of the most widely regarded and cited publications on clinical judgment are Neisworth (1990) and Meisels and Atkins-Burnett (2000). The only readily available source of its type on clinical judgment in early intervention is the special issue of *Topics in Early Childhood Special Education* devoted to "judgment-based assessment" (JBA; Neisworth, 1990). This issue contains nine position papers and literature reviews on clinical judgment and JBA and thus represents the predominant type of descriptive treatment of this topic in the literature. As the special issue states, clinical judgment is widely practiced and valued in assessment for early intervention, especially for children with significant disabilities, and to enable parents to function as partners with professionals on interdisciplinary teams.

ESSENTIAL PRACTICE CHARACTERISTICS FOR ACCURATE CLINICAL JUDGMENT

Within the relevant research literature, five practice characteristics emerge as essential and common features that have some evidence base to support the use of clinical judgment in early childhood intervention. Across the literature, clinical judgments were based on the collection and synthesis of functional data about the child's overall interactions within his or her physical and social environments—the child's developmental ecology. These five practice characteristics were present in at least 80% of the studies. I strongly recommend their implementation in order to ensure reliable, valid, and practical use of clinical informed opinion in the field.

Construct Operational Definitions of Attributes under Focus

Operational definitions of the constructs and functional domains to be appraised must be created. These include such areas of child status and functioning as cognitive, language, motor, social, adaptive, physical, temperament, self-regulation, and neurobehavioral development. Beyond the theoretical construct under consideration (e.g., early language skills, early motor skills), operational definitions provide structure at the most basic level of measurement by specifying the particular dimensions or attributes being appraised. This structure helps ensure that parents, professionals, and other caregivers, using ratings, classify various attributes under consideration using similar lenses.

Use Structured Rating Formats to Record Informed Opinions

Structuring the rating of informed opinion in conjunction with using operational definitions further ensures reliable assessment ratings by guiding how specific attributes are to be quantitatively or qualitatively rated. Rating formats vary in terms of mode (e.g., written scales, interviews, archival data coding), rating scheme (e.g., qualitative and quantitative scales, open-ended responses), and level of detail. Most studies support the use of *Likert* scale rating formats (i.e., scales of 3-1 or 5-1 levels most often) or functional classification profiles (i.e., typical, at risk, mild, moderate, severe).

Gather Data from Multiple Sources: Settings, Individuals, Methods

It is important to gather comprehensive and ecological information about children's functioning in the home, at school, and in the community to foster accurate judgments and decisions about needs and services. Teachers, psychologists, and speech, occupational, and physical therapists often operated within the school setting. However, each brought unique perspectives given the specific nature of their assessments and as such each was judged as constituting a distinct setting or assessment contribution. Information should mostly be gathered and synthesized from a combination of clinical judgment tools, curriculum-based measures, file reviews of traditional scale results, and interviews. Similarly, parents' perspectives about child functioning must be viewed as offering a unique source of information (e.g., sleep, eating, behavior, play, attachment, self-care, temperament) that is indispensable to accurate and representative decision making.

Establish Consensus Decision-Making Processes

Consensus decision making entails the integration and synthesis of information from multiple individuals and sources to facilitate sound and appropriate diagnostic and planning decisions. Ideally, information is obtained from four or more individuals (Suen, Bagnato, Lu, & Neisworth, 1993) and informational sources may include medical records, educational records, and prior assessments. In every study, integrating all (as opposed to some) informational sources provided the most reliable and accurate snapshots of children's development. In addition, best practice is supported when a standard process and set of procedures exist to resolve differences in judgments and to reach collaborative decisions about the needs of children.

Provide Training to Facilitate Reliable Ratings

Position papers (Danaher, Shackelford, & Harbin, 2004; Hemmeter, Joseph, Smith, & Sandall, 2001; Sandall, McLean, & Smith, 2000) strongly support the need for training and modeling to guide the formation of accurate judgments and decisions. In fact, the training of raters is described in the manuals of some of the most effective clinical judgment and team decision-making instructions, including The System to Plan Early Childhood Services (SPECS; Bagnato & Neisworth, 1990) the ABILITIES Index (Simeonsson, 2002), and the International Classification of Functioning: Children and Youth Version (ICF; Simeonsson, 2002).

PARENT–PROFESSIONAL TEAMWORK

Models

Working as a team has become synonymous with early intervention. Professionals recognize that serving young children with special needs and their families is a complex venture that demands a multispecialist approach. No one profession or discipline "owns" a developmental domain or disorder. Development is interactive and so is effective early intervention. Neuromotor dysfunctions, for example, distort progress in several interrelated developmental domains: play, motor, socialization, and self-care. The various team members (e.g., physical therapist, communication specialist, early educator, psychologist, and parents) must coordinate their goals and methods to assess and promote progress for children with neuromotor impairments. Federal and state laws and regulations recognize the need for cross-disciplinary work and so mandate a multidimensional and multidisciplinary approach to assessment, evaluation, and intervention. It targets both the broad and narrow needs of children in the physical, cognitive, speech–language, psychosocial, self-help, and social behavior domains. Laws and best practices also emphasize the family's priorities and needs for various things—information, financial resources, help in coping with stress, and services matched to their own circumstances. The law specifies that professionals must be available for assessment and intervention, including educators, language specialists, physical and occupational therapists, vision and hearing specialists, psychologists, social workers, physicians, nurses, and nutritionists. The parent, however, is a *crucial* member of the team who provides and gains information to help the child thrive. In short, the team approach to assessment and intervention represents best practice and is institutionalized by legislation.

The very existence of *teaming* as a service technique underscores that a child's problems are the result of complex biological and environmental interactions and that collaboration among specialists is necessary. "Teamwork," however, is a buzzword often used to give the illusion of collaboration in the absence of any team identity or coordinated efforts. Teams evolve their own styles based upon shared purposes, aims, and methods; yet, the social chemistry between every person on the team is the true measure of team identity or "groupness." To be effective as a team, parents and interdisciplinary professionals must trust one another, respect each other's legitimate roles and expertise, be ready to freely share judgments in a problem-solving process, be receptive to allow others to assume and share part of their typical role responsibilities, and accept structuring from a permanent or rotating team coordinator.

Three models of teamwork are recognized by the early intervention field, each with its own distinguishing characteristics, but in practice some are better than others and no one "pure" version of any model exists; hybrid versions are apparent in everyday applications.

Multidisciplinary Model

The most widely used but, frankly, inadequate model is the multidisciplinary team (MDT). MDTs use several professionals, who emphasize their own disciplinary perspectives in assessing particular developmental domains in an independent manner. Collaboration between the several specialists is infrequent. Thus, the diagnostic picture of child and family functioning that emerges is most often fragmented and often faulty. The MDT model does not promote a "whole-child," interactive view. The most tangible evidence of this fragmentation is the diagnostic report that is completed at the end of an MDT evaluation. This report is usually an unintegrated collection of the separate reports of each professional stapled together into one report. Most importantly, the recommendations are typically redundant and offer a nonunified and confusing list of goals and directives for the parent. Worse, sometimes recommendations actually conflict. For the program, MDT evaluations perpetuate interventions that are discipline specific and unorchestrated. One is reminded of the old parables about the several blind men who each examined a different part of an elephant and then provided very different descriptions of the beast. Actually, research demonstrates that reliable and valid clinical judgments are less likely when parents and professionals act in isolation and at a distance as "members" of multidisciplinary teams. Actually, the MDT model only masquerades as a team approach and thus is not recommended in early intervention.

Interdisciplinary Model

Interdisciplinary teams (IDT) share unifying views and practices. IDTs assume a "whole-child" perspective and stress the integral involvement of parents as partners on the team by a process of *collaborative goal-setting*. They enable team members and parents to integrate their assessment and intervention efforts by organizing services around functional skills or developmental domains (e.g., cognitive, language, perceptual/fine motor, social–emotional, gross motor, self-care) rather than by the discipline that provides those services. Authentic curriculum-based systems and structured clinical judgment formats are most often used by IDTs as common tools to focus services and to link assessment, program goal-planning, and progress evaluation (Bagnato & Neisworth, 1999a). While IDTs rarely "release" role responsibilities, team members place a high premium on frequent consultation so that a unified view about child and family needs is created. Intervention goals are designed so that common goals are integrated into each discipline's therapy. For example, language goals are included as central features in the activities of the child with a communication disorder within the early childhood special education classroom. Opportunities for social and object play are integrated into physical therapy routines. The IDT model exemplifies a real team approach, but members must constantly work at reducing conflict and ensuring coordination of services. Reports produced by IDTs are integrated and seldom contain conflicting views. The cross-talk among members, familiarity with each other, and acquaintance with each discipline's role help to yield comprehensive, coordinated assessment and reporting.

Most research supports the accuracy and utility of clinical judgments generated by interdisciplinary teams of parents and professionals.

Transdisciplinary Model

Clinical judgment has not been widely studied on transdisciplinary teams. Procedures that enable team members to share or "release" assessment and therapeutic expertise with each other characterize the transdisciplinary team model (TDT). TDT models are built upon an interactive approach to service delivery. TDT formats minimize disciplinary boundaries and promote team consensus. Team members and parents work actively together with the child in dyads or triads. The emphasis is upon play-based and modified arena-style assessments and consultation with designated team members who deliver instruction and therapy based on plans that integrate goals from all disciplines. The parent and family are central partners who eventually learn and assume primary responsibilities as collaborative decision makers and cotherapists for their child. TDT models are most successful when team members have worked together for a long period and have perfected a give-and-take chemistry that encourages each team member to feel valued even though consultation rather than direct service delivery becomes their primary model of operation.

Prominent Team Members

Unlike school settings, the team approach in early childhood intervention settings is distinctive in three ways: (1) greater numbers of professionals involved, (2) the style of team collaboration, and (3) the central role of parents as partners. Interdisciplinary and transdisciplinary team approaches are the most frequently employed structures for planning and delivering services (especially with infants). Team specialists thrive upon conjoint interactions for assessment and instruction or therapy. Common goals and methods in the form of curriculum-based procedures are the benchmarks of preschool teaming. Finally, parents do more than merely attend individualized education plan (IEP) meetings during the preschool years. Rather, parents are integral team members who have a central voice in designing and implementing child and family plans that fit their particular life circumstances. Parents and professionals in early childhood settings must be familiar with each other's roles. The following discussion identifies and portrays these core team members.

Early Childhood Educators

With the movement toward inclusion in regular early childhood settings, various early childhood educators (ECE), including early care and education providers and child development professionals, care for and instruct young children both without and with developmental delays and disabilities. Whether credentialed or not, ECE observe, assess, judge, plan, and intervene with children having delays and disabilities. Their authentic assessment, care, and instruction practices are guided by the professional standards of the National Association for the Education of Young Children (NAEYC). Most often, Early Head Start and Head Start settings are the inclusion settings and their inclusion procedures and practices in assessment and intervention are guided by the Head Start Performance Standards. Increasingly, early intervention consultative and direct services are provided in family child care homes, private early care and education classrooms, and other group care arrangements. In many instances, ECE have the strongest relationship with parents and other family members. ECE are integral members of the early intervention team

Early childhood special educators (ECSE) are the primary interventionists on the team; their professional practices for assessment and intervention are guided by the Division for Early Childhood (DEC) of the Council for Exceptional Children. They combine developmental content and behavioral methods to help young children learn in both individual and group settings, whether home or center based. In many programs, the educator, the parent, and the speech–language specialist make up the interdisciplinary team. The teacher works to integrate team member goals into the classroom instructional and therapeutic plan using both consultation and direct service modes and to balance efforts across developmental domains.

Speech–Language Pathologist

Speech–language difficulties are the most frequently observed problems in early childhood. Thus, the speech–language specialist is an essential member of the early intervention team. The professional guides the team in understanding the child's ability to use language pragmatically for social communication and helps to integrate language goals into ongoing classroom routines. As needed, the language specialist also helps the team to use signing and assistive communication devices. Speech–language pathologists are skilled in using a combination of traditional methods, natural environment language samples, and clinical judgment methods to diagnose the severity of communication difficulties.

Occupational and Physical Therapists

For preschoolers with neuromotor dysfunctions, the services of occupational therapists (OT) and physical therapists (PT) are invaluable on the interdisciplinary team. For example, proper positioning by neuromotor therapists enables psychologists, teachers, and other team members to obtain more accurate assessments of young children with cerebral palsy. OTs and PTs help the team and parents to understand the impact of motor impairments on other areas of competence. Often, the neuromotor thera-pist is the member most likely to be selected to implement the team's inter-vention plan for children who have neurological and multiple impairments.

Care Coordinator

The care coordinator (CC) or family support specialist, often a social worker, enables the team to appraise and incorporate family issues as a central concern in early intervention programming and service delivery. The CC is a parent advocate who emphasizes the characteristics of the family and home environment to facilitate quality care and stimulation for the young child with special needs. These characteristics include level of stress within the family, economic concerns, the home environment, need for information, social support, and parenting skills. Most often in the 0–3 system, the CC helps the parent to become an integral partner and collaborative decision maker on the interdisciplinary team and em-phasizes the parent's priorities to coordinate services among multiple community agencies. Using clinical judgment approaches, the CC helps the parent to define the extent of services that will be needed to help their child best.

Primary Care Physician and Pediatric Nurse Practitioner

Each child's primary care physician (PCP) has become a more active con-sultant to the early intervention team. The PCP helps clarify relationships among the young child's medical needs, developmental competencies, and endurance for program participation. Similarly, the PNP often consults directly with early intervention programs and provides on-site in vivo sup-port on such issues as asthma care, seizure monitoring, use of portable res-pirators, care of gastrostomy tubes, and diagnosis of attention disorders (Bagnato et al., 2004). Also, many PCPs and PNPs are parent advocates and can contribute judgments on mother–infant interaction and family his-tory and coping style. PCPs and PNPs are skilled in using clinical judgment for diagnostic decision making and the earliest referrals for early interven-tion services.

Applied Developmental Psychologist

Over the last decade, psychologists with training as applied developmen-tal psychologists (ADPs) are providing services and support in diverse early childhood intervention settings. Often with state school psychology credentials, ADPs both consult and provide individualized support to teachers, parents, and other team members on managing challenging behaviors, preventing maladaptive behavior patterns, linking health and education concerns, and conducting specialized assessments to guide eligibility determination. Enlightened and nontraditional "developmental school psychologists" in some states are providing an invaluable resource to early intervention programs in many roles including serving as team leader to facilitate parent–professional team consensus decision making (Bagnato, Neisworth, Paget, & Kovaleski, 1987; Bagnato, 1999).

Clinical Judgment and Team Decision Making

Studies examining the contributions of parents, professionals, and teams to the assessment, diagnosis, and planning for young children with delays and disabilities (see Table 7.1) demonstrate that (1) parents' judgments are integral to accurate and representative assessments of their children's abilities; (2) teams that include parents make accurate judgments about the needs of young children with developmental delays and disabilities; (3) team decisions using the collaborative judgments of four professionals and a parent produce the most reliable assessments of infants, toddlers, and preschoolers for high-stakes decisions; and (4) clinical judgment measures correspond well with more structured measures of developmental status.

EXEMPLARY CLINICAL JUDGMENT INSTRUMENTS

System to Plan Early Childhood Services

The System to Plan Early Childhood Services (SPECS) was designed to provide a structured format for gathering clinical judgment data from parents and professionals on an interdisciplinary team and applying the data for early detection and assessment (Developmental Specs), team decision making (Team Specs), and program planning, service delivery, and progress evaluation (Program Specs) involving the needs of children from 2 to 6 years of age. The national field-validation research on SPECS is reported in two technical resource manuals (Bagnato & Neisworth, 1990; Bagnato, Neisworth, & McCloskey, 1994).

Rating–rerating reliability studies on the Developmental Specs were conducted among early childhood educators and paraprofessional aides (n = 163) with correlation coefficients ranging from .60 to .87 across the 19 developmental dimensions.

Concurrent validity studies were conducted between the Developmental Specs ratings across the clusters of communication, sensorimotor, physical, self-regulation, cognitive, and self-social, and 12 different formal and observational scales to document the comparability of the assessments and

TABLE 7.1. Research Foundations for Using Clinical Judgment (Informed Clinical Opinion) for Early Intervention Eligibility: Study Focus and Practice Characteristics

Study reference	Study focus	Defined characteristics	Structured opinions	Multiple settings or individuals	Multisource consensus decisions	Training to structure opinions
Bagnato (1984)	Parent–professional congruence	x	x	x	x	x
Bagnato & Neisworth (1985a)	Parent–professional congruence	x	x	x		
Bagnato & Neisworth (1990)	Judgment-based scales and formats	x	x	x		x
Bagnato & Neisworth (1999a)	Judgment-based scales and formats	x	x	x		x
Blacher-Dixon & Simeonsson (1981)	Parent–professional congruence	x	x	x		
Casey, McIntire, & Leveno (2001)	Judgment-based scales and formats	x	x		x	
Glascoe (1991)	Early detection and classification	x		x		
Gradel, Thompson, & Sheehan (1981)	Parent–professional congruence	x	x	x		
Gresham, Reschly, & Carey (1987)	Judgment-based scales and formats	x	x	x	x	
Henderson & Meisels (1994)	Early detection and classification	x	x	x	x	
Kochanek, Kabacoff, & Lipsitt (1990)	Early detection and classification	x		x	x	
Records & Tomblin (1994)	Early detection and classification	x	x	x	x	
Sampers, Cooley, & Shook (1996)	Early detection and classification	x	x		x	
Suen, Bagnato, Lu, & Neisworth (1993)	Judgment-based scales and formats	x	x	x	x	x
Suen, Logan, Neisworth, & Bagnato (1995)	Judgment-based scales and formats	x	x	x	x	x
Percentage of studies incorporating each practice characteristic		100%	87%	80%	53%	47%

outcomes for children. The percentage of agreement among scales was moderate to high in all domains.

Discriminant function analyses were conducted on typical and atypical child data for various disability categories (e.g., delay, mental retardation, neuromotor impairment, communication disorder, hearing impairment, behavioral/emotional disorder, autism/PDD) and among various rater groups (e.g., parent, early childhood special educator teacher, speech–language pathologist, social worker, regular early childhood educator, paraprofessional aide, psychologist, occupational therapist). Analyses focused upon determining the classification accuracy of Developmental Specs ratings and SPECS decisions about services for a mean of 594 children with typical development and a mean of 118 children with atypical development (range = 11–392). Analyses also focused on classification accuracy by rater group for over 200 team members. Overall mean correct classification by disability category was 84.8% (range = 75% for developmental delay to 96% for hearing impairment). Overall mean correct classification by rater group was 76.8% (range = 66% for psychologist to 90% for early childhood special educator).

Overall, the SPECS system has the necessary psychometric rigor for accurate and sensitive team decisions for eligibility determination, program planning, and progress monitoring.

ABILITIES Index

The ABILITIES Index was designed to provide a noncategorical classification format for describing the functional capabilities of individuals with diverse developmental disabilities. ABILITIES uses a rating scale format (1–6) to classify a functional capability range from normal to profound difficulty. Cross-cultural research has been conducted to document the reliability of the ABILITIES index for use in making disability classification decisions (Bailey, Simeonsson, Buysse, & Smith, 1993; Simeonsson, Bailey, Smith, & Buysse, 1995). Studies involved 254 children, 213 parents, 133 teachers, and 135 interdisciplinary professionals.

Interrater agreement studies among 133 teachers and 135 specialists (total number of agreements/agreements + disagreements) showed that 86% of the ratings of one rater were within one point of those of the second rater. Correlations among raters were low to moderate with an average of .60 across raters. Lower ratings and levels of agreement were observed on less well-defined and complex categories (i.e., social skills, inappropriate behavior, intellectual functioning, communication, and health).

A study of the stability of ratings was conducted with 44 teachers on ratings conducted one month apart. Agreement within one point was documented in 91% of the instances with kappas in the moderate range (.77).

Temperament and Atypical Behavior Scale

The Temperament and Atypical Behavior Scale (TABS) is a judgment-based method for recording observations in the natural environment and recollections about the presence or absence of atypical temperament and self-regulatory behaviors in children 11 to 71 months of age. The TABS was designed specifically as a functional and noncategorical method to screen and determine eligibility for early intervention and support services by young children who are at risk for later developmental delays and disabilities. The TABS is one of the few judgment-based instruments with national norms that has been field validated for specific early intervention purposes.

National normative research on the TABS (Bagnato, Neisworth, Salvia, & Hunt, 1999; Bagnato & Neisworth, 1999b) was conducted in 33 states with a pooled norm group of children with typical (n = 621) and atypical (n = 212) development . Factor analytic studies on the full 55-item TABS Assessment resulted in four distinct and empirically derived factors with associated eigenvalues: detached (.52–.66); underreactive (.55–.66); hypersensitive/active (.55–.69; and dysregulated (.46–.61). These studies confirmed and validated the regulatory disorders conceptualization in Zero to Three's diagnostic classification system (DC: 0–3; Zero to Three, 1994).

The stability of TABS Assessment ratings was studied with a sample of 157 children over a 2–3 week period. All participated in early intervention programs, home and center based. Coefficients showed excellent stability ranging from .73 to .94.

Sensitivity and specificity studies on the TABS show strong support for the TABS screener. Of the 833 children in the pooled sample, 83% were correctly classified as normal or atypical by the screener. Of the 17% incorrectly classified, only 2.4% were false negatives and these were all children identified as at risk but not with disabilities. Approximately 14.5% of the children incorrectly classified were false positives; only 6% of these children showed disabilities. Therefore, a conservative estimate of the accuracy of the TABS screener is 72% correct classification.

Ages and Stages Questionnaire: Social–Emotional

The Ages and Stages Questionnaire: Social–Emotional (ASQ: SE; Squires, Bricker, & Twombly, 2002; Davis & Squires, 2002) is a norm-referenced observation-based rating scale designed to collect judgments about the social–emotional capabilities of infants, toddlers, and preschool children. Initial research on the ASQ: SE supports its reliability, validity, and overall technical adequacy as a screening and assessment instrument for use by parents and professionals in early intervention

Normative data were based on over 3,000 rating scales and validity studies were based on ratings for over 1,000 children. Parent test–retest reliability over a 1- to 3-week period was .94. Screening accuracy studies indicated overall sensitivity (correctly detecting delays or atypical development) at only 78% and overall specificity (correctly identifying typical development) at 94%. Concurrent validity comparisons between the ASQ: SE and other measures such as TABS and Brief Infant Toddler Social Emotional Assessment (BITSEA; Briggs-Gowen & Carter, 2002) on 90 children and mothers corroborate the normative studies on sensitivity and specificity.

Adaptive Behavior Assessment System II

While not described as a clinical judgment tool, the Adaptive Behavior Assessment System II (ABAS) is, arguably, the most comprehensive and technically adequate authentic observation and judgment-based rating scale available to professionals. The ABAS is a norm-referenced, multidomain, continuous measure of adaptive behavior competencies for individuals from birth to 89 years of age. The content of the ABAS is aligned with the *Diagnostic and Statistical Manual of Mental Disorders* (DSM-IV) and American Association on Mental Retardation (AAMR) systems. Raters include anyone, professional or layperson, who knows the individual best and can provide a representative appraisal of skills across multiple domains of functioning. For young children from birth to age 5, the domains include communication, community use, functional preacademics, home living, health and safety, leisure, self-care, self-direction, social, and motor. Caregiver raters respond through a 0–3 rating scale: 0 = is not able; 1 = never when needed; 2 = sometimes when needed; 3 = always when needed.

For children ages birth to 5 years, the standardization sample comprised 2,100 individuals representative of the U.S. population. The ABAS II results in scores including a general adaptive composite (GAC) having a mean of 100 and standard deviation of 15 and skill-area standard scores with a mean of 10 and standard deviation of 3, and critical values within 90% and 95% confidence intervals. Reliability studies included interrater, test–retest, and internal consistency analyses. Perhaps the most unique feature of the ABAS II is the broad scope of validity studies comparing each atypical sample with a matched "typical" control group. The studies were conducted during development across individuals who had at least 15 types of developmental disabilities and disorders (e.g., autism, learning disabilities, early developmental delays [*n* = 126], Alzheimer's disease, neuromotor impairments). Concurrent validity studies were conducted with most of the major psychoeducational measures used by professionals. The validity study with children showing early developmental delays included a matched control group sample of typically developing children.

Table 7.2 summarizes the essential and operational information for these exemplary clinical judgment systems.

TABLE 7.2. Measures Utilizing Clinical Judgment

Instrument	Author	Publisher	Age range	Domains	Sample	Technical adequacy
SPECS (System to Plan Early Childhood Services) • Infant • Developmental • Team • Program	Bagnato & Neisworth (1990)	American Guidance Service	Birth–24 months 24–72 months	Communication, Sensorimotor, Physical, Self-regulation, Cognition, Self-social Developmental support, Behavioral, Communication, Gross/Fine motor support, Vision, Hearing and medical support, Special, Transition support and teamwork	1,300 children, .31 typical and .69 had developmental problems	Acceptable reliability for all 19 dimensions. Test–retest reliability Content and construct validity Classification accuracy
ABILITIES Index	Simeonsson & Bailey (1991)	University of North Carolina	Birth–21 months	Audition, Behavior and social skills, Intellectual function, Limbs, Intentional communication, Tonicity, Integrity of physical health, Eyes, Structural status	254 children, 213 parents, 133 teachers and 135 interdisciplinary professionals	
TABS (Temperament and Atypical Behavior Scale)	Bagnato, Neisworth, Salvia, & Hunt (1999)	Paul H. Brookes	11–71 months	Detached, Hyper-sensitive/active, Underreactive, Dysregulated	621 typical and 212 atypical developing children	Internal consistency Reliability: .95 in at-risk sample, .88 children not at risk, Content and construct validity
Ages and Stages Questionnaire (ASQ)	Bricker & Squires (1999)	Paul H. Brookes	4 months–5 years	Communication, Gross motor, Fine motor, Problem solving, Personal–social	~1,000 children	Test–retest reliability, Construct validity .86 specificity overall
ABAS (Adaptive Behavior Assessment System)	Harrison & Oakland (2003)	Psychological Corporation	0–89 years	Communication, Community use, School/home living, Functional preacademics, Health and safety, Leisure, Self-care, Self-direction, Social, Motor	2,100 children Validity studies included 126 children with at least 15 types of developmental disabilities	Internal consistency, Interrater reliability, Construct validity, Convergent and discriminant validity

SPECS: A CLINICAL JUDGMENT MODEL TO GUIDE PARENT–PROFESSIONAL TEAM DECISION MAKING

Interdisciplinary team procedures are the key to the effectiveness of pre-school service delivery efforts. Team procedures are mandated by the new law and must synchronize the work of developmental, educational, medical, and mental health professionals, parents, and paraprofessionals (IDEIA, 2004).

Despite advancements in child tests, curricula, and methods, programs are typically without an organizing structure for interdisciplinary team appraisal that can synthesize multisource assessment information about children and families, translate data into a blueprint for service delivery, and gauge child progress as a function of planned intervention. Early interventionists as well as program administrators repeatedly declare that instead of more tests and more curricula they need to have some sort of organizational format that allows them to coordinate team decision making; they need a streamlined way to reach consensus about child and family needs and program components.

Research on team functioning identifies three important issues: (1) team activities rarely reflect the use of a "planned, systematic and functional decision-making process"; (2) structured team decision-making models are much more effective than unstructured ones; and (3) teacher and team member judgments are often just as effective for diagnostic and program planning purposes as standardized test-based criteria.

Effectiveness should be judged in practical and tangible terms: broader coverage of developmental, behavioral, and family needs; numbers of team members actively participating in group decision making; increased involvement of parents in team negotiations; increased options for service delivery; wider consideration of program features; relationship between scope of child and family needs and program "intensity."

SPECS (Bagnato & Neisworth, 1990, 2005) is an authentic assessment system that relies on clinical judgment and team decision-making strategies to link interdisciplinary assessment and intervention. The SPECS system encompasses all five practice characteristics that define accurate use of clinical judgments for valid and effective decision making in early childhood intervention.

Purposes and Features of SPECS

SPECS offers common tools for team decision making to generate a consensus about child and family needs. This consensus offers the team a method for translating assessment data directly into plans for education and therapy. Finally, SPECS offers an economical method for evaluating child progress and program effectiveness. Thus, SPECS serves clinical purposes—

assessment, service delivery planning, progress/program evaluation—as well as administrative purposes, including team organization, case coordination, staff allocation, and program impact.

SPECS uses structured clinical judgment ratings to appraise the functional competencies of children 24 to 72 months of age in 6 domains and 19 developmental and behavioral subdomains. Judgment-based assessment provides the most natural vehicle for team collaboration if the rating scales are structured. Based upon a functional, noncategorical approach, SPECS incorporates data from multiple sources (e.g., tests, curricula, interviews, observation, parents, team members, several settings) so that team members can "cross-talk" through consistent and readily understood language and ratings about child needs. SPECS uses a consensus rating system to help the team determine the type and extent of therapy services that will be provided to each child and family. This consensus also enables team members to pose specific questions about needed program requirements that are scored to generate a "program intensity profile" encompassing 10 separate dimensions.

SPECS Components

SPECS consists of three interrelated components that link team assessment and intervention. Developmental Specs (D-Specs) is the primary child appraisal instrument in the system. It uses numerous 5-point Likert rating scales to record the judgments of parents and team members about the child's developmental and behavioral capabilities and needs across 19 developmental areas. Traditional areas are surveyed, for example, gross motor skills and receptive language abilities; in addition, emphasis is placed upon several important but difficult to assess characteristics that are crucial in program planning: attention, normalcy, temperament, self-control, social competence, and motivation.

The second SPECS component, Team Specs (T-Specs), organizes team and parent judgments to enable the team to determine "consensus" ratings of each developmental area that can be profiled. This consensus is then cross-referenced with 10 therapy options (e.g., speech–language therapy, behavior therapy, transition services, physical therapy) and scored to generate decisions regarding the types of services needed (e.g., consult, direct therapy).

Program Specs (P-Specs), the third component, translates the T-Specs consensus data about type of therapy into specific decisions about the content, methods, and strategies that should make up the child's service plan. Specific questions organized and weighted by the "intensity" of the intervention option selected by the team give the 10 service areas more detail. These questions are summed to determine subarea and overall "program intensity ratings" by quartiles (25th = low intensity, 50th = medium, 100th

= high) in each of the 10 areas, which include Adaptive Services, Early Education, Physical Therapy, Transition Needs, and Medical Needs. P-Specs enables the team and administrative personnel to compare beginning-of-the-year and end-of-the-year intensity ratings to determine progress. Data from D-Specs, T-Specs, and P-Specs are used to chart child progress and program impact.

Use of SPECS for Team Meetings

Figure 7.1 illustrates the flow of activities for team decision making using SPECS. The psychologist often assumes the role of interdisciplinary team coordinator and can promote and model best practices through cross-talk and collaboration among team members and parents by virtue of special expertise in group processes. You can facilitate more collaborative efforts among professionals and parents by following the five steps described below.

Step 1: Have All Team Members Contribute to the Assessment. A child is referred to your program initially for possible identification of special needs and enrollment for intervention. After an observation or actual assessment by team member(s) and an interview with the parent, each professional and the parent can contribute ratings or observational and test data. The D-Specs is a common tool that maps the results of any assessment (whether formal or informal) onto a 5-point continuum that facilitates cross-talk among the parent and other team members. Ideally, D-Specs is completed by the teacher, speech therapist, psychologist, parent, social worker, and any other member to profile judgments of the preschooler's capabilities and needs in 20 developmental and behavioral areas. No one team member "owns" a particular developmental domain. The D-Specs enables each team member to contribute judgments in all functional areas.

Step 2: Determine Team Consensus. Convene the team to discuss the child's status and service delivery/therapy needs. Use a natural give-and-take style of negotiation. This style encourages the parent, paraprofessionals, and professionals to present their judgments and the reasons for them. The team coordinator helps the team to reconcile discrepancies in perceptions. Then, the coordinator guides the team to establish a consensus rating of the child's status in each developmental domain; this is graphed on the T-Specs.

Step 3: Establish the Level of Service Needed. Using these consensus ratings, the team coordinator completes the T-Specs, which enables the team to cross-reference the team ratings with the therapies and service

COMMUNICATION

RECEPTIVE LANGUAGE

Understanding information as shown in various ways, such as following directions and identifying objects and pictures.

5 Typically understands information, especially speech and gestures, as well as or better than most children of the same age.

4 Usually understands most information expected of a child about the same age.

③ Sometimes comprehends speech and gestures, but shows observable problems in understanding.

2 Only occasionally understands; generally fails to comprehend most speech and gestures.

1 Rarely shows any understanding of surrounding events.

EXPRESSIVE LANGUAGE

Communication of thoughts, feelings, and needs in various ways, including gestures, signs, body positions, sounds, words, and sentences.

5 Typically communicates in a meaningful way as well as or better than most children of the same age.

4 Usually expresses thoughts, feelings, and needs in a meaningful way as well as children of the same age.

3 Sometimes communicates to others in a meaningful way, but shows obvious problems in expression.

② Can communicate only occasionally in a meaningful way; others generally fail to understand what the child thinks, feels, or needs.

1 Almost never communicates meaningfully.

SENSORIMOTOR

HEARING

Usefulness of hearing; skill in activities requiring hearing, such as listening and identifying sounds. (If the child wears a hearing aid, the rating should be based on hearing with the aid.)

⑤ Typically performs tasks involving hearing as well as or better than most same-age children.

4 Shows satisfactory skill in hearing, although minor efforts to aid hearing may be necessary.

3 Shows definite problems or limitations in hearing; requires some help or special arrangements.

2 Requires a hearing aid and special help to learn (for example, gestures, visual cues).

1 Requires continual help and supervision to cope with surroundings; is unresponsive to sound except at extreme levels.

SENSORIMOTOR (cont.)

VISION

Usefulness of vision; skill in activities requiring vision, such as eye-hand coordination and sight recognition. (If the child wears glasses, the rating should be based on his or her vision with the glasses.)

⑤ Typically performs tasks involving vision as well as or better than most same-age children.

4 Shows satisfactory skill in vision, although minor efforts to aid sight may be necessary.

3 Shows definite problems or limitations in vision; requires help or special arrangements.

2 Requires frequent help and alternative ways to see and learn (for example, touching, sound cues).

1 Requires continual help and supervision to cope with surroundings; is unresponsive to light except at extreme levels.

GROSS MOTOR

Skill in moving around (for example, crawling, walking, running, jumping), keeping balance, throwing, and kicking.

⑤ Typically moves around, balances, and shows coordination as well as or better than most same-age children.

4 Usually moves around, balances, and shows coordination, but not as well as most same-age children.

3 Shows some clumsiness and problems in moving around, balancing, and coordinating; requires more help or special arrangements than same-age children.

2 Shows serious problems in moving around, balancing, or coordinating; requires frequent assistance and special devices.

1 Needs continual assistance and special devices to achieve any purposeful movement.

FINE MOTOR

Skill in activities requiring grasping and handling, such as stacking blocks, assembling, pouring, drawing, and writing.

5 Typically grasps and handles objects as well as or better than most same-age children.

④ Usually grasps and handles objects, but not as well as most same-age children.

3 Shows some problems in grasping and handling; requires more help than most same-age children.

2 Shows serious problems in grasping and handling; requires frequent help and special arrangements.

1 Needs continual assistance and special arrangements to grasp and handle objects.

FIGURE 7.1. Example of D-Specs rating scales.

delivery options that are indicated. For example, speech–language services are cross-referenced with the developmental areas of expressive language, receptive language, and basic concepts. Thus, the team can determine if the child's problems warrant a consultation (closer look by the therapist) or whether the child should be placed in therapy immediately.

Step 4: Determine the Needed "Program Intensity" on the P-Specs. After establishing a team consensus and determining extent of individual therapy needs, your team coordinator uses the P-Specs to guide the members in answering questions regarding the type and intensity of programming for your child in such areas as behavior therapy, adaptive arrangements, speech–language therapy, and medical services. Answers to these questions are weighted by scores that reflect the effort, intrusiveness, and restrictiveness of the decision option chosen. Then, an overall Program Intensity Score is calculated to reflect the team's perception about the extent of services that will be needed in this child's individualized program.

Step 5: Repeat SPECS to Monitor Progress. The psychologist on the early intervention team is perhaps in the best position to advocate for economical ways to monitor child progress and program impact. Your team must recognize that progress evaluation is not only best practice but also mandated by federal law. A progress/program evaluation system helps the team to gauge effective and ineffective intervention goals and methods, to inform parents of their child's gains, and to ensure accountability to administrative groups and funding agencies. SPECS is a synchronized or "linked" system in which assessment, intervention, and evaluation are interrelated operations.

You can reconvene the team at regular intervals (e.g., semiannually) to reevaluate the child and the parent(s) or family using the SPECS components. In particular, the P-Specs can be rescored at the end of the year in each of the 10 intervention areas to determine decreases in amount of services needed and thus program intensity. Increases in developmental competence (higher D-Specs levels) correspond to decreases in program intensity (lower P-Specs percentages). When this judgment-based team data is congruent with the child's actual progress on the program's developmental curriculum and norm-based measures, the preschool program will have powerful evidence of learning and behavior change that has generalized across people, settings, and materials. You can document and validate the program's instructional and therapeutic effectiveness.

A Case Vignette of Team Collaboration

Sam is a 24-month-old infant, the younger of two children in the Potter family. Mrs. Potter was induced at 41 weeks and reported a difficult delivery. Sam had a brain hemorrhage at birth and suffers from febrile seizures. Sam is not talking yet and his parents have behavioral concerns.

Their pediatrician referred the family to the county's early intervention provider that serves children from birth to 3 years of age. Mary Shaw, the service coordinator and child development specialist, began to assess Sam's development, using a battery of measures including the Battelle Developmental Inventory (Newborg, 2005) and the Adaptive Behavior Assessment System (Harrison & Oakland, 2003). Once this profile was completed, Ms. Shaw prepared to report the assessment results and her impressions to the other members of the interdisciplinary early intervention team. Ms. Shaw translated her findings, observations, and opinions into D-Specs ratings (see Figure 7.1) and profiled these ratings on the individual rater profile sheet (see Figure 7.2).

Based on direct assessment, observation, and parental interview, she rated Sam as having mild developmental deficits overall. Important variations are evident, however, such as near average sensorimotor skills. Sam's scores are disclosed in Figure 7.2. Significant concerns are apparent in the areas of communication and self regulation. Using these ratings, Ms. Shaw conveys her perceptions of the extent of Sam's deficits and strengths to other team members at the meeting.

At this point, the team decides that other members will complete assessments in various ways before the next meeting. The speech therapist will evaluate Sam's home routine and communication needs. The occupational therapist will assess self-regulatory and sensory issues. The social worker, the team's parent advocate, will visit the Potter home and conduct an interview and observation of Sam in his natural environment. In addition, the parents will provide their insights into Sam's strengths and weaknesses. The results of all their appraisals by a range of formal or informal methods will be translated into the terminology of the D-Specs rating scale. Ms. Shaw encourages all team members to attempt to rate Sam in all areas.

In the next stage, the team meets again to discuss and compare their individual assessments through the common language of the D-Specs rating scale. Figure 7.3 presents the T-Specs team summary form, which contrasts team member ratings. Note the generally high agreement among team members. Major discrepancies are evident only in Mrs. Potter's lower score on self-control but higher ratings of Sam's social skills.

Ms. Shaw, the service coordinator, finally guides the team in negotiating a consensus about Sam's developmental and behavioral capabilities (see Figure 7.4). Note that team consensus ratings are ascertained through discussion and shared perceptions; they are not merely the mathematical average of individual ratings. "Interdisciplinary decisions are more than the sum of thinking of professionals and parents; shared perspectives lead to more accurate observations and evaluations, and more appropriate and thoughtful recommendations" (Healy, Keese, & Smith, 1989, p. 73).

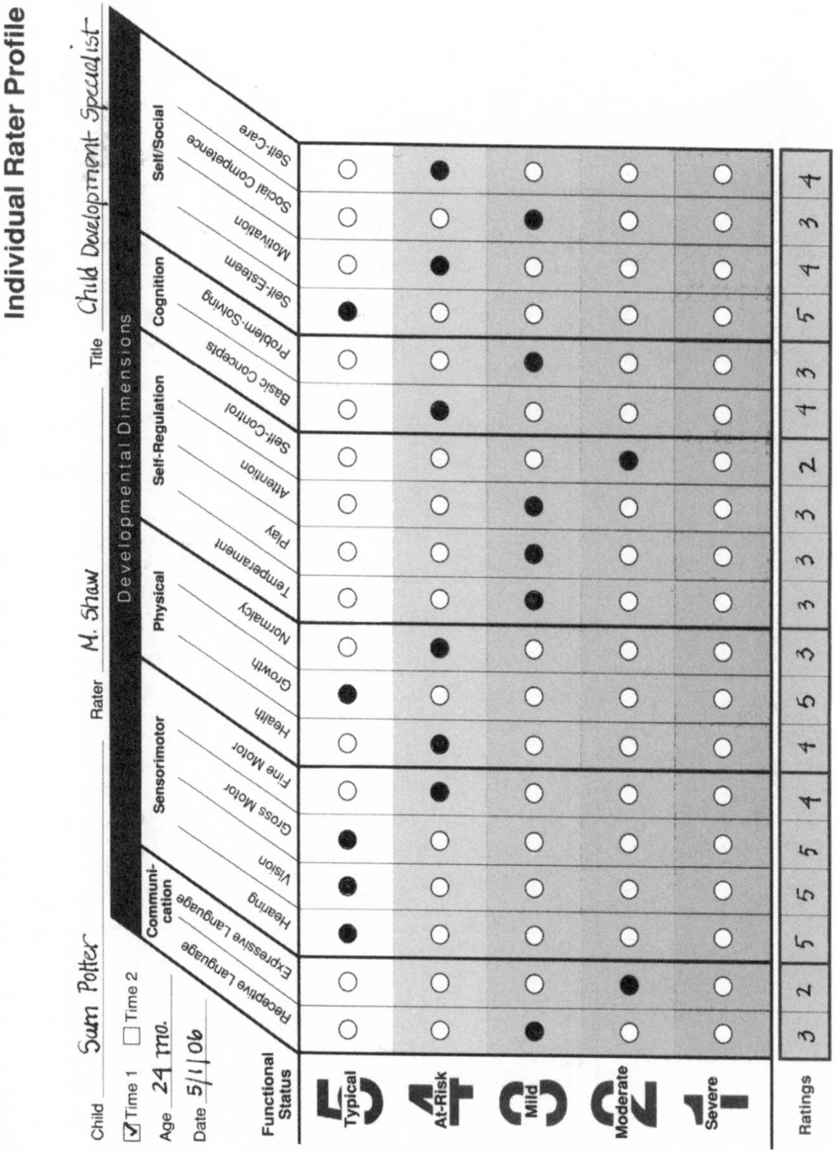

Individual Rater Profile

FIGURE 7.2. Individual rater profile.

Team Summary

Child **Sam Potter**   ☑ Time 1 ☐ Time 2   Age **24 mo.**   Date **5/1/06**

Record each member's ratings, determine the range, and discuss discrepant ratings to reach a consensus.

Team Member	Communication				Sensorimotor			Physical				Self-Regulation			Cognition			Self/Social	
	Receptive Language	Expressive Language	Hearing	Vision	Gross Motor	Fine Motor	Health	Growth	Normalcy	Temperament	Play	Attention	Self-Control	Basic Concepts	Problem-Solving	Self-Esteem	Motivation	Social Competence	Self-Care
Parent	2	1	4	5	5	5	4	5	4	2	4	3	1	4	3	5	5	5	3
Early Childhood Educator																			
Paraprofessional Aide																			
Speech/Language Therapist	2	2	5	5	5	5	5	4	2	3	2	2	3	2	5	4	3	4	
Preschool Program Supervisor																			
Developmental School Psychologist																			
Social Worker	2	2	5	5	5	4	5	3	3	3	2	3	4	3	4	5	4	4	4
Physical Therapist	3	2	5	5	5	4	5	4	3	4	3	2	4	3	5	5	4	4	
Occupational Therapist	3	1	5	5	4	4	5	4	3	3	3	2	4	2	4	4	4	3	
Hearing Specialist																			
Vision Specialist																			
Nurse/Pediatrician																			
Other	3	2	5	5	5	4	5	4	3	3	3	3	4	2	5	4	3	4	
Range (Low to high)	2-3	1-2	4-5	0	4-5	4-5	0	3-4	2-3	3-4	2-3	1-3	3-4	2-3	4-5	4-5	3-5	3-4	
TEAM CONSENSUS*	3	2	5	5	4	4	5	3	3	3	2	4	3	4	4	3	4		

*Transfer these ratings to the Service Matrix below.

FIGURE 7.3. T-Specs team summary form.

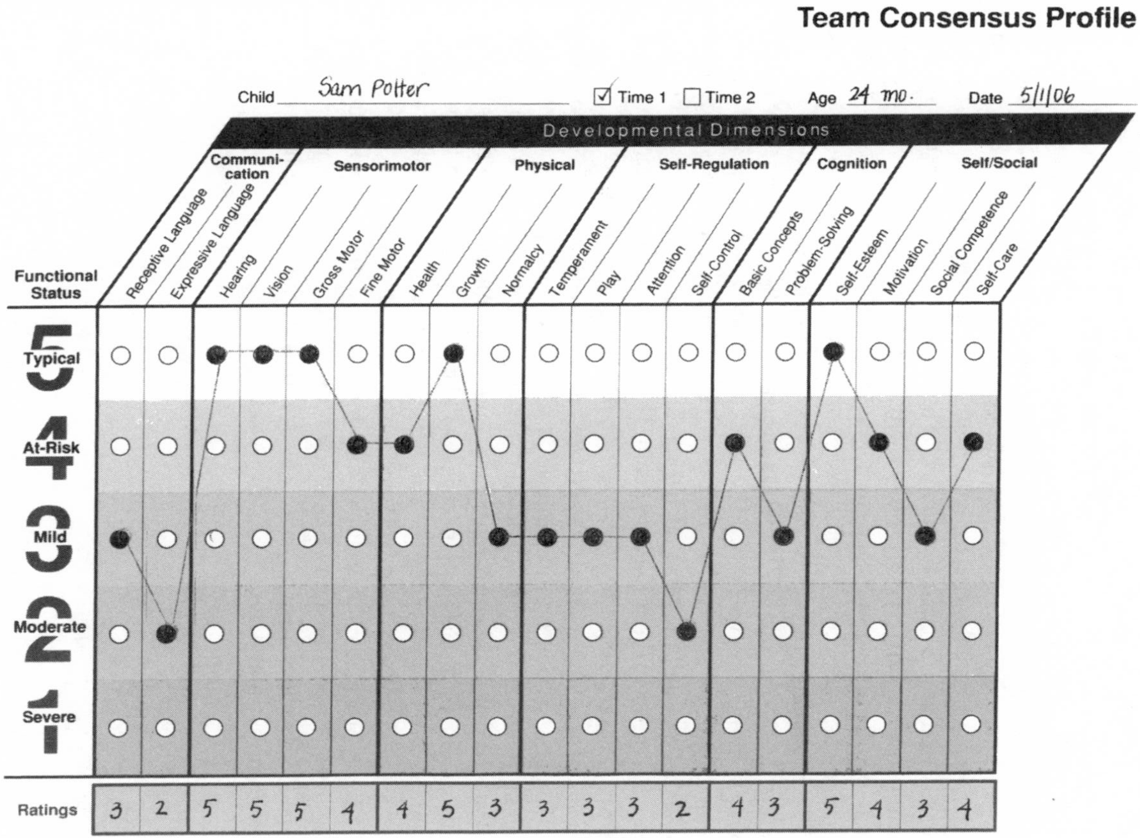

FIGURE 7.4. T-Specs consensus profile.

The T-Specs consensus ratings enable the team to complete the P-Specs service matrix shown in Figure 7.5. In the area of communication, for instance, the sum of the team's ratings indicates that Sam requires direct services to help with receptive and expressive language difficulties.

Finally, the P-Specs pose a series of specific questions that the team completes in each of the 10 intervention/service areas, guided by Ms. Shaw. For example, the moderate level of need in the area of receptive and expressive communication (Figure 7.6) results in the decision to recommend speech therapy to help Sam begin to follow verbal directions and communicate his needs in a positive manner. The team agrees that increasing his communicative capabilities is also likely to result in decreasing problem behaviors. Pictures and basic sign language will be introduced to augment communication. Needs are similarly exposed in the area of behavior. Ms. Shaw graphs these ratings on the P-Specs Program Intensity Ratings Profile (Figure 7.7). Sam requires no vision, hearing, or physical therapy services. Intensity ratings at the 10 to 20% level are observed for early education, occupational therapy, and medical services. Behavior therapy is needed at the 25% level, and the most intense services are required in speech and language therapy, at the 55% level. Sam's IEP will now be written based on the SPECS team assessment and service delivery program results..

It must be emphasized that arriving at a consensus in assessment and deciding on service options and a program plan are jobs that must be accomplished by the team. Some system has to be employed to arrive at and record team consensus regarding child status and program design. It is likely that other models and materials will be developed to meet team needs as interdisciplinary services for children expand. SPECS is a way to standardize, simplify, and speed the necessary decision making.

Team procedures are mandated by federal legislation in early intervention. SPECS complies with Public Law 99-457 in design, content, and use. Table 7.3 provides a summary of the essentials of the law and how SPECS matches those mandates.

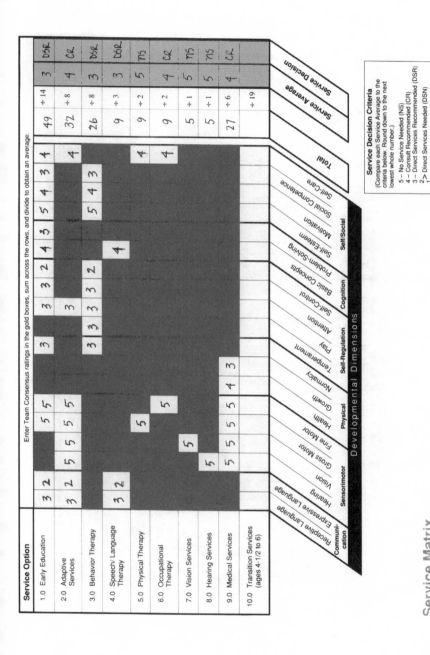

FIGURE 7.5. P-Specs service matrix.

169

4.0 SPEECH/LANGUAGE THERAPY

INTENSITY
RATINGS

Time 1   Time 2

From Team Specs: Service Average _____

Service Decision _____

4.1 What types of communication needs are most notable for this child?
(Check each that applies.)

Time 1   Time 2

☐ ☐ None (0)

☐ ☐ Articulation (1)

☑ ☐ Receptive skills (1)

☑ ☐ Expressive skills (1)

☑ ☐ Pragmatic/social skills (1)

☐ ☐ Voice quality (1)

☐ ☐ Fluency (1)

☐ ☐ Other (1): _____

(Sum values of all
options checked
under 4.1)

4.1 | 3 | |

4.2 What is the best setting for speech/language therapy?

Time 1   Time 2

☐ ☐ Not needed (0)

☐ ☐ Within classroom activities (1)

☐ ☐ Separate small groups (2)

☑ ☐ Individual sessions (3)

4.2 | 3 | |

4.3 How much speech/language therapy is needed?

Time 1   Time 2

☐ ☐ None (0)

☐ ☐ Consultation (1)

☑ ☐ Direct Service sessions per week:

Time 1   Time 2

☐ ☐ One (1)

☑ ☐ Two (2)

☐ ☐ Three (3)

☐ ☐ Four (4)

☐ ☐ Five (5)

4.3 | 2 | |

Briefly describe any additional speech/language therapy concerns or needs.

_____

_____

_____

(Sum scores for
items 4.1–4.3)

4.0 SPEECH/LANGUAGE THERAPY
Intensity Ratings Sum (IRS)

| 8 | |

FIGURE 7.6. P-Specs service intensity example.

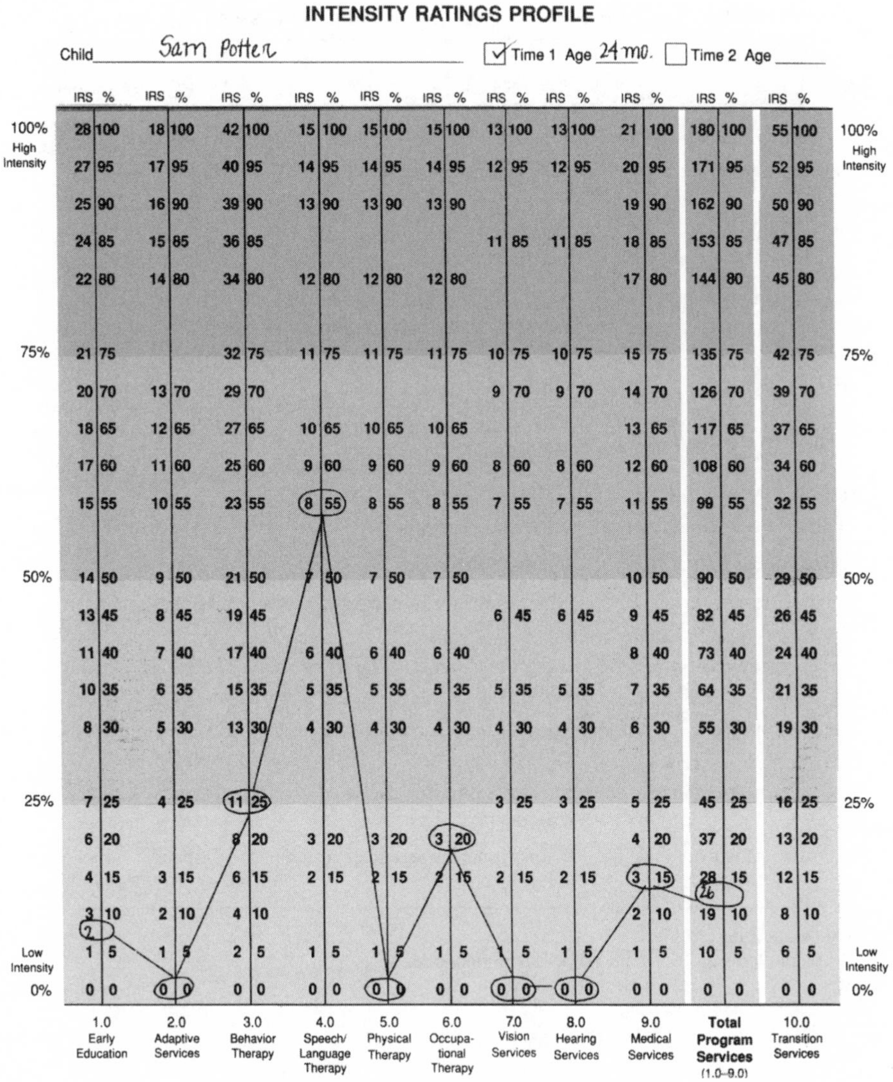

FIGURE 7.7. P-Specs program intensity ratings profile.

TABLE 7.3. SPECS Features Corresponding to Public Law 99-457 Provisions

Public Law 99-457 Mandate	SPECS feature	SPECS component
Noncategorical diagnosis	5-point functional ratings	D-Specs, T-Specs
Developmental delay definitions	Five classification levels	D-Specs[a]
Objective criteria	Operational definitions and scoring	D-Specs, T-Specs, P-Specs
Team evaluation	Team consensus ratings and collaborative program decisions	D-Specs, T-Specs[c], P-Specs
Developmental whole-child focus	Six domains, 19 developmental dimensions	D-Specs, T-Specs
Individual child/family plan	45 instruction and therapy questions	P-Specs
Case management	Case coordination	P-Specs
Explicit service linkages	10 service options	T-Specs, P-Specs
Service delivery intensity	Intensity ratings	P-Specs
Child plan with family focus	Child and family program needs	P-Specs
Parent participation	Integrated parent judgments and goals	D-Specs, T-Specs
Program/progress evaluations	Time 1/time 2, child program monitoring	D-Specs, T-Specs, P-Specs
Interagency coordination	Interdisciplinary case management decisions	T-Specs, P-Specs
Program transitions	Transition competencies and needs	P-Specs[b]

[a]Individual Rater Profile.
[b]Program Options, Transition Services Questionnaire.
[c]Service Matrix, Team Consensus Profile.

BEST-PRACTICE GUIDEPOINTS

♦ Know state regulations for use of clinical judgment in early intervention, especially for eligibility determination.

♦ Recognize that informed clinical opinion is particularly important when standardized measures are inappropriate or unavailable.

♦ Use clinical judgment systems to detect capabilities in children that are inconsistent or low threshold in their expression.

♦ Rely upon clinical judgment systems to unify and facilitate team decisions about child characteristics and specific programmatic and intervention needs.

♦ Emphasize clinical judgment methods to enable parents to be active and integral participants in the assessment process.

♦ Recognize that judgments based on intuition, prior experiences, observations, and anecdotal information occur widely in the field and are unavoidable components of the assessment process.

♦ *Operationally define* the attributes to be judged.

♦ Use *rating formats* to guide and structure how specific attributes are classified by various people.

♦ Select exemplary *clinical judgment scales* to standardize the decision making.

♦ Ensure that individuals providing clinical judgments have undergone *training* in the use of the clinical judgment instrument and decision-making process.

♦ Ensure clinical judgment data is derived from *multiple settings*.

♦ Collect clinical judgment data from *parents and professionals and other caregivers*.

♦ Generate *consensus decision making* via a structured process of resolving differences in clinical judgments and in reaching agreement on child/family needs.

♦ Advocate for the use of the term *informed opinion* as the most communicable terminology regarding the use of judgments in assessment and decision making.

♦ Recognize that both parents and professionals can and do render decisions or judgments based on vital impressions, perceptions, intuitions, recollections, and observations, which are not clinical in nature.

♦ Act upon informed opinions based on personal life factors that are important in themselves in the decision making process in early intervention.

| BEST-PRACTICE EVIDENCE |

Allen, K. E., Holm, V. A., & Schiefelbusch, R. L. (1979). *Early intervention: A team approach*. Baltimore: University Park Press.

Bagnato, S. J. (1984). Team congruence in developmental diagnosis and intervention: Comparing clinical judgment and child performance measures. *School Psychology Review, 13*(1), 7–16.

Bagnato, S. J. (1996). Psychology in education as developmental healthcare: A proposal for fundamental change and survival. In R. Talley, T. Kubiszyn, M. Brassard, & R. J. Short (Eds.), *Making psychology in schools indispensable: Critical issues and emerging perspectives* (pp. 125–128). Washington, DC: American Psychological Association.

Bagnato, S. J. (1999). *Efficacy of collaborative developmental healthcare support in inclusive early childhood programs—Final research report of HealthyCHILD*. Washington, DC: Children's Hospital of Pittsburgh, Early Childhood Partnerships, U.S. Department of Education, Office of Special Education and Rehabilitative Services.

Bagnato, S. J., Blair, K., Slater, J., McNally, R., Matthew, J., & Minzenberg, R. (2004). Developmental healthcare partnerships in inclusive early childhood intervention settings: The HealthyCHILD model. *Infants and Young Children, 17*(4), 301–317.

Bagnato, S. J., Fevola, A., Smith-Jones, J., & Matesa, M. (2004). *The evidence for clinical judgment in early intervention: A research synthesis*. Pittsburgh, PA: TRACE Center, Puckett Institute.

Bagnato, S. J., Fleischer, K. H., Belgredan, J. H., & Ogonosky, A. B. (1990). An overview of judgment-based assessment. *Topics in Early Childhood Special Education, 10*(3), 13–23.

Bagnato, S. J., Minzenberg, B., Blair, K., Silex-Fireman, K., & McNally, R. (2004). Developmental healthcare partnerships in inclusive early childhood settings: The HealthyCHILD model. *Infants and Young Children, 17*(4), 301–317.

Bagnato, S. J., & Neisworth, J. T. (1985a). Assessing young handicapped children: Clinical judgment versus developmental performance scales. *Journal of Partial Hospitalizations, 3*(11), 13–21.

Bagnato, S. J., & Neisworth, J. T. (1985b). Efficacy of interdisciplinary assessment and treatment for infants and preschoolers with congenital and acquired brain injury. *Analysis and Intervention in Developmental Disabilities, 5*(1–2), 107–128.

Bagnato, S. J., & Neisworth, J. T. (1990). *System to Plan Early Childhood Services* (SPECS; Manual for a team assessment/intervention system). Circle Pines, MN: American Guidance Service.

Bagnato, S. J., & Neisworth, J. T. (1991). *Assessment for early intervention: Best practices for professionals*. New York: Guilford Press.

Bagnato, S. J., & Neisworth, J. T. (1999a). Collaboration and teamwork in assessment for early intervention. *Child and Adolescent Psychology Clinics of North America, 8*(2), 347–363.

Bagnato, S. J., & Neisworth, J. T. (1999b). Normative detection of early regulatory disorders and autism: Empirical confirmation of DC:0–3. *Infants and Young Children, 12*(2), 98–106.

Bagnato, S. J., Neisworth, J. T., & McCloskey, G. (1994). *Technical manual for the Sys-*

tem to Plan Early Childhood Services (SPECS). Circle Pines, MN: American Guidance Service.

Bagnato, S. J., Neisworth, J. T., Paget, K. D., & Kovaleski, J. (1987). The developmental school psychologist: Professional profile of an emerging early childhood specialist. *Topics in Early Childhood Special Education, 7*(3), 75–89.

Bagnato, S. J., Neisworth, J. T., Salvia, J., & Hunt, F. (1999). *Temperament and Atypical Behavior Scale (TABS)*. Baltimore: Brookes.

Bailey, D. B., Simeonsson, R. J., Buysse, V., & Smith, T. (1993). Reliability of an index of child characteristics. *Developmental Medicine and Child Neurology, 35*, 806–815.

Benner, P., & Tanner, C. (1987, January). Clinical judgment: How expert nurses use intuition. *American Journal of Nursing, 87*(1), 23–34.

Biro, P., Daulton, D., & Szanton, E. (1991). *Informed clinical opinion* (NECTAC Notes No. 4). Chapel Hill: University of North Carolina, FPG Child Development Institute, National Early Childhood Technical Assistance Center.

Blacher-Dixon, J., & Simeonsson, R. J. (1981). Consistency and correspondence of mothers' and teachers' assessments of young handicapped children. *Journal of the Division for Early Childhood, 3*, 64–71.

Bricker, D. (Ed.). (2002). *Assessment, Evaluation and Programming System for Infants and Children* (2nd ed.). Baltimore: Brookes.

Briggs-Gowen, M. J., & Carter, A. S. (2002). *Brief Infant–Toddler Social and Emotional Assessment (BITSEA) Version 2.0*. New Haven, CT: Yale University.

Casey, B. M., McIntire, D. D., & Leveno, K. J. (2001). The continuing value of the Apgar score for the assessment of newborn infants. *New England Journal of Medicine, 344*(7), 467–471.

Danaher, J., Shackelford, J., & Harbin, G. (2004). Revisiting a comparison of eligibility policies for infant/toddler programs and preschool special education programs. *Topics in Early Childhood Special Education, 24*(2), 59–67.

Davis, M. S., & Squires, J. (2002, December). *Comparing three recently developed social–emotional screening instruments*. Paper presented at the meeting of the Division for Early Childhood (DEC), San Diego, CA.

Dawes, R. M., Faust, D., & Meehl, P. E. (1989). Clinical versus actuarial judgment. *Science, 243*(4899), 1668–1674.

Glascoe, F. P. (1991). Can clinical judgment detect children with speech–language problems? *Pediatrics, 87*(3), 317–322.

Glascoe, F. P., & Dworkin, P. H. (1993). Obstacles to effective developmental surveillance: Errors in clinical reasoning. *Journal of Developmental and Behavioral Pediatrics, 14*(5), 344–349.

Golin, A. K., & Ducanis, A. J. (1981). *The interdisciplinary team*. Rockville, MD: Aspen Publishers.

Goodnow, J. J. (1988). Parents' ideas, actions, and feelings: Models and methods from developmental and social psychology. *Child Development, 59*(2), 286–320.

Gradel, K., Thompson, M. S., & Sheehan, R. (1981). Parental and professional agreement in early childhood assessment. *Topics in Early Childhood Special Education, 1*(2), 31–39.

Greener, D. (1988). Clinical judgment in nurse-midwifery. A review of the research with implications for education. *Journal of Nurse Midwifery, 33*(6), 261–268.

Gresham, F. M., Reschly, D. J., & Carey, M. P. (1987). Teachers as "tests": Classification accuracy and concurrent validation in the identification of learning disabled children. *School Psychology Review, 16*(4), 543–553.

Grove, W. M., Zald, D. H., Lebow, B. S., Snitz, B. E., & Nelson, C. (2000). Clinical versus mechanical prediction: A meta-analysis. *Psychological Assessment, 12*(1), 19–30.

Harrison, P., & Oakland, T. (2003). *Adaptive Behavior Assessment System* (2nd ed.). San Antonio, TX: The Psychological Corporation.

Hayes, A. (1990). The context and future of judgment-based assessment. *Topics in Early Childhood Special Education, 10*(3), 1–12.

Healy, A., Keese, P., & Smith, R (1989). *Early services for children with special needs: Transactions for family support* (2nd ed.). Baltimore: Brookes.

Hemmeter, M. L., Joseph, G. E., Smith, B. J., & Sandall, S. (2001). Program assessment: Improving practices for young children with special needs and their families. In S. Sandall, M. B. McLean, & R. J. Smith (Eds.), *DEC Recommended Practices*. Longmont, CO: Sopris West.

Henderson, E. L., & Meisels, J. S. (1994). Parental involvement in the developmental screening of their young children: A multiple-source perspective. *Journal of Early Intervention, 18*(2), 141–154.

Hresko, W. P., Miquel, S. A., Sherbenou, R. J., & Burton, S. D. (1994). *Developmental Observation Checklist System*. Austin, TX: PRO-ED.

Individuals with Disabilities Education Act, 20 U.S.C. § 1432(5), 1435(a)(1) (1997).

Individuals with Disabilities Education Improvement Act, 20 U.S.C. § 1414(b) (6) (50a) (2004).

Iscoe, I., & Payne, S. (1972). Development of a revised scale for the functional classification of exceptional children. In E. P. Trapp & P. Himelstein (Eds.), *Readings on exceptional children* (pp. 3–29). New York: Appleton-Century-Crofts.

Kochanek, T. T., Kabacoff, R. I., & Lipsitt, L. P. (1990). Early identification of developmentally disabled and at-risk preschool children. *Exceptional Children, 56*(6), 528–538.

Meehl, P. E. (1954). *Clinical versus statistical predictions: A theoretical analysis and review of the evidence*. Minneapolis: University of Minnesota Press.

Meisels, S. J., & Atkins-Burnett, S. (2000). The elements of early childhood assessment. In J. P. Shonkoff & S. Meisels (Eds.), *Handbook of early childhood intervention* (pp. 231–257). Cambridge, UK: Cambridge University Press.

Miller, J. A., Bagnato, S. J., Dunst, C. J., & Mangis, H. (2006). Psychoeducational interventions in pediatric neuropsychiatry. In C. E. Coffey & R. A. Brumback (Eds.), *Textbook of pediatric neuropsychiatry* (2nd ed., pp. 701–714). Washington, DC: American Psychiatric Press.

Neisworth, J. T., & Bagnato, S. J. (2004). The mismeasure of young children: The authentic assessment alternative. *Infants and Young Children, 17*(3), 198–212.

Newborg, J. (2005). *Battelle Developmental Inventory* (2nd ed.). Itasca, IL: Riverside.

Records, N., & Tomblin, B. (1994). Clinical decision making: Describing the decision rules of practicing speech–language pathologists. *Journal of Speech and Hearing Research, 37*(1), 144–156.

Records, N., & Weiss, A. L. (1990). Clinical judgment: An overview. *Journal of Childhood Communication Disorders, 13*(2), 153–165.

Sampers, J., Cooley, G., & Shook, L. (1996). Utilizing clinical judgment in the early identification of premature infants with motor difficulties. *Infant–Toddler Intervention, 6*(2), 117–124.

Sandall, S., McLean, M. E., & Smith, R. J. (2000). *DEC recommended practices in early intervention/early childhood special education.* Longmont, CO: Sopris West.

Shackelford, J. (2002). *Informed clinical opinion* (NECTAC Notes No. 10). Chapel Hill: University of North Carolina, FPG Child Development Institute, National Early Childhood Technical Assistance Center. Available at http://www.nectac.org

Simeonsson, R. J., & Bailey, D. B. (1991). *The ABILITIES Index.* Chapel Hill, NC: Frank Porter Graham Development Center, University of North Carolina.

Simeonsson, R., Bailey, D., Smith, T., & Buysse, V. (1995). Young children with disabilities: Functional assessment by teachers. *Journal of Developmental and Physical Disabilities, 7*(4), 267–284.

Squires, J., Bricker, D., & Twombly, E. (2002). *Ages and Stages Questionnaires: Social–Emotional.* Baltimore: Brookes.

Suen, H., Bagnato, S. J., Lu, C., & Neisworth, J. T. (1993). Measurement of team decision making through generalizability theory. *Journal of Psychoeducational Assessment, 11,* 120–132.

Suen, H. K., Logan, C. R., Neisworth, J. T., & Bagnato, S. J. (1995). Professional congruence: Is it necessary? *Journal of Early Intervention, 19*(3), 243–252.

Suen, H., Logan, C. R., Neisworth, J. T., & Bagnato, S. J. (1996). Parent–professional congruence: Is it necessary? *Journal of Early Intervention, 19*(3), 243–252.

Ysseldyke, J. E., Thurlow, M., Graden, J., Wesson, C., Algozzine, B., & Deno, S. (1983). Generalizations from five years of research on assessment and decision making: The University of Minnesota Institute. *EEQ, 4*(1), 75–93.

Zero to Three. (1994). *Diagnostic classification of mental health and developmental disorders of infancy and early childhood (DC: 0–3).* Washington, DC: Author.

CHAPTER 8

◆ ◆ ◆

How Can We Effectively Assess for Severe Disabilities?

◆

with PAMELA S. WOLFE *and* RICHARD KUBINA

BEST-PRACTICE ISSUES

◆ How are IQ tests inappropriate for young children with severe disabilities?

◆ How do the professional definitions of severe disabilities highlight the need for authentic assessment?

◆ Why are adaptive assessment instruments optimal for both diagnosis and intervention for severe disabilities?

◆ What are the advantages of developmental task analysis in early childhood assessment for severe disabilities?

◆ Are ecological evaluations essential to assessment for severe disabilities?

Janice is a personable girl attending her neighborhood elementary school. At age 5, she is just beginning kindergarten in an inclusive classroom. Before entry into public school, she attended a preschool in a classroom of children with severe disabilities. Janice was identified at birth as having severe medical and cognitive issues. The family physician referred her family to local early intervention services. Subsequent testing by various professionals (including a psychologist, physician, physical therapist, and feeding expert) found that Janice had severe cognitive disabilities;

Pamela S. Wolfe, PhD, is Associate Professor in the Department of Educational and School Psychology, and Special Education, at The Pennsylvania State University.

Richard Kubina, PhD, is Associate Professor in the Department of Educational and School Psychology, and Special Education, at The Pennsylvania State University.

her IQ has been estimated to be 35. Further, she was diagnosed has having poor fine motor skills, but adequate gross motor skills and is able to walk independently. Janice also was found to be prone to grand mal seizures that are only partially controlled by medication. The seizures seem to occur when she is tired or overstimulated by noise or lights.

The speech–language therapist has been working with Janice and her family to identify a communication system as Janice currently communicates through vocalizations. The vocalizations are distinct enough for the family to discern; however, both her parents and teachers want to give her a consistent way to communicate her wants and needs to others in her class and the community. Janice also experiences difficulty with eating. Although her eating issues began at an early age, they appear to have no physiological basis. However, her parents and teachers have noticed that Janice has trouble chewing and swallowing foods of certain textures and often gags or vomits. She is able to feed herself with some assistance but is unable to use the toilet independently. Everyone agrees that Janice has a winning personality and is quick to laugh or smile at peers. After 3 months at her new school, she is still adjusting to the classroom. The teachers have noted that Janice gets frustrated with tasks that are difficult for her and she occasionally vocalizes loudly and becomes noncompliant. Right now, the staff at school has been providing a great deal of assistance to Janice (along with a classroom paraprofessional), but they are working on giving her more independence in the classroom. Her adjustment has been helped by Janice's personality, which has made her popular with several students in the class. Many of her peers are quick to volunteer to be her "peer buddy." However, her parents are concerned that with peers in a helping role, "true friendships" might be hard to establish.

WHO ARE PERSONS WITH SEVERE DISABILITIES?

What might seem an easy question is actually a difficult one. Individuals such as Janice who have severe disabilities are an extremely heterogeneous group presenting a number of strengths and challenges. Such individuals typically have a number of deficits that make learning and community living difficult. Persons who traditionally have been categorized as having a severe disability include those who are severely or profoundly mentally disabled, autistic, or have multiple disabilities (such as a combination of mental and physical disabilities). Obviously the range and variation in disabilities can vary widely, making characterization of the group difficult. A number of definitions have been commonly used with persons having severe disabilities, including the TASH definition and the American Association on Mental Retardation (AAMR) definition. TASH defines severe disabilities as pertaining to

> individuals of all ages who require extensive ongoing support in more than one major life activity in order to participate in integrated community settings

and to enjoy a quality of life that is available to citizens with few or no disabilities. Support may be required for life activities such as mobility, communication, self-care, and learning as necessary for independent living, employment, and self-sufficiency. (Adopted by TASH, December 1985, revised November 1986; reprinted in Meyer, Peck, & Brown, 1991, p. 19)

The AAMR definition is used with persons who have severe cognitive deficits. The most recent definition of mental retardation is as follows:

a disability characterized by significant limitations both in intellectual functioning and in adaptive behavior as expressed in conceptual, social, and practical adaptive skills. This disability originates before age 18. (American Association on Mental Retardation, 2002)

Common to both definitions is an emphasis on a severity of disability that can result in significant limitations in life functioning. Further, both definitions highlight deficits in adaptive skill areas such as communication, learning, mobility, and social interactions. Because of their variety of needs, students with severe disabilities will likely interact with a number of specialists, educators, and other professionals who can assist in implementing assessment and intervention plans.

ASSESSMENT ISSUES RELATED TO YOUNG CHILDREN WITH SEVERE DISABILITIES

Perhaps with no other population is the need for authentic assessment more clearly evidenced than with students having severe disabilities. Given the nature and extent of their disabilities, traditional assessment procedures have been largely unsuccessful for students with severe disabilities. Traditional standardized assessments, such as those designed to ascertain intelligence quotients (IQs), frequently cannot be used with students with severe disabilities because these students are often not able to comply with test administration protocols (e.g., verbally state an answer, provide a written response). Further, few, if any standardized IQ tests include students having severe disabilities in their normative samples (Sigafoos, Cole, & McQuarter, 1987). Because IQ tests often cannot accurately assess intellectual functioning, the information they yield offers little meaningful information related to instructional programming. Functional assessment, or assessment that informs instruction, can provide educators and parents with information related to what and how to teach based on the student's performance in natural environments. Knowing that a child's IQ is 24 tells very little. However, knowing that a child has difficulty with fine motor tasks such as putting on her coat and hat in the morning guides educators in deciding what skills should be addressed at home and in the school.

Before entering the public school system, Janice was given an IQ test by a school psychologist. The score obtained was 35, putting Janice in the category of students with severe cognitive disabilities. However, both the school psychologist and her parents believed that the score obtained really didn't reflect Janice's true strengths and weaknesses. As her kindergarten teacher stated, the score gave no direction for Janice's educational programming and how to plan for the future.

ASSESSMENT STRATEGIES

When initiating assessments for students with severe disabilities, it must be determined who will conduct an assessment, and when and where the assessment will occur. Assessments will yield valid outcomes only if they are conducted in a purposeful manner with a clearly defined outcome.

Who Should Assess Students with Severe Disabilities?

Due to the cognitive, motor, communication, and social skill deficits that many students with severe disabilities display, a number of professionals may be involved in assessment. Physicians may be involved in neurological assessments or for other screening procedures to detect whether a severe disability is present (although it is often detected at birth). Dieticians may be called upon to assess students with feeding or eating issues. Physical and occupational therapists may be involved in assessment of motor difficulties and sensory issues. Speech–language therapists may assess students to determine whether there are communication difficulties and how the child's needs should be addressed. These professionals may conduct ongoing assessment of a child to determine if assistive technology is needed, what vocabulary will be used, and if and when assistive technology should change as the child matures. Within the school system, teachers and school psychologist are likely to be involved in evaluation for the individualized education plan (IEP). Finally, parents will be integrally involved in the assessment of their child. Not only will they work with myriad professionals, parents themselves may conduct formal and informal assessments of their child's functioning. Parental assessment is particularly critical for students with severe disabilities given the need to identify functional skills pertinent to the home and community settings.

When and Where to Assess

When assessment occurs will, of course, depend on why the assessment was initiated. Assessments conducted for diagnosis and placement may occur when the child with severe disabilities is initially referred for services. However, many assessments will be conducted on an ongoing basis to determine how well the student is progressing in various skills and curricula. *Where* assessment will occur also depends on why the assessment was initiated.

Standardized tests may be conducted in carefully structured testing environments. However, given the poor applicability of standardized tests to students with severe disabilities, most authentic assessments will be conducted in the very settings in which the skills should be displayed. For example, feeding difficulties may be assessed at home during mealtime or at school during a snack. Physical therapists may conduct assessments related to gross motor functioning as the student moves about the school or community. Speech–language therapists may assess communication skills when the child is at home playing with a sibling or at preschool during circle time. Parents may assess fine motor skills when their child is getting dressed in the morning by observing how well he or she is able to button a jacket or tie a shoelace. By conducting assessment in natural environments, parents and professionals will be able to determine how well the student will perform where the actual skill will be used. The assessment results can then be used to develop socially valid instructional goals and objectives.

Janice already has interacted with a psychologist for an initial diagnosis. Currently, specialists at a feeding clinic are assessing Janice to determine if any physiological basis exists for her eating difficulties. The staff at the feeding clinic includes a physician, a dietician, and a behavior specialist who are working as a team to identify issues and change her eating habits to include a broader range of textures. Another physician also is working with Janice and her family to determine a pattern in her seizure activity. The physician is tracking the effects of her medication on the seizure activity and has asked the family to systematically observe what occurs before and after each seizure, and how long each seizure lasts. Based on the data, the physician can detail the options available to Janice (which might include surgery or other medications).

How to Assess

How assessment occurs will vary greatly depending on the characteristics of the child and the types of skill(s) that have been targeted. There are several suggested approaches that can be used to collect data for alternate/authentic assessments of student performance (Ysseldyke & Olsen, 1997), including observation, recollection, and record review.

Observation

Observation can include systematic or nonsystematic procedures. In systematic observation, an observer records data on precisely defined (operational) behaviors. The observer can record the frequency, magnitude, or duration of a behavior or complete a checklist of previously identified behaviors. In nonsystematic observations, an observer can record behavior by using an anecdotal record. Other methods of observation can include videotaping and audiotaping. Observations are only as accurate as the observers themselves; systematic observations should include reliability measures of multiple observers. Janice's team is using direct observation in a number of assessment situations. For example, the feeding clinic is videotaping her eating at various meal times. Further, the speech–language therapist is observing Janice in a number of settings (including the home) to see what vocabulary might be needed for a new communication system. Finally, the IEP team has suggested that an extended observation be conducted of Janice in her natural settings to determine why she may be displaying noncompliant behavior. Specifically, the team will be conducting a functional behavior assessment (see Chapter 9) to determine whether her vocalizations and noncompliant behavior serve a purpose for her. If a purpose or function is identified, the team will work on establishing "replacement" behaviors for Janice.

Recollection

Recollection can also be used to collect data on student performance. This can include the use of interviews, surveys, or rating scales in which people who are familiar with the student are asked to recall his or her performance. Janice's team is also using recollection in their assessment strategies. The speech–language pathologist is asking the parents and past teachers to identify vocabulary for her communication system through a structured interview. Also, Janice's teachers have used the AAMR Adaptive Behavior Scale School 2 to identify functional skills that should be included in her IEP. The teachers have asked the parents, as well as past and current school personnel, to complete the checklist of adaptive skills.

Record Review

Another source of data is existing information or record review. This can include school cumulative records, school databases, student products, anecdotal records, and nonschool records. One critical record to review is the IEP. Although it is difficult to aggregate data from IEPs for group analysis (due to variability in how they are written), the IEP provides information from a variety of sources and professionals on student progress. When Janice transitioned from preschool to kindergarten, educators from both settings reviewed past individualized family service plans (IFSPs) to see what goals and objectives might be appropriate to target during her transition. Review of her past records indicated that the family had some respite care issues that the kindergarten staff felt were relevant to discuss with them.

PURPOSES AND METHODS OF ASSESSMENT
FOR YOUNG CHILDREN WITH SEVERE DISABILITIES

There are a number of reasons why an assessment may be initiated, including diagnosis, curriculum or IEP development, and instructional evaluation.

It is important to remember that in many cases assessment is an ongoing process that will continue as the student progresses through life.

Diagnosis and Placement

To receive services within the educational system, children with severe disabilities typically must obtain a diagnosis. Once a diagnosis has been established, the student can begin to receive educational and related services needed including speech–language therapy, occupational and physical therapy, adaptive physical education, and/or therapeutic support services. How diagnosis and placement occur will vary within each school district.

Adaptive Scales

IQ is a standardized measure often used in diagnosis and placement decisions. However, due to the poor applicability of such tests for this population, IQ often yields only a gross approximation of the student's abilities. As supported by both the TASH and AAMR definitions of severe disabilities, emphasis is placed on the use of adaptive skill measures to determine diagnosis and, particularly, placement. Adaptive behavior can be defined as the manner in which individuals adapt themselves to the demands of their physical and social environment (Schmidt & Salvia, 1984). How adaptive a behavior is will depend on the physical environment in which the individual operates, social and cultural expectations, age, and context (Salvia & Ysseldyke, 2004). Adaptive scales typically involve commercially available checklists or scales designed to measure criteria such as self-care skills, community use, or functioning in specific domain areas such as motor or social skills. Further, adaptive scales can be either norm or criterion referenced. Generally, results from adaptive scales can be used to portray a student's overall strengths and weaknesses rather than specific skill attainment. There has been some criticism of the use of adaptive scales, primarily because the concept of adaptation is vague and difficult to measure and scales cannot assess an individual's ability to adapt to changing circumstances (Brown & Snell, 2000). Generally, assessment of adaptive behavior does not require direct observation, but rather the cumulative observations of individuals who know the student well; no formal training is required to administer an adaptive checklist or scale. The scale's usefulness will depend largely on the number of items it includes and the types of items in relation to the person being evaluated. Not all scales are specific enough to be used for instructional planning, but most can be reorganized into life skills categories (e.g., motor, communication, functional academics) and relevant domains (e.g., personal hygiene, safety, eating, and toileting) to aid in programming decisions. Five factors (Cone, 1987) should be considered when using an adaptive behavior scale for instructional programming decisions:

1. The scale should be relevant to different environments.
2. It should have a comprehensive listing of behaviors.
3. It should have items linked to instructional activities.
4. The items and ratings should be specific enough to determine initial programming decisions.
5. The instrument should be helpful in determining the scope sequence, and content of instruction (p. 129).

Table 8.1 contains a listing of adaptive scales that can be used for young children with severe disabilities. Tables 8.2, 8.3, 8.4, and 8.5 list

TABLE 8.1. Adaptive Scales for Use with Children Having Severe Disabilities

Instrument	Author/publisher	Ages	Domain areas assessed
AAMR Adaptive Behavior Scale School 2 (ABS-S2)	Nihira, Leland, & Lambert (1993a, 1993b)	3–21 years	Independent and Responsible Functioning; Physical Development; Language Development; Socialization Behaviors; Personal–Social Responsibility
Adaptive Behavior Inventory (ABI)	Brown & Leigh (1986a, 1986b)	6 years– 18 years, 11 months	Self-Care Skills; Communication Skills; Social Skills; Academic Skills; Occupational Skills
Autism Screening Instrument for Educational Planning, Second Edition (ASIEP-2)	Krug, Arick, & Almond (1993)	Language and social age of 3– 49 months	Sensory Behaviors; Relating; Body and Object Use; Language; Social/Self-Help
Behavior Assessment System for Children (BASC)	Reynolds & Kamphaus (1992)	4–18 years	Adaptive Behaviors; Adjustment to Teachers, Students, and New Situations; Problem Behaviors; Internalizing and Externalizing Behaviors
Checklist of Adaptive Living Skills (CALS)	Morreau & Bruininks (1991)	Infants to adults	Adaptive Behavior; Self-Care; Personal Independence; Social Functioning; Work Community; Residential
Inventory for Client and Agency Planning (ICAP)	Bruininks, Hill, Weatherman, & Woodcock (1986)	Infants to adults	Adaptive Behavior Domains (Motor Skills, Social and Communication Skills, Personal Living Skills, Community Living Skills); Broad Independence; Maladaptive Behavior Indexes (Internalized, Asocial, Externalized, General); Service Level Index
Vineland Adaptive Behavior Scales (VABS)	Sparrow, Balla, & Cicchetti (1984a, 1984b)	3 years– 12 years, 11 months	Communication, Daily Living Skills, Socialization, Motor Skills, Maladaptive Behavior (27 minor and 9 more serious behaviors)

TABLE 8.2. Behavior Scales for Children with Severe Disabilities

Instrument	Author/publisher	Ages	Domain areas assessed
Behavior Evaluation Scale-2 (BES-2)	McCarney & Leigh (1990)	Grades K–12	Learning/Self-Control; Interpersonal/Social; Inappropriate Behavior under Normal Circumstances; Unhappiness/Depression; Physical Symptoms; Fears
Behavior Rating Profile-2 (BRP-2)	Brown & Hammill (1990)	6 years, 6 months– 18 years, 6 months	Emotional, Behavioral, Personal, or Social Adjustment Problems
Child Behavior Checklist and 1991 Profile for Ages 4–18	Achenbach & Edelbrock (1991)	4–18 years	Participation in Extracurricular Activities; Social Interactions; School Functioning; Internalizing Problems; Externalizing Problems; Social Problems; Thought Problems; Attention Problems; Sex Problems
Child Behavior Checklist and 1992 Profile for Ages 2–3	Achenbach & Edelbrock (1992)	2–3 years	Anxious/Withdrawn Behavior; Aggressive Behavior; Destructive Behavior; Sleep Problems; Somatic Problems
Direct Observation Form (DOF)	Achenbach (1986)	5–14 years	On-Task Behaviors; Problem Behaviors (internalizing and externalizing)
Systematic Screening for Behavior Disorders (SSBD)	Walker & Severson (1992)	Grades 1–6	Internal and External Problem Behaviors

TABLE 8.3. Motor Scales for Children with Severe Disabilities

Instrument	Author/publisher	Ages	Domain areas assessed
Bender Visual–Motor Gestalt Test II (BVMGT)	Bender & The American Orthopsychiatric Association, Inc. (2006)	5–11 years (Koppitz, 1975)	Visual–motor skills (9 geometric designs to be copied on paper)
Developmental Test of Visual Perception, Second Edition (DTVP-2)	Hammill, Pearson, & Voress (1993)	4–10 years	Eye–hand coordination, spatial relations, visual–motor speed, etc.

TABLE 8.4. Language Scales for Children with Severe Disabilities

Instrument	Author/publisher	Ages	Domain areas assessed
Comprehensive Assessment of Spoken Language (CASL)	Carrow-Woolfolk (1999a)	3–21 years	Subtests: Comprehension of Basic Concepts; Synonyms; Antonyms; Sentence Completion; Idiomatic Language; Syntax Construction; Paragraph Comprehension of Syntax; Grammatic Morphemes; Sentence Comprehension of Syntax; Grammaticality Judgment; Nonliteral Language Test, Meaning from Context; Inference Test; Ambiguous Sentences Test; Pragmatic Judgment
Comprehensive Receptive and Expressive Vocabulary Test—Second Edition (CREVT-2)	Wallace & Hammill (2002)	Receptive: 4–90 years; Expressive: 5–90 years	Receptive and Expressive Vocabulary
Test for Auditory Comprehension of Language—Third Edition (TACL-3)	Carrow-Woolfolk (1999b)	3 years–9 years, 11 months	Vocabulary; Grammatical Morphemes; Elaborated Phrases and Sentences—pointing, no oral response is required
Test of Language Development, Primary: Third Edition (TOLD-P:3)	Newcomer & Hammill (1999)	4 years–8 years, 11 months	Picture Vocabulary; Relational Vocabulary; Oral Vocabulary; Grammatic Understanding; Word Discrimination; Phonemic Analysis; Word Articulation

TABLE 8.5. Academic Scales for Children with Severe Disabilities

Instrument	Author/publisher	Ages	Domain areas assessed
Cognitive Abilities Scale—Second Edition (CAS/2)	Bradley-Johnson & Johnson (2001)	3–47 months	Infant Form (3–23 months): • Exploration of Objects • Communication with Others • Initiation and Imitation Preschool Form 24–47 months): • Oral Language • Reading • Mathematics • Handwriting • Enabling Behaviors—abilities that aid effective learning
Young Children's Achievement Test (YCAT)	Hresco, Peak, Herron, & Bridges (2000)	Preschool–grade 1	General Information (common and practical concepts); Reading; Mathematics; Writing; Spoken Language

(continued)

TABLE 8.5. (*continued*)

Instrument	Author/publisher	Ages	Domain areas assessed
Complex Scales			
Battelle Developmental Inventory (BDI)	Newborg, Stock, Wnek, et al. (1988)	Birth–8 years	Five domains: • Personal–Social Domain—abilities to engage in meaningful social interaction; abilities to express feelings and emotions; development of self-awareness and self-worth; coping skills • Adaptive Domain—independent functioning and attention; ability to assume responsibility • Motor Domain—muscle control, body coordination, perceptual–motor functioning • Communication Domain—receptive language skills; expression of information, thoughts and ideas • Cognitive Domain—ability to discriminate objects; memory; reasoning and judgment; concept development
Bayley Scales of Infant Development, Second Edition (BSID-ll)	Bayley (1993)	1–42 months	Three subscales: • Mental Scale—memory, problem solving, conceptualization, language, social skills • Motor Scale—fine/gross motor • Behavior Rating Scale—(test-taking behavior) arousal/attention, orientation/engagement, emotional regulation, quality of movement
Denver Developmental Screening Test II (DDST)	Frankenburg, Dodds, et al. (1990)	Birth–6 years	Four general areas: • Personal–Social Development • Fine Motor Development • Gross Motor Development • Language Development
Developmental Indicators for the Assessment of Learning—Third Edition (DIAL-3)	Mandell-Czudnowski & Goldenberg (1990)	3 years–6 years, 11 months	Subtests: Motor; Concepts; Language; Self-Help; Social Development (successful relationships with family and peers)
Developmental Profile ll (DP-ll)	Alpern, Boll, & Shearer (1984)	Birth–9 years, 6 months	Five subscales: • The Physical Scale—39 items that assess gross and fine motor skills • The Self-Help Scale—39 items that assess survival and self-care

(continued)

TABLE 8.5. *(continued)*

Instrument	Author/publisher	Ages	Domain areas assessed
Developmental Profile ll (DP-ll) *(cont.)*			• The Social Scale—39 items that assess "expression of needs and feelings, interactions with others, sense of identity, and adherence to rules and regulations" • The Academic Scale—34 items that assess cognitive functioning (e.g., perception, memory, categorization) • The Communication Scale—38 items that assess verbal and nonverbal expression and language comprehension
Behavior Evaluation Scale (BES)	McCarney (1992)	36–72 months	Academic Progress (performs tasks independently); Social Relationships; Personal Adjustment
Early Screening Inventory—Revised (ESI-R); preschool and kindergarten versions	Meisels, Marsden, Wiske, & Henderson (1997)	ESI-P: birth–4½ years; ESI-K: 4 years, 5 months–6 years	Visual-Motor/Adaptive, • Language and Cognition, • Gross-Motor Skills and Abilities
Infant Mullen Scales of Early Learning (IMSEL)	Mullen (1989)	Birth–36 months	Five subtests: • Gross Motor Base • Visual Receptive Organization • Visual Expressive Organization • Language Receptive Organization • Language Expressive Organization
Kaufman Assessment Battery for Children (K-ABC)	Kaufman & Kaufman (1983)	2 years, 5 months–12 years, 5 months	Designed to assess the way children process information and the amount of information they have obtained, compared with others of similar age and background. Subscales: Sequential Processing Scale; Simultaneous Processing Scale; Achievement Scale; Nonverbal Scale
Mullen Scales of Early Learning (MSEL)	Mullen (1995)	21–63 months	Four subtests: • Visual Receptive Organization • Visual Expressive Organization • Language Receptive Organization • Language Expressive Organization

(continued)

TABLE 8.5. (*continued*)

Instrument	Author/publisher	Ages	Domain areas assessed
Preschool Evaluation Scale (PES)	McCarney (1992b)	Birth–35 months; 36–72 months	Domains: • Large Muscle • Small Muscle • Cognitive Thinking • Expressive Language • Social/Emotional • Self-Help Skills
Pyramid Scales	Cone (1984)	Birth–adult	Sensory (Tactile Responsiveness, Auditory Responsiveness, Visual Responsiveness); Primary (Gross Motor, Eating, Fine Motor, Toileting, Dressing, Social Interaction, Washing–Grooming, Receptive Language, Expressive Language); Secondary (Recreation–Leisure, Writing, Domestic Behavior, Reading, Vocational, Time, Numbers, Money)
Scales of Independent Behavior—Revised (SIB-R)	Bruininks, Woodcock, Weatherman, & Hill (1996)	Infants–90 years	Fine and Gross Motor Skills; Social Interaction; Language Comprehension and Expression; Personal Living Skills; Self-Care Skills; Community Living Skills
Teacher's Report Form and 1991 Profile for Ages 5–18	Achenbach (1991b)	5–18 years	Academic Performance; Adaptive Characteristics; Problem Behaviors
Work Sampling System (WSS)	Meisels, Jablon, Marsden, Dichtelmiller, Dorfman, & Steele (1994)	Preschool–grade 5	Components: Developmental Guidelines; Developmental Checklist; Portfolios—data collected about: Personal and Social Adjustment; Language and Literacy; Mathematical Thinking; Scientific Thinking; Social Studies; Arts; Physical Development

adaptive scales that can be used in domain areas such as behavior, motor, language/communication, and academics, respectively.

CURRICULUM/IEP DEVELOPMENT

Assessment also can occur on an ongoing basis to guide instruction. One critical outcome of such assessment is the development of the IEP. The IEP serves to outline what goals and objectives will be targeted for instruction, and how such instruction will occur. It must be carefully developed to reflect meaningful goals for the student with severe disabilities in a variety of domain areas. Educators must also use assessment to determine how effectively a student is moving through instructional content. Instructional content can be informally determined or guided by the use of a published curriculum.

Curriculum-Based Assessment

Curriculum-based assessment (CBA) measures can be used to determine a student's current abilities, identify instructional goals, and track academic progress. Most curricula include a scope and sequence of skills that are appropriate for students at a given age. Curriculum based measures share three features: (1) proficiency is sampled from materials found in the student's curriculum; (2) assessment recurs over time; and (3) information from the assessment is used to formulate instructional decisions (Tucker, 1987). Some CBA measures for young children with severe disabilities are listed in Table 8.6.

TABLE 8.6. Curriculum-Based Measures for Students with Severe Disabilities

- *Behavioral Characteristics Progression (BCP)* (Office of the Santa Cruz Superintendent of Schools, 1997).

- *Carolina Curriculum for Infants and Toddlers with Special Needs* (Johnson-Martin, Jens, Attermeier, & Hacker, 1991)

- *The Carolina Curriculum for Preschoolers with Special Needs* (Johnson-Martin, Attermeier, & Hacker, 1990)

- *Assessment, Evaluation, and Programming System (AEPS: Measurement for Birth to Three Years* (Bricker, 1992)

- *Early Intervention Developmental Profile* (Schafer, Moersch, Rogers, et al., 1981)

- *Hawaii Early Learning Profile* (Furuno et al., 1984)

- *Syracuse Community-Referenced Curriculum Guide for Students with Moderate and Severe Disabilities* (Ford et al., 1989)

- *Choosing options and accommodations for children (COACH)* (Giangreco, Cloninger, & Iverson, 1993)

- *Callier–Azusa Scale* (Stillman, 1982)

- *Oregon Project for Visually Impaired and Blind Preschool Children* (Anderson et al., 1991)

- *Every Move Counts* (Korsten, Dunn, Foss, & Francke, 1993)

- *Developmental Programming for Infants and Young Children* (DPIYC) *(0–36 months) (Rev. ed.)* (Rogers & D'Eugenio, 1981)

- *Developmental Programming for Infants and Young Children* (DPIYC) *(3–6 years)* (Brown et al., 1981)

Environmental Assessment

Ecological inventories are assessments conducted in the child's natural environment to determine what skills and activities are required for participation. The ecological inventory, which is based on a top-down approach to skill development that focuses on the skills needed in the environment as the source of curriculum content (Brown et al., 1979), is seen by many as the most valid form of assessment for instruction of students with severe disabilities (Orelove & Sobsey, 1996). Ecological inventories are functional and individualized and offer flexible content, but they can be time consuming and determine a large number of needs, making prioritization of skills difficult. To begin an ecological inventory, the team (including parents and professionals) must first identify the environments in which the student operates. For a young child with disabilities this might include the home, community, and school. Next, the team identifies the activities undertaken in each environment. Once the activities have been identified through direct observation, the team determines whether the student has the skills to perform the activities required. The performance of students with disabilities is compared to that of students without disabilities to see if differences exist. If discrepancies are noted, educators then decide how to provide the student with the needed skill by either teaching the skill, teaching an adaptation, or modifying the environment so the student can perform the skill.

How to Conduct an Ecological Inventory

- Identify the appropriate curriculum domain (e.g., self-help, play, community, functional academics).
- Identify the setting/environment.
- Identify the subenvironments within the environment.
- Identify the activities that occur in the subenvironment.
- Determine whether the student has the skills to perform the activities required in the subenvironment.
- Teach the needed skills either by teaching the entire skill, developing an adaptation, or modifying the environment. (Falvey, 1995)

Figure 8.1 presents an example of an ecological inventory developed for Janice that is related to her morning routine. The inventory details what activities and skills are required when Janice first enters the classroom each morning. Janice's team may find that she needs assistance on some of the tasks that require fine motor skills such as hanging up her coat on the hook inside her locker or hanging up her backpack. If there are discrepancies in her performance on these skills, the teacher can decide to teach the skill, make an adaptation (e.g., have her put her coat and backpack on the floor of the locker), or modify the environment (e.g., enlarge or lower the hook in her locker).

Student: Janice   Domain: Community   Subenvironment: Hallway and classroom

Date: 3/15   Environment: School   Teacher: _____

Inventory for person without disabilities		Student inventory[a]	Discrepancy analysis	What-to-do options
Activity: Use locker	*Skills:* Find your locker			
	Open locker			
	Take off backpack			
	Take off coat			
	Hang up coat inside of locker			
	Close locker			
Activity: Enter classroom	*Skills:* Take velcro photo from locker door			
	Carry backpack to classroom			
	Find your classroom			
	Enter classroom and greet teacher			
	Put velcro photo on attendance chart			
	Find your desk			
	Hang up backpack on hook on the desk			
	Sit down at your desk and wait for teacher or assistant to come with daily schedule sheet			

[a]Code: [+] = correct response; [–] = incorrect response.

FIGURE 8.1. Ecological inventory for morning routine.

193

INSTRUCTIONAL EVALUATION

Another type of assessment centers on instructional evaluation, or how well a student is progressing on targeted skills. Task analyses and portfolios often are used to evaluate student progress. Further, assessments to identify reinforcer preferences are used to increase student participation and enhance instruction.

Task Analysis

A cornerstone of instruction of students with severe disabilities is the use of task analyses. A task analysis (TA) is a detailed description of each behavior required to perform a complex behavior (Alberto & Troutman, 1999). A task analysis breaks down specific activities within a cluster of skills. For instance, one could task analyze the specific activities required in a morning arrival routine at school. Specific activities might include entering the classroom, hanging up coat and backpack, washing and drying hands, and going to the designated play area. Task analysis can be used in assessment to illustrate how well a student performs an activity at each step. If the educator determines that the student is unable to perform an activity, he or she is then able to teach the necessary skill. Typically, a task analysis is developed from the results of an ecological inventory. The instructor performs the task and observes peers performing the task in natural settings. Then, the task analysis is developed into a data recording form. The steps of the TA are stated in terms of observable behavior and result in a visible change in the process or chain of behaviors. The steps are listed in the sequence in which they occur and stated so that they serve as the verbal prompt (e.g., wash your hands). Detail that is necessary for the assessment of performance is given in parentheses (e.g., wash your hands (front and back three times with hot water) (Brown & Snell, 2000). Figure 8.2 presents characteristics of a quality task analysis. Obviously the number of steps in the task analysis will vary depending on the task and the student. Some students with severe cognitive disabilities may need steps of a task broken down into the smallest possible components. Figure 8.3 presents a task analysis data recording form for Janice for the skill of putting on a sweater. The task analysis form used in Janice's class illustrates how graphing can be recorded directly on the form itself. In this case, the teacher records Janice's performance according to the key provided on the form. The teacher then consults the criteria specified for Janice to determine what responses are counted as correct. In Figure 8.3, all responses that are coded as independent or verbal prompts are counted as "corrects." The teacher then counts the number of "correct" responses and circles the corresponding number on the TA. Janice has a number of other skills that are broken down in task analyses. Other tasks include her lunchroom routine and a number of lei-

Teacher: _____

Scored by: _____

Characteristics	YES	NO	Comments
1. The target behavior is specified.			
2. Steps are stated in terms of observable behavior.			
3. Given client characteristics, steps are written with adequate detail (not too many or too few behaviors per step).			
4. Each step in the task analysis results in a visible change in the product or process.			
5. Each step states the verbal prompt to be used.			
6. The task analysis is listed on a data sheet with a recording key, date, and space for student's name.			
7. The instructional cue and materials to be used are listed on the data sheet.			
8. Criteria for task completion are stated in terms of percentage or number of steps and/or duration (e.g., within 5 minutes).			
9. Criteria for task completion specify the minimal number of days for which the student must maintain the target accuracy (e.g., 100% correct over 3 consecutive days).			
TOTAL			

FIGURE 8.2. Task analysis checklist. From M. E. Snell (1993). Reprinted by permission of Pearson Education, Inc., Upper Saddle River, NJ.

sure skills. The leisure activities were selected to ensure that Janice is an active participant in games or activities to enhance making friends.

Portfolio Assessment

Another form of authentic assessment used to track instructional progress is a portfolio. Assessment portfolios are a collection of evidence reflecting the development and learning of an individual over time. Originally developed to assess the learning and development of young children, portfolios are now being used with students of all ages and in all subject matters. The use of portfolios also has been used with students having severe disabilities (Kleinert & Kearns, 1999; Kampfer, Horvath, Kleinert, & Kearns, 2001). Portfolios

Student: Janice

Teacher: Mr. B.

Domain/Activity: Motor/Putting on split-front sweater

Criteria: Using system of least prompts, Janice will follow verbal prompts
(or be independent) 85% of the time, in five consecutive trials.

Prerequisites: Knowing directions in space, and some body parts.

Date	3/1	3/2	3/3	3/5	3/6	3/8				
Task Analysis	#1	#2	#3	#4	#5	#6	#7	#8	#9	#10
10. Adjust the waist of the sweater (so it lays flat and is comfortable).	M	M	M	V	V	V				
9. Adjust the neck of the sweater (so it lays flat and is comfortable).	P	M	M	M	(V)	(M)				
8. With your left hand, pull up right arm of sweater to free your right hand.	+	+	+	(+)	+	+				
7. With your right hand, pull up left arm of sweater to free your left hand.	V	V	(V)	+	+	+				
6. Spread your arms so your hands go through the arms of the sweater.	V	(V)	V	V	V	V				
5. Lift up your arms straight up above your head, let sweater flip behind you.	(M)	M	V	V	V	V				
4. Put your hands into the arm openings on each side (so they disappear in the arm).	M	V	V	V	V	V				
3. Find the arm openings close to the neck, on both sides.	V	V	V	V	V	V				
2. Lay sweater on the back side flat on the table in front of you (neck/label facing you).	M	M	M	M	M	V				
1. Look for the label in the neck of your sweater. (This is the back side.)	V	V	V	V	V	V				

Key: I = independent/no prompts; V = verbal prompts; M = model prompts; P = physical prompts.

FIGURE 8.3. Completed task analysis for Janice for putting on a sweater.

should go beyond simply presenting a display of a student's work; they are intended to facilitate judgments about a student's performance—what the student has done and what he or she is capable of doing. The following six elements are commonly highlighted in the literature. Portfolio assessment:

1. Targets valued outcomes for assessment.
2. Uses tasks that mirror work in the real world.
3. Encourages cooperation among learners and between teacher and student.
4. Uses multiple dimensions to evaluate student work.
5. Encourages student reflection.
6. Integrates assessment and instruction (Salvia & Ysselydyke, 2004, p. 256).

Of particular importance for students having severe disabilities is the inclusion of tasks used in real world activities. An example of a portfolio assessment for young children with disabilities is the Work Sampling System (WSS; Marsden, Meisels, Jablon, & Dichtelmiller, 1994). The WSS uses portfolios of students' work samples and developmental checklists to assess children's skills before transition to kindergarten.

Although portfolio assessment is gaining in practice, there are several criticisms of its merit. Concerns center on what to include in the portfolio and how to accurately assess what is included. It is suggested that items included in the portfolio be tied to the individualized goals and objectives of each student as outlined in the IEP. Further, items should be related to the school, district, and state objectives, goals, and benchmarks. Examples of information that could be included in portfolios may encompass:

1. Samples of student written work
2. Photos of work products
3. Anecdotal records
4. Videotapes of students engaged in activities
5. Checklists of adaptive behavior
6. Charts or graphs of progress
7. Schedule of student activities (e.g., weekly schedule)
8. Daily log
9. Incident records (for problem behaviors) (Meisels & Steele, 1991; Meyer & Janney, 1989; Wesson & King, 1996).

Data should be collected a minimum of one to two times per month and can be selected by both the teacher and student.

The second issue related to portfolio assessment is how to accurately assess the contents. Two questions should guide the evaluation of a portfolio: (1) is the student making adequate progress? and (2) if the portfolio is being used as an alternate assessment, is there sufficient evidence that the student is achieving the standards outlined by the school, district, or state? One of the most critical concerns centering on the evaluation of portfolios is how it can be objective (Salvia & Ysselydyke, 2004). Objective evaluation can be improved if educators prespecify what the evidence should look like. Further, two independent observers or judges can score the portfolio to make evaluation less subjective. Various states have undertaken the use of portfolio assessment for students with severe disabilities. Research into the outcomes of such assessment have indicated that although there has been some value in the use of portfolios, the amount of time required to assemble them is a major issue (e.g., teachers said they spent 25–35 hours outside of their instructional day to complete one portfolio). Further, teachers stated that the subjective scoring was of concern, as well as the validity of the portfolio for assessing the effectiveness of a program (Kampfer et al., 2001). Thus, although the use of portfolio assessment holds promise, more work is needed to continue to refine the process for use in assessment. Although portfolio assessment often is valued by parents for its social validity, it may not be dependable for guiding instruction.

Assessing Student Preferences

Educators working with students having severe disabilities also must assess student preferences. Determining preferences and identifying reinforcers for students have been shown to decrease undesirable behavior and increase behaviors desired for task completion (Brown & Snell, 2000). Identification of reinforcing activities and tangibles often is the first step in assessment and instruction. Obviously, one of the easiest ways to determine preferences is to directly ask (interview) students about their likes and dislikes. However, because many students with severe disabilities experience difficulties with communication, assessment of preferences may need to be conducted in ways other than interview. When assessing for preferences, educators and parents need to remember that what is reinforcing for one student may not be for another. Further, the same child's reinforcement preferences may vary from day to day.

One way to assess preferences for young children is to interview individuals who know the child well. To be most effective, interviews should be combined with direct observation methods to identify reliable preferences (Green, Reid, White, Halford, Brittain, & Gardner, 1988). Other methods of assessing preferences include observations of approach/avoidance behavior (which should be operationally defined for each student); observations of forced choice items (e.g., two items are placed before the student to see which the student prefers); and reinforcer sampling (e.g., several items are offered to the student to see which is preferred). Figure 8.4 presents an example of a reinforcer survey that can be used to determine student prefer-

Name: _____ Age: _____

Date: _____

1. The things I like to do after school are _____

_____

2. If I had ten dollars I'd _____

_____

3. My favorite TV programs are _____

_____

4. My favorite game at school is _____

_____

5. My best friends are _____

_____

6. My favorite time of day is _____

_____

7. My favorite toys are _____

_____

8. My favorite record is _____

_____

9. My favorite subject at school is _____

_____

10. I like to read books about _____

_____

11. The places I'd like to go in town are _____

_____

12. My favorite foods are _____

_____

13. My favorite inside activities are _____

_____

14. My favorite outside activities are _____

_____

15. My hobbies are _____

_____

16. My favorite animals are _____

_____

17. The three things I like to do most are _____

_____

FIGURE 8.4. Reinforcer survey form. The reinforcer survey may be given to one student or a group of students. If the students cannot read, the survey is read to them. If they cannot write their answers, the answers are given orally.

ences. Parents, peers, siblings, or others who know the student well can fill out the survey. Figure 8.5 illustrates a form for reinforcer sampling. In this case, reinforcers could be systematically assessed to determine preference.

When Janice first entered preschool, teachers had a difficult time determining what Janice found reinforcing. Her teachers used several techniques to determine reinforcers, including interviewing her parents, observing Janice during free time activities, and conducting a forced-choice sample. All strategies indicated that Janice found peer and teacher attention reinforcing, as well as use of her tape recorder to play music and playing with adaptive toys. Using the identified reinforcers, the teachers were able to create a list of rewards for Janice that could be used across the day. The kindergarten team now working with Janice can refer to the established list but will also conduct their own assessments because they are aware that Janice's preferences will likely change.

PRIORITIZING ASSESSMENT RESULTS FOR STUDENTS WITH SEVERE DISABILITIES

Authentic assessments conducted for students with severe disabilities typically will yield many skills that need to be addressed. How do you decide what skills or activities should be targeted? First, targeted skills should be those skills needed in current and future environments. Further, the skills should be identified as a priority by IEP team members including the family, the students themselves, and school personnel such as the teacher, occupational or physical therapist, or speech–language pathologist. Skills should be chronologically age appropriate and socially valid. If the student has medical or life threatening issues, these too should be addressed, (e.g., learning routines centered on use of a feeding tube or taking medication, or decreasing dangerous behaviors that pose a risk to the students themselves or those around them, such as self-injurious behavior identified through a functional behavior assessment).

SUMMARY

Students such as Janice present a number of challenges that must be addressed across the life span. Undoubtedly Janice and her family will continue to interact with a number of professionals who may initiate various assessments. Like other individuals with severe disabilities, Janice will benefit from assessments that yield functional skills useful in her daily life. Authentic assessment is critical for students such as Janice to assure that skills are functional and derived from "real life" environments. Without authentic assessment, important instructional time may be wasted.

Forced-Choice Reinforcement Selection

Student: _____ Date: _____

Environment: _____ Tester: _____

Latency for Selection: _____

Trials	Items Used	Comments
1		
2		
3		
4		
5		
6		
7		
8		
9		
10		
11		
12		

Summary:

Item	# Times Chosen	Percentage

FIGURE 8.5. Reinforcer sampling form.

BEST-PRACTICE GUIDEPOINTS

♦ Use a functional and adaptive approach to assess the strengths and limitations of children with severe disabilities..

♦ Use alternative authentic assessment strategies instead of IQ tests to meet the requirement of documenting significant deficits in cognitive capabilities.

♦ Rely on both parents working together with specific professionals (e.g., physical therapist, speech–language pathologist) in a natural setting to best assess the child's functional competencies.

♦ Focus the assessment process on identifying functional goals and strategies for intervention.

♦ Emphasize an ecological assessment of the child's and family's environment as the "core" of best practices with severe disabilities.

♦ Implement a process of conducting frequent observational assessments based on sequential curricular competencies to document small increments of change in the child's behavior.

BEST-PRACTICE EVIDENCE

Achenbach, T. M. (1986). *Direct Observation Form (DOF)*. Burlington, VT: University of Vermont, Department of Psychiatry.

Alberto, P. A., & Troutman, A. C. (1999). *Applied behavior analysis for teachers* (5th ed.). Upper Saddle River, NJ: Prentice Hall.

American Association on Mental Retardation. (2002). *Mental retardation: Definition, classification, and systems of supports* (10th ed.). Washington, DC: Author.

Bradley-Johnson, S., & Johnson, M. C. (2001). *Cognitive Abilities Scale* (2nd ed.). Austin, TX: PRO-ED.

Bricker, D. D. (1992). *Assessment, Evaluation, and Programming System (AEPS): Measurement for Birth to Three Years*. Baltimore: Brookes.

Browder, D. M. (1991). *Assessment of individuals with severe disabilities: An applied behavior approach to life skills assessment* (2nd ed.). Baltimore: Brookes.

Brown, F., & Snell, M. E. (2000). Meaningful assessment. In M. E. Snell & F. Brown (Eds.), *Instruction of students with severe disabilities* (5th ed., pp. 67–114). Upper Saddle River, NJ: Merrill.

Brown, L., Branston, M. B., Hamre-Nietypski, S., Pumpian, I., Certo, N., & Gruenewald, L. (1979). A strategy for developing chronological-age-appropriate and functional curricular content for severely handicapped adolescents and young adults. *Journal of Special Education, 13*(1), 81-90.

Brown, L., & Hammill, D. (1990). *Behavior Rating Profile* (2nd ed.). Austin, TX: PRO-ED.

Brown, L., & Leigh, J. (1986a). *Adaptive Behavior Inventory*. Austin, TX: PRO-ED.

Brown, L., & Leigh, J. (1986b). *The Adaptive Behavior Inventory manual*. Austin, TX: PRO-ED.

Brown, S., D'Eugenio, D., Drew, J., Haskin, S., Whiteside Lynch, E., Moersch, M., et al.

(1981). *Developmental Programming for Infants and Young Children (DPIYC): Developmental programming for infants and young children (3–6 years)*. Ann Arbor: University of Michigan Press.

Bruininks, R. H., Hill, B. K., Weatherman, R. F., & Woodcock, R. W. (1986). *Inventory for client and agency planning*. Chicago: Riverside.

Carrow-Woolfolk, E. (1999a). *Comprehensive assessment of spoken language*. Circle Pines, MN: American Guidance Service.

Carrow-Woolfolk, F. (1999b). *Test for auditory comprehension of language—Third edition*. Austin, TX: Pro-Ed.

Cone, J. D. (1987). Intervention planning using adaptive behavior instruments. *Journal of Special Education, 21*(1), 127-148.

Falvey, M. (1995). *Inclusive and heterogeneous schooling: Assessment, curriculum, and instruction*. Baltimore: Brookes.

Ford, A., Schnorr, R., Meyer, L., Davern, L., Black, J., & Dempsey, P. (1989). *The Syracuse Community-Referenced Curriculum Guide for Students with Moderate and Severe Disabilities*. Baltimore: Brookes.

Giangreco, M. F., Cloninger, C. J., & Iverson, V. S. (1993). *Choosing options and accommodations for children: A guide to planning inclusive education*. Baltimore: Brookes.

Green, C. W., Reid, D. H., White, L. K., Halford, R. C., Brittain, D. P., & Gardner, S. M. (1991). A comprehensive evaluation of reinforcer identification processes for persons with profound multiple handicaps. *Journal of Applied Behavior Analysis, 24*(3), 537–552.

Johnson-Martin, N. M., Attermeier, S. M., & Hacker, B. J. (1990). *The Carolina curriculum for preschoolers with special needs*. Baltimore: Brookes.

Johnson-Martin, N. M., Jens, K. G., Attermeier, S. M., & Hacker, B. J. (1991). *The Carolina curriculum for infants and toddlers with special needs* (2nd ed.). Baltimore: Brookes.

Kampfer, S. H., Horvath, L. S., Kleinert, H. L., & Kearns, J. F. (2001). Teachers' perceptions of one state's alternate assessment: Implications for practice and preparation. *Exceptional Children, 67*(3), 361–374.

Kleinert, H. L., & Kearns, J. F. (1999). A validation study of the performance indicators and learner outcomes of Kentucky's alternate assessment for students with significant disabilities. *Journal of the Association for Persons with Severe Handicaps, 24*(2), 100–110.

Korsten, J. E., Dunn, D. D., Foss, T. V., & Francke, M. K. (1993). *Every move counts*. San Antonio, TX: Therapy Skill Builders/Psychological Corporation.

Krug, D. A., Arick, J. R., & Almond, P. A. (1993). *Autism Screening Instrument for Educational Planning* (2nd ed.). Austin, TX: PRO-ED.

Marsden, D. B., Meisels, S. J., Jablon, J. R., & Dichtelmiller, M. L. (1994). *Work Sampling System: Kindergarten development guidelines*. Ann Arbor, MI: Rebus Planning Associates.

McCarney, S. B., & Leigh, J. E. (1990). *Behavior Evaluation Scale—2*. Columbia, MO: Hawthorne Educational Services.

Meisels, S. J., & Steele, D. M. (1991). *The early childhood portfolio collection process*. Ann Arbor: University of Michigan, Center for Human Growth and Development.

Meyer, L. H., & Janney, R. (1989). User friendly measures of meaningful outcomes: Evaluating behavior interventions. *Journal of the Association for Persons with Severe Handicaps, 14*(4), 263–270.

Meyer, L. H., Peck, C. A., & Brown, L. (Eds.). (1991). *Critical issues in the lives of people with severe disabilities.* Baltimore: Brookes.

Morreau, L. E., & Bruininks, R. H. (1991). *Checklist of Adaptive Living Skills.* Chicago: Riverside.

Newborg, J., Stock, J. R., Wrek, L., Guidubaldi, J. G., & Sviricki, J. (1988). *Batelle Developmental Inventory.* Itasca, IL: Riverside.

Nihira, K., Leland, H., & Lambert, N. (1993a). *AAMR Adaptive Behavior Scale—School* (2nd ed.). Austin, TX: PRO-ED.

Nihira, K., Leland, H., & Lambert, N. (1993b). *Examiner's manual, AAMR Adaptive Behavior Scale—Residential and Community* (2nd ed.). Austin, TX: PRO-ED.

Orelove, F. P., & Sobsey, D. (1996). *Educating children with multiple disabilities* (3rd ed.). Baltimore: Brookes.

Parks, S. (1992). *Hawaii Early Learning Profile.* Palo Alto, CA: Office of the Santa Cruz Superintendent of Schools.

Reynolds, C. R., & Kamphaus, R. W. (1992). *Behavior Assessment System for Children.* Circle Pines, MN: American Guidance Service.

Rogers, S. J., & D'Eugenio, D. B. (1981). *Developmental Programming for Infants and Young Children* (DPIYC; Vol. 2). Early intervention developmental profile (EIDP). Ann Arbor: University of Michigan Press.

Salvia, J., & Ysseldyke, J. E. (2004). *Assessment in special and inclusive education* (9th ed.). Boston: Houghton Mifflin.

Schmidt, M., & Salvia, J. (1984). Adaptive behavior: A conceptual analysis. *Diagnostique, 9*(2), 117–125.

Sigafoos, J., Cole, D. A., & McQuarter, R. J. (1987). Current practices in the assessment of students with severe handicaps. *Journal of the Association for Persons with Severe handicaps, 12*(4), 264–273.

Snell, M. E., & Brown, F. (2000). *Instruction of students with severe disabilities* (5th ed.). Upper Saddle River, NJ: Merrill.

Sparrow, S., Balla, D., & Cicchetti, D. (1984a). *Vineland Adaptive Behavior Scales: Interview edition, expanded form.* Circle Pines, MN: American Guidance Service.

Sparrow, S., Balla, D., & Cicchetti, D. (1984b). *Vineland Adaptive Behavior Scales: Interview edition, survey form manual.* Circle Pines, MN: American Guidance Service.

Stillman, R. (1986). *The Callier-Azusa Scale: G Edition.* Dallas, TX: Callier Center for Communication Disorders.

Tucker, J. (1987). Curriculum-based assessment is no fad. *Collaborative Educator, 1*(4), 4–10.

Office of the Santa Cruz Superintendent of Schools. (1997). *Behavioral Characteristics Progression (BCP).* Palo Alto, CA: Author.

Walker, H. M., & Severson, H. H. (1992). *Systematic screening for behavior disorders* (2nd ed.). Longmont, CO: Sopris West.

Wesson, C. L., & King, R. P. (1996). Portfolio assessment and special education students. *Teaching Exceptional Children, 28*(2), 44–48.

Westling, D. L., & Fox, L. (2004). Meeting the needs of young children. In D. L. Westling & L. Fox (Eds.), *Teaching students with severe disabilities* (3rd ed., pp. 500–527). Upper Saddle River, NJ: Pearson.

Ysseldyke, J. E., & Olsen, K. (1997). Putting alternate assessment into practice: What to measure and possible sources of data. *Exceptional Children, 65*(2), 175–185.

CHAPTER 9

◆ ◆ ◆

How Can We Do Functional Behavioral Assessment with Preschoolers?

◆

with RICHARD KUBINA, PAMELA S. WOLFE,
and DEVENDER R. BANDA

BEST-PRACTICE ISSUES

◆ Do all challenging behaviors require assessment using functional behavior assessment?

◆ Why is it important to determine the cause of early childhood behavior problems?

◆ Do teachers and caregivers need to operationally define such common behaviors as "playing"?

◆ Can parent reports of behavior problems be used in functional behavior assessment?

◆ Are there assessment packages that make direct observation of behavior less time consuming?

An exasperated teacher confides in a colleague, "Every time I tell Mandy to play with friends she starts to cry. The more I encourage her to play the louder she cries. I have tried everything! Mandy probably misses

Devender R. Banda, PhD, is Assistant Professor of Special Education in the Department of Educational Psychology and Leadership at Texas Tech University.

her mom but she needs to learn to make friends and play. What should I do?" The teacher's colleague responds with empathy and concern, "You might want to try a play buddy, that worked well with Sharon. Or you could try to give her a sticker for playing with a friend. Once Mandy gets used to school she will probably outgrow this phase."

Professionals may deem Mandy's behavior a problem serious enough to warrant a behavior change program. Her apparent refusal to play interferes with her ability to play with others and become more independent. If Mandy continues to cry during playtime her teachers will no doubt try different interventions to stop the problem behavior. They may ultimately resort to intrusive or punitive measures after exhausting all of their positive interventions. Without knowing the cause of the behavior, Mandy's teachers select interventions based on their experience and professional knowledge. Such approaches to solving behavior problems can often lead to the wrong intervention. For example, the first time she cried the teacher may have comforted Mandy by giving her hugs and playing a game. The attention could have reinforced Mandy's crying. Teaching her alternative methods to obtain the teacher's attention could replace her crying behavior and also serve as an opportunity to involve Mandy in playtime activities. Analyzing the reason why the behavior occurs before implementing a behavior change program falls under the domain of functional behavioral assessment (FBA).

OVERVIEW OF FUNCTIONAL BEHAVIORAL ASSESSMENT

In the professional literature and in practice, the terms *functional behavioral assessment*, *functional assessment*, and *functional analysis* have appeared as synonyms for one another (O'Neill, 2005). Both functional assessment and FBA can be thought of as umbrella terms referring to a number of strategies acquiring assessment information. The term "functional behavioral assessment" refers to a systematic process of gathering information that helps practitioners determine the cause of a behavior. In regard to outcomes, O'Neill (2005) lists five main objectives:

1. Creating operational definitions detailing the extent of the targeted problem behaviors.
2. Ascertaining events or stimuli that give rise to targeted problem behaviors.
3. Uncovering outcomes or events that may maintain or reinforce targeted problem behaviors.
4. Integrating the assessment information and coming up with summary statements or concise hypotheses.
5. Collecting and synthesizing observational data to verify or refute summary statements or hypotheses.

Each of these outcomes assists the practitioners to collect and interpret data in an orderly and effectively way to "maximize the effectiveness and efficiency of behavioral support" (O'Neill, Horner, Albin, Storey, & Sprague, 1997, p. 3). The FBA outcomes help guide programming and interventions.

Operational Definitions

Operational definitions offer very specific depictions of a behavior (Alberto & Troutman, 2003). For example, "Sally plays with friends" does not specifically describe what qualifies as the target behavior. Operationally defining "playing" may involve specific categories of play, such as playing with "movement toys" versus "reactive toys." Or the play may involve imaginative play with single or multiple peers. Operational definitions describe the topography of the behavior, or what it looks like, as well as the measurable dimensions manifested in its occurrence. These include frequency, rate duration, latency, topography, force, and locus (Alberto & Troutman, 2003).

After identifying the operational definitions of the target behaviors the practitioners then must determine if the behaviors share a relationship (O'Neill, 2005). If the behaviors share effects of punishment or reinforcement, produce a similar function, or are comparable along a dimension, the term *response class* applies (Malott & Trojan-Suarez, 2004). A child who yells in a room full of other children to obtain adult attention demonstrates an example of a response class. Also, the child may hit another child and gain adult attention. Although the two behaviors differ topographically, they both serve the same function. Therefore yelling and hitting may be said to be in the same response class.

Triggers or Antecedents

The determinants of a behavior include events and stimuli that precede a behavior and those events that follow a behavior. In identifying the antecedent occasions for a behavior, the behavior or response itself, and the outcomes of the behavior a practitioner observes a behavioral contingency—a highly predictable pattern of behavior (Malott & Trojan-Suarez, 2004). Specifically, when certain antecedent conditions evoke a behavior a particular outcome immediately follows the behavior. A behavioral contingency is said to have three components or terms: Antecedents, Behaviors, and Consequences (Kazdin, 2001). Through observation and analysis, behavioral contingencies allow practitioners to examine why problem behaviors occur and also to seek socially acceptable alternative behaviors that may serve a similar function in achieving a particular outcome.

As noted above, events or stimuli immediately preceding a behavior are called antecedents (Kazdin, 2001). A teacher tells a child that she must pick up her toy. The demand from the teacher represents an antecedent event. If the antecedent event reliably occurs immediately before a behavior, such as the child tantrum, the practitioners can better understand one of the important relations in the occurrence of a problem behavior. If a temporally contiguous stimulus (i.e., preceding the behavior) shows a high probability of triggering or evoking a behavior the antecedent is called a discriminative stimulus. A discriminative stimulus, technically noted as S^D, receives its evocative power because in the past a behavior occurring in its presence produced reinforcement or punishment (Malott & Trojan-Suarez, 2004). A child turning the crank on a jack-in-the box offers an example of an S^D. The crank on the toy serves as the discriminative stimulus for the behavior of turning the crank because in the past the behavior of turning the crank resulted in producing an effect.

Another set of factors that influence antecedents falls under the class of establishing operations or motivative operations (Michael, 1982, 1988, 1993, 2000). It momentarily changes the effectiveness of a reinforcer. A motivative operation may serve to make a reinforcer more salient and it may also increase the probability of the occurrence of other behaviors associated with the initial behavior. Satiation and deprivation demonstrate the altering effects of two common motivative operations. In the example above, if a child had played with a jack-in-the-box for 10 minutes, presenting another, different jack-in-the-box with an array of new toys may affect the relevance of the S^D. The child may be less likely to turn the crank of the new jack-in-the-box because he has satiated his play behavior with that particular type of toy.

Reinforcement and Punishment

Consequential events that follow a behavior can serve to increase or decrease its probability of occurrence. The technical terms *reinforcement* and *punishment* depict the contingent relationship between a behavior and the subsequent effects of consequences. Positive reinforcement means that a behavior immediately followed by the presentation of a reinforcer will result in an increased probability of the behavior occurring (Kazdin, 2001). Depressing the button on a water fountain produces water. Positive reinforcement predicts that a person's button-pushing behavior will increase in future instances of encountering water fountains (provided the student is thirsty—the motivative operation of water deprivation momentarily alters the effectiveness of the S^D). Negative reinforcement occurs when a behavior is immediately followed by the termination of a negative reinforcer. A child who covers his ears when a sibling cries demonstrates the effects of negative reinforcement. The behavior, covering ears, terminates the negative reinforcer of the loud crying. Both positive and negative reinforcers are defined by their effects on behavior (Kazdin, 2001). Thus, even though an adult may think M&M's serve as a positive reinforcer for a child's behavior, the candies may turn out to have no effect, thus we would not use the term positive reinforcer. Regardless what type of reinforcement contingency is in effect, the effect on the behavior is the same: a future increase in the behavior.

Punishment expresses the relationship between consequences and the resulting decreased probability of occurrence for a behavior. Punishment happens in two forms: Type I, positive or just punishment, and Type II, negative punishment or penalty. The immediate presentation of an aversive condition following a behavior that results in a decreased probability of the behavior is called punishment (Malott & Trojan-Suarez, 2004). A young child who sips Tabasco sauce from a bottle (behavior) will show a decreased probability of her sipping behavior in the future due to the presentation of the aversive condition (strong taste). The sipping from the Tabasco sauce behavior is punished. Penalty, the other form of punishment, is the "immediate, response-contingent removal of a reinforcer resulting in a decreased frequency of that response" (Malott & Trojan-Suarez, 2004, p. 85). A penalty contingency is in effect when a child loses "goody tickets" (e.g., tickets that can be exchanged for "goodies" at the end of the day) immediately following the behavior of calling a peer a mean name.

Summary Statements and Hypotheses

The information obtained during the FBA process should be summarized to create summary statements and behavioral hypotheses (O'Neill, 2005). A summary statement takes into account (1) relevant motivative operations, (2) antecedents, (3) operationally defined behavior(s), and (4) consequences. A diagram, as shown in Figure 9.1, containing the summary of these four pieces of information helps pull together all of the information from the FBA (O'Neill et al., 1997). Several statements may emerge for the same student, indicating that the behavior may have multiple functions (O'Neill, 2005).

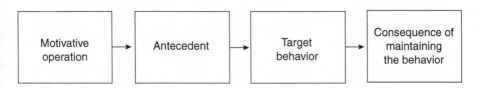

FIGURE 9.1. Diagram showing how a summary statement might be formed. Adapted from O'Neill, Horner, Albin, Storey, and Sprague (1997). Copyright 1997 by Wadsworth. Reprinted with permission of Wadsworth, a division of Thomson Learning: www.thomsonrights.com. Fax 800-730-2215.

Observational Data

The last objective of an FBA may be thought of as "bringing it all together." By gathering observation data the practitioner has the ability to ether confirm or disconfirm the hypotheses made regarding the target behavior. An FBA yields important information that can then be used for developing a robust behavioral intervention to help a child decrease inappropriate behaviors or learn or increase new and adaptive behaviors.

CONDUCTING A FUNCTIONAL
BEHAVIORAL ASSESSMENT

Conducting a functional assessment is similar to conducting other assessments. Information on the target behavior is collected from several sources. A single source of information may not be sufficient to provide meaningful behavioral interventions for children with behavioral problems. In an FBA, teachers and practitioners should gather information from a variety of sources and environments to get the function of a problem behavior. Conducting an FBA is time consuming—it requires trained personnel, facilities, and parental and staff support. Practitioners need to use behavioral strategies such as reinforcement, modification of the environment, and modified instruction. Several methods may be used to conduct an FBA, including informant methods, direct observation, and the use of functional analysis (O'Neill et al., 1997). Each of these is described briefly below, with examples.

Informant Methods

Informant methods are indirect measures that depend heavily on the information provided by parents, peers, and other adults who have knowledge about the child. Family members, teachers, and peer groups can provide significant information about the child's environment and the motivative operations, antecedents, and consequences related to a problem behavior. Informant assessments give practitioners an idea of the settings and environments in which a problem behavior occurs. The most commonly used informant methods are interviews and rating scales.

Interview

Interviews can be structured or unstructured. Structured interviews provide specific information required to obtain the function of problem behavior. Often, practitioners may gather information from parents that is not relevant to the intervention. For instance, knowing the child's birthday and zodiac sign may be interesting, but will not necessarily prove germane to understanding the problem behavior. Structured interviews provide a guide so that pertinent information is collected. A structured interview involves information on a child's daily routines, in schedule of activities, sleeping and eating habits, home and school environments, and on the environments in which the target behavior occurs. It also helps the examiner to focus on information that is required in finding the function of the behavior. The interview, if conducted systematically, should allow the practitioner to gather as much information as possible about the various antecedents and consequences that are maintaining the behavior targeted for intervention.

Functional Analysis Interview Guide

A functional analysis interview (FAI) guide was developed by O'Neill and his colleagues (1997) based on several years of experience with children and families. The structured interview format is designed to help practitioners effectively obtain relevant information from parents, teachers, and other interviewees. The interview format asks questions related to problem behavior that help paint a picture of the following factors:

- Motivative operations
- Antecedents
- Frequency, intensity, and duration of the behavior
- Maintaining consequences
- Possible functions of the behavior

Stated differently, the FAI is geared toward asking questions which generate answers that will help provide detailed information regarding the problem behavior and present a starting point for direct observation. Figure 9.2 is an example, adapted from O'Neill et al., 1997, of a part of the FAI that helps the interviewer begin to gain an understanding of what communicative functions a behavior may have.

Motivational Assessment Scale (MAS)

The Motivational Assessment Scale (MAS) developed by Durand and Crimmons (1991), is a quick measure often used with other functional assessments including interviews and functional analyses. It consists of 16 items grouped into four categories of reinforcement: sensory stimulation, escape, attention, and tangibles. The MAS scale provides a tentative function of the target behavior. It has been found to be a reliable and valid measure when used with other functional assessments, particularly with functional analyses, and can be used by parents and teachers. The MAS has been empirically validated as an informant procedure in functional assess-

Assessed Purpose	Aggression	Self-injury	Facial Expression	Staring/Fixed Gaze	Moves Away	Moves Closer	Increased Movement	Offers Object	Grabs/Reaches	Nods/Shakes Head	Leads	Points	Single Signs	Complex Signs	Attempts Vocalization	Echolalia	Single Word	Multiple-Word Phrases	Complex Speech
								Means of Communication											
Request attention																			
Request help																			
Request preferred item																			
Request preferred activity																			
Request break																			
Show you something																			
Indicate physical pain																			
Indicate confusion or unhappiness																			
Protest or reject situation or activity																			

FIGURE 9.2. Form for hypothesizing possible communicative functions of a behavior. Adapted from O'Neill, Horner, Albin, Storey, and Sprague (1997). Copyright 1997 by Wadsworth. Reprinted with permission of Wadsworth, a division of Thomson Learning: www.thomsonrights.com. Fax 800-730-2215.

ment. However, the function determined by the MAS does not always match with the functions identified by the functional analyses. Therefore the results of the MAS should be regarded with caution.

Direct Observation

Direct observation is the most effective way to collect information about the function of the behavior. Unlike the informant methods, direct observation calls for physically observing a behavior as opposed to relying on conjecture and interviewees' memories and biases. Several techniques for direct observation are available to assess the function of problem behaviors.

ABC (Antecedent–Behavior–Consequence) Recording

An *anecdotal report* is "as complete a description as possible of a student's behavior in a particular setting or during an instructional period" (Alberto & Troutman, 2003, p. 96). Perhaps one of the most common forms of anecdotal reporting is ABC recording. An ABC record collects and structures information for a selected behavior. In ABC recording the observer records all events that occur prior to and after the occurrence of behavior. ABC records examine the relationship between antecedents (events that occur immediately before the behavior), problem behavior (the child's observable behavior), and the consequences that follow the problem behavior (events that occur immediately after the behavior). An example of ABC recording appears in Figure 9.3.

Student: Rachel   Observer: Mrs. Jones

Date: 04/06/2005   Activity: Language Arts with three peers

Time: 10:45 to 11:15 A.M.

Antecedent (What happened before the behavior?)	Behavior (What did the child do? Describe in observable terms.	Consequence (What happened after the behavior?)
Mrs. Burder shows a new word with picture to Rachel: "Say *cup*."	Rachel turns away. Rachel pulls the picture from Mrs. B. Rachel screams. Rachel throws all picture cards. Rachel starts hitting teacher.	Mrs. B: "Rachel, look here." Mrs. B: "Rachel, stop it." Mrs. B: "Don't scream: you are disturbing others." Mrs. B ignores. Mrs. B puts Rachel in time-out.

FIGURE 9.3. Example of an ABC record.

Functional Analyses

In some cases, interviews and direct observation may not provide enough information to determine the functions of behaviors. A functional analysis, often part of an FBA, will supply empirical information that can confirm or disconfirm hypotheses of a behavior's function. The term "functional analysis" means that a practitioner will (1) determine the *function* of a behavior by examining the effects the behavior has on the environment and (2) through *analysis* identify if a causal relationship exists between the behavior and reinforcement (Wacker, Berg, & Harding, 2005).

Young children's learning repertoire is often limited, and it is likely that one behavior might serve several purposes (e.g., Nathan may cry to get attention and also to escape a reading activity). Also, behavioral functions may change from time to time (e.g., Randy will throw an object to avoid a task and later throw objects to gain attention). Therefore, systematically manipulating various environmental events is necessary. The most common way of systematically manipulating the environment is to conduct *analogue* sessions. Each analogue session would have a condition that puts the child in a different situation and the practitioner would carefully observe how the behavior changes. Free play, solitary play, responding to a directive, requesting and seeking attention represent the most common analogue conditions (Wacker, Berg, & Harding, 2005).

Functional analyses with analogue sessions are the most efficient and effective ways to determine the function of a behavior. In the functional analysis either antecedents or consequences are systematically manipulated to see the potential effects of the manipulations on target behavior. Functional analyses require time and staff support, but they may be the only appropriate method for determining the function of some behavioral problems. They are more accurate than any other form of assessment (i.e., informant methods, direct observation methods) because they are the only method that clearly demonstrates a relation between environmental events and challenging behaviors. Although all behaviors do not necessarily require a functional analysis, for situations where they are appropriate practitioners can feel reasonably confident that the resulting evidence surrounding behavioral functions is accurate.

Functional assessment is particularly useful when the function (such as the wish for escape, attention, tangible item, or sensory input) maintaining the child's behavior isn't clearly defined. For example, suppose a child displays stereotypical behavior whenever tasks are presented and when attention is not provided. There may be two or more functions involved in the behavior. A practitioner can determine the function of the behavior by presenting one condition and withholding or controlling the other conditions. First, to determine whether escape, attention, or sensory function is controlling the behavior, a practitioner sets up an environment where no attention is given (attention condition) and observes the effect on the stereotypical behavior. In the second condition, the practitioner presents several tasks to the child (demand condition) and observes the effects of the behavior. In the third condition, the child is left alone (alone condition) for a determined period of time and the stereotypical behavior is recorded. If the stereotypical behavior is high during the attention condition, the practitioner can assume that attention is maintaining the behavior. If the stereotypical behavior is high during the escape, the practitioner can assume that escape (i.e., negative reinforcement) is controlling the behavior. When the stereotypical behavior is high during the sensory condition, it may be assumed that the sensory factor is maintaining the behavior. Systematic manipulation during the analogue conditions helps the practitioner empirically validate the function of behavior through presentation and control of antecedents and consequences. An example of functional analysis analogue conditions is also provided in Figure 9.4.

Time	Activity	Mon 04/05	Tue 04/06	Wed 04/07	Thu 04/08	Fri 04/09
9:00–9:40	Music					
9:50–10:30	Language					
10:40–11:20	Reading		■	■		■
11:30–12:20	Lunch					
12:30–1:10	English	■			■	
1:20–2:00	Math concepts			■		
2:10–2:50	Recess					
3:00–3:30	Speech session					

Student: Jacob   Behavior: <u>Pulls objects from others</u>

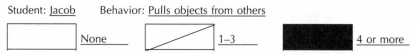

None   1–3   4 or more

FIGURE 9.4. Example of analogue conditions in a functional analysis.

Scatterplot

Touchette, McDonald, and Lager (1985) developed scatterplots to record when problem behaviors occur in time. A scatterplot is a chart where an observer records an event or series of events that take place during specified periods of time. A scatterplot provides a visual record of target behaviors across various time intervals and settings. Data from the scatterplot show the temporal relationship between time period and the behavior. In the example of a blank scatterplot provided in Figure 9.5, the black squares show when the problem behavior most frequently takes place: it emerges during the time periods for reading, English, and math concepts. The scatterplot signals that something during those periods might be associated with the problem behavior, telling the observer to closely examine these periods. Conversely, information regarding when the behavior is not happening may also yield important information as to the function of the behavior. Although a scatterplot does offer compelling clues as to a behavior's purpose, the association of the behavior with a specified time period does not provide causal evidence and should therefore be viewed as a part of a body of accumulating evidence, not as the sole evidence.

CONCLUSION

An FBA can take a number of forms. Informant methods foster a beginning understanding of a behavior's function. Observational methods bring the behavior under closer scrutiny and generate more confidence regarding its function. And finally, functional analysis produces empirical outcomes that bring the function of the behavior firmly into view. All or some of the

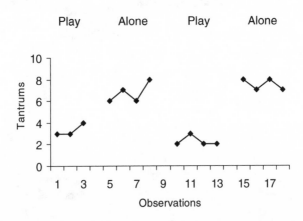

FIGURE 9.5. Example of a completed scatterplot.

investigational methods in an FBA can provide practitioners with effective and efficient procedures for determining the function of a behavior so the next step of behavioral programming can occur.

BEST-PRACTICE GUIDEPOINTS

♦ Challenging behavior (oppositional, stereotypical, self-abuse, etc.) is often amplified and maintained by the child's circumstances.

♦ Behavior, desirable and undesirable, is influenced by its consequences: if the outcome is reinforcing, the behavior will become stronger.

♦ Aspects of the child's setting can become "triggers" that set off undesirable behaviors; they become triggers if they are reliably present when undesirable behaviors are reinforced.

♦ Challenging behaviors have a function; that is, they serve a purpose for the child.

♦ Research has helped us classify four main functions of challenging behavior: gaining attention, accessing tangible reinforcers, escaping from demands, and sensory self-stimulation.

♦ Behaviors may be quite different but serve the same function; different maladaptive behaviors (e.g., screaming, hitting, crying) may lead to the same outcome (e.g., release from an instructional demand).

♦ Functional behavior assessment (FBA) procedures allow us to identify the triggers and consequences that support challenging behavior.

♦ Interview methods may be initially helpful in identifying suspect triggers and consequences; direct observation helps to further determine the responsible antecedents (triggers) and consequences.

♦ Conducting an analogue session, where variables are manipulated, is clearly the best procedure for finding the function(s) of the behavior.

♦ The goal of an FBA is to find the function of the unwanted behavior so that a *developmentally appropriate alternative* can be taught: a socially acceptable behavior that serves the same function or purpose for the child.

BEST-PRACTICE EVIDENCE

Achenbach, T. M. (1991b). *Teacher's Report Form and 1991 Profile for Ages 5–18.* Burlington: University of Vermont.

Achenbach, T. M., & Edelbrock, C. (1991). *Manual for Child Behavior Checklist and Revised Child Behavior Profile, Ages 4–18.* Burlington: University of Vermont.

Achenbach, T. M., & Edelbrock, C. (1992). *Manual for Child Behavior Checklist and Revised Child Behavior Profile, Ages 2–3.* Burlington: University of Vermont.

Alberto, P. A., & Troutman, A. C. (2003). *Applied behavior analysis for teachers* (6th ed.). Upper Saddle River, NJ: Merrill.

Alpern, G. D., Boll, T. J., & Shearer, M. S. (1984). *Developmental Profile II*. Los Angeles: Western Psychological Services.

Anderson, S., Boigon, S., & Davis, K. (1991). Self-help teaching activities. In S. Anderson, V. Simmons, D. Brown, J. Methvin, S. Boigon, & K. Davis (Eds.), *Oregon project for visually impaired and blind preschool children*. Medford, OR: Jackson Education Service District.

Bayley, N. (1993). *Bayley Scales of Infant development* (2nd ed.). San Antonio, TX: The Psychological Corporation.

Bender, L., & the American Orthopsychiatric Association. (2006). *Bender Visual–Motor Gestalt Test (Bender Gestalt II), second edition*. Upper Saddle River, NJ: Pearson Education.

Bruininks, R. H., Woodcock, R. W., Weatherman, R. F., & Hill, B. K. (1996). *Scales of Independent Behavior—Revised*. Itaska, IL: Riverside.

Carrow-Woolfolk, E. (1996). *Test for Auditory Comprehension of Language—Third Edition*. Austin, TX: PRO-ED.

Cone, J. D. (1984). *Pyramid scales*. Austin, TX: PRO-ED.

Frankenburg, W. K. et al. (1990). *Denver Developmental Screening Test, Second Edition*. Denver, CO: Denver Developmental Materials.

Functional behavioral assessment (FBA) worksheet. (n.d.). Retrieved March 18, 2006 from http://www.pattan.k12.pa.us/resources/request.aspx?UniqueID=02661

Functional behavioral assessment (n.d.). Retrieved March 18, 2006 from http://cecp. air.org/fba/default.asp

Furuno, S., O'Reilly, K. A., Hosaka, C. M., Inatsuka, T. T., Allman, T. L., & Zeisloft, B. (1984). *Hawaii Early Learning Profile and Activity Guide*. Palo Alto, CA: VORT Corporation.

Hammill, D., Pearson, N., & Voress, J. (1993). *TPV Developmental Test of Visual Perception*. Austin, TX: PRO-ED.

Hresko, W. P., Peak, P. K., Herron, S. R., & Bridges, D. L. (2000). *Young Children's Achievement Test*. Austin, TX: PRO-ED.

Iwata, B. A., Dorsey, M. F., Slifer, K. J., Bauman, K. E., & Richman, G. S. (1982). Toward a functional analysis of self-injury. *Analysis and Intervention in Developmental Disabilities, 2*(11), 3–20.

Kaufman, A. S., & Kaufman, N. L. (1983). *Kaufman Assessment Battery for Children*. Circle Pines, MN: American Guidance Service.

Kazdin, A. E. (2001). *Behavior modification in applied settings* (6th ed.). Belmont, CA: Wadsworth/Thomson Learning.

Luiselli, J., & Cameron, M. (Eds.). (1998). *Antecedent control: Innovative approaches to behavioral support*. Baltimore: Brookes.

Malott, R. W., & Trojan-Suarez, E. A. (2004). *Principles of behavior* (5th ed.). Upper Saddle River, NJ: Merrill.

Mandell-Czudnowski, C., & Goldenberg, D. (1990). *Developmental Indicators for the Assessment of Learning—Revised*. Circle Pines, MN: American Guidance Service.

McCarney, S. B. (1992a). *Early Childhood Behavior Scale*. Columbia, MO: Hawthorne Educational Services.

McCarney, S. B. (1992b). *Preschool Evaluation Scale*. Columbia, MO: Hawthorne Educational Services.

Meisels, S. J., Jablon, J. R., Marsden, D. B., Dichtelmiller, M. L., Dorfman, A. B., & Steele, D. M. (1994). *Work sampling system*. Ann Arbor, MI: Rebus.

Meisels, S. J., Marsden, D. B., Wiske, M. S., & Henderson, L. W. (1997). *Early Screening Inventory—Revised*. Ann Arbor, MI: Rebus.

Michael, J. (1982). Distinguishing between discriminative and motivational functions of stimuli. *Journal of the Experimental Analysis of Behavior, 37*(1), 149–155.

Michael, J. (1988). Establishing operations and the mand. *Analysis of Verbal Behavior, 6,* 3–9.

Michael, J. (1993). Establishing operations. *Behavior Analyst, 16*(2), 191–206.

Michael, J. (2000). Implications and refinements of the establishing operation concept. *Journal of Applied Behavior Analysis, 33*(4), 401–410.

Mullen, E. (1989). *Infant Mullen Scales of Early Learning*. Cranston, RI: T.O.T.A.L. Child.

Mullen, E. (1995). *Mullen Scales of Early Learning*. Circle Pines, MN: American Guidance Service.

Newcomer, P. L., & Hammill, D. D. (1999). *Test of Language Development—Primary* (3rd ed.). Austin, TX: PRO-ED.

O'Neill, R. E. (2005). Functional behavioral assessment of problem behavior. In G. Sugai & R. Horner (Eds.), *Encyclopedia of behavior modification and cognitive behavior therapy: Vol. 3. Educational applications* (pp. 1322–1329). Thousand Oaks, CA: Sage.

O'Neill, R. E., Horner, R. H., Albin, R. W., Storey, K., & Sprague, J. R. (1997). *Functional assessment and program development for problem behavior: A practical handbook* (2nd ed.). New York: Brooks/Cole.

Reichle, J., & Wacker, D. P. (Eds.). (1993). *Communicative alternatives to challenging behavior*. Baltimore: Brookes.

Repp, A., & Horner, R. (1999). *Functional analysis of problem behavior: From effective assessment to effective support*. Belmont, CA: Wadsworth.

Rogers, S. J., & D'Eugenio, D. B. (1981). *Developmental programming for infants and toddlers: Early intervention developmental profile* (Vol. 2). Ann Arbor: University of Michigan Press.

Schafer, S. D., et al. (1981). *Early Intervention Developmental Profile*. Ann Arbor, MI: University of Michigan Press.

Starin, S. (n.d.). *Functional behavioral assessments: What, why, when, where, and who?* Retrieved March 25, 2006 from http://www.wrightslaw.com/info/discipl.fab. starin.htm

Touchette, P. E., MacDonald, R. F., & Langer, S. M. (1985). A scatter plot for identifying stimulus control of problem behavior. *Journal of Applied Behavior Analysis, 18*(4), 343–351.

Wacker, D. P., Berg, W. K., & Harding, J. W. (2005). Functional analysis. In G. Sugai & R. Horner (Eds.), *Encyclopedia of behavior modification and cognitive behavior therapy: Vol. 3. Educational applications* (pp. 1317–1322). Thousand Oaks, CA: Sage.

Wallace, G., & Hammill, D. D. (2002). *Comprehensive Receptive and Expressive Vocabulary Test* (2nd ed.). Austin, TX: PRO-ED.

CHAPTER 10

♦ ♦ ♦

What Are Proper Approaches to Detect, Classify, and Intervene for Temperament and Self-Regulatory Behavior Problems in Young Children?

♦

BEST-PRACTICE ISSUES

♦ Why should the use of the DSM be discouraged for children below the age of 5?

♦ Why is developmental psychopathology not a developmentally appropriate framework for classifying early childhood behavior problems?

♦ Is temperamental style the most stable predictor of children's social and self-regulatory behavior?

♦ Why should competence in prosocial and self-control behaviors be the target of early detection rather than diagnosis of psychopathology?

♦ Does the increased incidence of serious early childhood behavior problems not signal the need for increased mental health diagnoses?

♦ Why are more intervention-based classification frameworks for behavioral health support needed in early childhood?

♦ Are there authentic measures to guide early detection, classification, and behavioral health supports for young children?

For more than a decade, researchers, policy makers, and agency professionals have decried the increased incidence of serious social behavior problems among young children raised in high-risk environments. Epidemiological research estimates an 18% incidence in extreme behavior problems among high-risk children. Knitzer (2000a) reports an incidence of 25–33% for clinically significant social behavior problems among Head Start children. Consistent research demonstrates that the reason young children "fail" in kindergarten is not primarily the lack of preacademic competency, but rather the lack of basic social skills and self-regulatory behaviors. It is clear that early detection linked with effective behavioral and family support is necessary to help young children and the parents and professionals who care for them in early childhood settings.

BEST PRACTICES IN EARLY BEHAVIOR DETECTION AND SUPPORT

Various early childhood professional organizations and research centers (i.e., National Association for the Education of Young Children; Division for Early Childhood of the Council for Exceptional Children; Center for the Social–Emotional Foundations of Early Learning) promote developmentally appropriate practices (DAP) for both assessing and intervening to build prosocial and self-control behaviors with preschool children. The following dimensions highlight the major objectives of this DAP approach:

- Use authentic and direct observation methods to describe child behavior in real-life circumstances.
- Describe strengths in child behavior as building blocks to develop more mature skills.
- Use positive behavior support methods to reduce interfering behaviors and foster the acquisition of prosocial competencies.
- Use functional classification systems that enable teams to plan effective behavioral support plans.
- Target the development of the social–emotional prerequisites for early school success: prosocial behaviors with peers and adults, resiliency and coping behaviors, and self-control skills, including waiting, sharing, turn taking, following directions, attention, using words instead of actions, perspective taking, and conflict resolution.
- Practice prevention through a continuum of graduated consultative and intervention supports delivered to teachers, parents, and children on-site and *in vivo*.
- Encourage systems reform to foster linkages among health, education, and human services.

TEMPERAMENT AND SELF-REGULATION: DEVELOPMENTALLY APPROPRIATE AND EVIDENCE-BASED FOUNDATION FOR EARLY DETECTION, CLASSIFICATION, AND INTERVENTION

When young children are well behaved, we ascribe positive attributes to them—curious, inquisitive, impish, happy, attentive, and playful. In contrast, misbehavior results in negative attributions and de facto diagnoses—aggressive, inattentive, hyperactive, defiant, emotionally labile, explosive, odd, and unpredictable. These characterizations obscure the child's positive qualities, reflect the variable tolerance of adults for the "disturbing" behaviors, and function as a self-fulfilling prophecy to encourage the exclusion of children with behavior problems from many early childhood programs. A national study on exclusion and suspension from early childhood programs alludes to many of these consequences (Gilliam & Shahar, 2006).

It is absurd that "oppositional defiant disorder" (ODD) is arguably the most frequently used mental health diagnosis for young children 2–5 years of age. When psychologist colleagues and child psychiatrists refer parents and children to me for ODD, I often state that I am more worried if they *do not* have the "disorder" at these ages. Obviously, the trouble with psychopathological labels for young children is that they are based on an adult-oriented medical, not developmental, model; a medical model presumes that the problem resides within the child and reflects some underlying disease or disorder in "mental" or personality functioning.

In contrast, toddlers and preschoolers are expected normatively to show increasing independence, limit testing, and separation from adults as they grow and develop their skills and abilities. Rather than internal diseases, behavior difficulties in young children are the result of reactions to interactions with peers, adults, and the physical environment. If the environment does not positively support emerging prosocial and self-control competencies then problem behaviors occur; the behaviors reach a level of concern based upon the frequency, duration, and intensity of the actions. Misbehavior in young children is not a mental disease; misbehaviors in young children represent extremes of temperamental styles and differences in acquiring effective self-control behaviors based upon developmental expectancies. Behavioral health (not mental health) in young children results from rewarding and self-perpetuating prosocial and self-regulatory behaviors and nurturing environments.

Temperament has been defined as "biologically rooted individual differences that can be observed longitudinally as early appearing and relatively stable dimensions of behavior" (Bates, 1989, p. 4). Temperament and self-regulation are clearly linked in the process of development: nurturing environments support stable and effective temperaments and self-regulation. Nonsupportive and unhealthy environments disrupt the process of development and result in extremes in temperament and dysfunctions in self-regulation.

Five types of "core" behavioral characteristics have been identified as common and consistent dimensions throughout decades of research on early childhood temperament and behavioral style:

1. Negative reactivity: Fearfulness and distress displayed with new people and situations.
2. Negative reactivity: General irritability and distress when confronting frustrating situations.
3. Positive affectivity: Prosocial emotional behavior expressed with peers and adults and in play with objects.
4. Gross motor activity/energy expense: General "on the go" physical activity level.
5. Attentional persistence: Selective and sustained attention, task orientation, and task engagement.

Similarly, research over the past 20 years has defined the interrelationship between temperament and self-regulatory competencies, especially through the work of Kopp (1982) documenting the five developmental phases of self-regulation in infants, toddlers, and preschoolers through natural observational studies:

1. *Phase 1: Neurophysiological modulation (0–3 months).* Emerging organization of behavior through biological maturation and interaction with the environment resulting in arousal, activation, and regulation of basic functions (sleep; wakefulness; coordinating sucking, swallowing, and feeding; orientation to people and objects; crying)
2. *Phase 2: Sensorimotor modulation (3–9 months).* Emerging "understanding" of the world regarding one's own capability to operate on one's world (cause–effect and means–end behaviors in how toys work, and contingencies between child behavior and adult behavior)
3. *Phase 3: Control (12–18 months).* Emerging social behavior with siblings, peers, and adults; discovering social rules that govern behavior, and the beginnings of self-monitoring (playing by self, parallel play with others, turn taking with adults, responding to "no")
4. *Phase 4: Self-control (24–36 months).* Emerging capability to understand social rules, respond to verbal directives, and to delay behavior (not touching a hot stove, going to bed at a set time each night, not hitting or biting when distressed)
5. *Phase 5: Self-regulation (36–60 months).* Emerging capability to modify behavior based on situational rules (active play on the playground/sitting and paying attention in class)

DeGangi (1991) used Kopp's developmental phases research to organize a similar framework applied to young children with developmental delays and disabilities. This work outlined the developmental consequences of neurobiological conditions and negative environments that occur or co-occur at each of the five stages and interact to produce mild to severe disruptions in self-regulation, or regulatory disorders (e.g., sensory sensitivities, problems expressing emotions, overactive behavior, detachment, underreactive behavior, and state dysregulation).

Thus, temperament and self-regulation are intertwined and synchronized in the developmental course of all young children. Temperament and self-regulation offer a developmentally appropriate and evidence-based "roadmap" for assessment, early detection, and intervention for infants, toddlers, and preschool children with challenges in acquiring prosocial and self-control behaviors.

CLASSIFICATION FOR EXTREMES OF TEMPERAMENT AND PROBLEMS IN SELF-REGULATION

Within the past decade, early childhood researchers, policy makers, practitioners, and parents have combined their efforts to champion early detection and classification frameworks for social behavior problems in young children that are developmentally appropriate, sensible, practical, and aligned with both professional standards and research.

Arguably the best and most useful classification framework that has emerged is the *Diagnostic Classification of Mental Health and Developmental Disorders of Infancy and Early Childhood* (DC: 0–3; Zero to Three, 2005). DC: 0–3 was developed through expert consensus and focus groups based on both clinical experience and subsequent prospective, empirical national research (Bagnato & Neisworth, 1999). The major purposes of DC: 0–3 are:

1. To provide an early behavioral classification framework that is developmentally appropriate and based upon a self-regulatory model.
2. To use early behavioral classification as the gateway to effective early intervention.
3. To implement effective early interventions before early deviations in social and self-regulatory behavior become consolidated into maladaptive patterns that limit development and daily functioning.

Perhaps the most relevant dimension of DC: 0–3 is the "Regulatory Disorders" classification. Regulatory disorders are defined as "difficulties in regulating emotions and behaviors as well as motor abilities in response to sensory stimulation that lead to impairment in development and functioning" (p. 28). The above definition underscores the interrelationships among temperament and self-regulatory processes in development. By combining the DC: 0–3 classification framework and appropriate measures of temperament, early social behavior, and self-regulation, professionals and parents can gather authentic information on children that can simultaneously guide early detection, assessment, and intervention.

Related to early classification is the practical construct of *neurobehavioral phenotypes (NP)*. NP are defined as recurring patterns or clusters of behavioral symptoms (i.e., "markers") that may distinguish certain neurological and genetic syndromes and neurodevelopmental disabilities. Nationwide researchers speculate that neurobehavioral markers of self-regulatory difficulties can be observed in young children with specific neurodevelopmental disorders (e.g., autism spectrum disorder or fragile X syndrome) and can exemplify problems in the development of self-regulation. They may also offer early predictors of later disorders and may be used to distinguish among types of disorders.

However, much research much be conducted to confirm these speculations. Clearly, initial research in this area is supportive. Researchers have examined aggression, social ineptness, and poor social communication in adolescents with fragile X and have begun to explore and define precursors in preschoolers with the syndrome. For young children with autism spectrum disorder, researchers have documented early self-regulatory problems in the lack of imitation, pretend play, joint focus of attention, and social communication as sensitive indicators for the disorder. Conspicuously, attention deficits and hyperactivity are so commonly identified and reported as coexisting in various disorders (e.g., autism spectrum disorder, fragile X syndrome, drug and alcohol exposure, early seizure disorders) that the value of these descriptions for differential diagnoses in young children is suspect.

EVIDENCE-BASED ASSESSMENT OF SELF-REGULATION IN EARLY CHILDHOOD: THE TEMPERAMENT AND ATYPICAL BEHAVIOR SCALE

The Temperament and Atypical Behavior Scale (TABS; Bagnato, Neisworth, Salvia, & Hunt, 1999b) is an authentic observation scale designed to detect the presence of specific problems or "markers" of dysfunctions in self-regulatory behavior, temperament, or behavioral style in typical daily routines. The primary purpose of TABS is to document atypical self-regulatory behavior in order to quickly qualify children for early intervention services, particularly when developmental delays are not assessed but are likely with the continued impact of challenging and/or atypical behaviors on developmental progress. The second major purpose of TABS is to classify the type of regulatory disorder so as to guide intervention planning. TABS is sensitive to improvements during and resulting from individualized intervention.

The TABS system is nationally standardized and normed on a pooled sample (621 typically developing children; 212 children with delays or disabilities) of nearly 1,000 infants, toddlers, and preschoolers from 4 months to 71 months of age. The TABS system is composed of three major products:

1. *TABS Screener*: 15-item scale designed to conduct individual or large-scale surveillance to detect the risk status for regulatory behavior dysfunctions; strong sensitivity and specificity (false negatives = 2.4%; false positives = 14.59%; 83% screening accuracy) data based on the normative sample.

2. *TABS Assessment Scale*: 55-item scale of atypical behavioral indicators divided into a four-factor structure of regulatory disorder types: Detached; Underreactive; Hypersensitive–Active; and Dysregulated; results in normative diagnostic assessment (no-categorical) of a "regulatory disorder" based on standard scores (Temperament and Regulatory Index: mean = 100; SD = 15; Factor scores: T = 50; SD = 10; percentiles). The TABS is completed by both parents and professionals separately or in collaboration and is phrased at a fifth-grade reading level; *it* is scored by a Yes, No, and Needs Help option structure (enables parents and professionals to highlight priorities for social validation and goal-planning purposes).

3. *TABS Assessment and Intervention Manual*: Contains standardization information, normative data, technical studies, and field-validated behavioral strategies for clusters of the 55 related indicators on the TABS to guide intervention planning.

TABS has been endorsed by the American Academy of Pediatrics (AAP) as a preferred screening and assessment instrument for young children (2001). TABS use is supported by strong reliability and validity studies. The TABS factor structure is particularly strong (especially the Detached and Hypersensitive–Active subscales, which can stand alone). TABS prospective research provided national empirical data to confirm the four types of regulatory disorders cited in DC: 0–3. Figure 10.1 displays the Detached subscale of the TABS, illustrated by such items as "seems to be in own world; overly interested in toy or object; stares at lights; overexcited in crowded places."

Table 10.1 shows the TABS means and standard deviations for the typical sample and the atypical sample. The display makes clear that for typically developing children detached, underreactive, and dysregulated behavioral indicators are rare (raw score range = 0.35–0.63). Overall mean

DETACHED	No	Yes	Need Help
1. Consistently upset by changes in schedule	☐	☐	☐
2. Emotions don't match what is going on	☐	☐	☐
3. Seems to look through or past people	☐	☐	☐
4. Resists looking you in the eye	☐	☐	☐
5. Acts like others are not there	☐	☐	☐
6. Hardly ever starts on own to play with others	☐	☐	☐
7. Moods and wants are too hard to figure out	☐	☐	☐
8. Seems to be in "own world"	☐	☐	☐
9. Often stares into space	☐	☐	☐
10. "Tunes out," loses contact with what is going on	☐	☐	☐
11. Plays with toys in strange ways	☐	☐	☐
12. Plays with toys as if confused by how they work	☐	☐	☐
13. Makes strange throat noises	☐	☐	☐
14. Disturbed by too much light, noise, or touching	☐	☐	☐
15. Overexcited in crowded places	☐	☐	☐
16. Stares at lights	☐	☐	☐
17. Overly interested in toy/object	☐	☐	☐
18. Flaps hands over and over	☐	☐	☐
19. Shakes head over and over	☐	☐	☐
20. Wanders around without purpose	☐	☐	☐
Detached Raw Score ⟶		☐	

FIGURE 10.1. Sample TABS Detached factor subscale and items.

TABLE 10.1. TABS Means and Standard Deviations for Typical and Atypical Samples

Factor	Typical[a]	Atypical[b]
Detached	0.63(1.26)	5.02(4.69)
Hypersensitive–Active	1.62(2.13)	5.37(4.83)
Underreactive	0.35(0.85)	2.16(2.67)
Dysregulated	0.35(0.79)	1.29(1.64)
TRI	2.95(3.40)	13.84(9.85)

[a] $n = 621$.
[b] $n = 212$.

for the typical sample is 2.95 (standard score = 100). Nevertheless, Hypersensitive–Active behavioral indicators demonstrate their commonality and frequency in typical child development. This raises questions about the high threshold that must be used to diagnose attention-deficit/hyperactivity disorder in young children and the inappropriate overreliance on this diagnosis by physicians and psychologists when such behaviors are common among young children. In contrast, Table 10.1 demonstrates that the fewest children demonstrate the highest number of these atypical behaviors. Nevertheless, for children with assessed developmental delays and disabilities, atypical behaviors are much more common, with raw scores ranging from 1.29 to 5.02. Overall mean for the atypical sample is 13.84 (standard score = 55). Interdisciplinary professionals can use the TABS cutoff scores for at-risk status and disorder to declare eligibility for early intervention and wrap-around behavioral support services. While TABS promotes a "services without labels" philosophy and best practices, professionals can and have used TABS to support the diagnosis of autism spectrum and other related disorders. TABS has been used in national research studies on autism and fragile X syndrome funded by the National Institutes of Health and foundations.

COMPLEMENTARY AUTHENTIC ASSESSMENT MEASURES OF EARLY CHILDHOOD BEHAVIOR

While the TABS and other similar measures use "atypical markers" as the focus of their assessments in order to facilitate early detection and early intervention, many other complementary authentic measures assess positive developmental "building blocks" for prosocial and self-control behaviors. The most effective and technically adequate of these measures are summarized in Table 10.2.

DEVELOPING A SYSTEM OF EARLY CARE

Currently, an "unsystem" of care exists for young children; there is no unified network that ensures family-friendly and accessible education, medical, and behavioral health services and supports for all children. Even in early care and education, there are different rules, regulations, philosophies, and missions—and, often, token integrations and inconsistent inclusion—among Early Head Start, Head Start, public and private center and family child care, school district prekindergarten, and early intervention programs. Simply, we have no universal access to early care and education in the United States. Services for children and families are based on restrictive eligibility criteria that require psychopathological diagnoses for access to

TABLE 10.2. Complementary Authentic Assessment Measures of Early Social and Self-Control Behavior

Measure	Publisher	Age range	Scoring	Domains (subdomains)	Administration	Reliability
Ages and Stages Questionnaire: Social–Emotional (ASQ-SE) (Squires, Bricker, Twombly, 2001)	Paul H. Brookes	6–60 months	Norm referenced; Provides raw scores to corresponding cutoff scores	Self-regulation, Compliance, Communication, Adaptive functioning, Autonomy (across 8 age intervals)	10–15 minutes	Overall internal consistency .86
Vineland Social–Emotional Early Childhood Scales (SEEC) (Sparrow, Balla, & Cicchetti, 1998)	American Guidance Service	Birth–71 months	Norm-referenced; Gives standard scores, percentile ranks, age equivalents	Communication, Daily Living Skills, Socialization, Motor Skills, Maladaptive Behavior	15–20 minutes	Overall internal consistency .86
Preschool and Kindergarten Behavior Scales (Merrell, 1994)	PRO-ED	3–6 years	Norm-referenced; Provides standard scores, percentiles and risk levels for composite and subscales	Social Skills (cooperation, interaction, independence) Problem Behavior (externalizing, internalizing)	8–12 minutes	Social Skills .88 to .96 Problem Behavior .78 to .97
Social Skills Rating System (Gresham & Elliott, 1991)	American Guidance Service	3–18 years	Norm-referenced; Provides standard scores, and percentile ranks	Social Skills (cooperation, assertion, responsibility, empathy self-control) Problem Behaviors (Externalizing problems, Internalizing problems, Hyperactivity) Academic Competence	25 minutes Multirater (teacher, parent, student forms)	Social Skills .90 Problem Behaviors .84 Academic Competence .95
Temperament Assessment Battery for Children (Martin, 1988)	PRO-ED	3–8 years	Norm-referenced Provides T scores and percentile ranks	Activity, Adaptability, Approach/Withdrawal, Emotional Intensity, Distractibility, Persistence	Parent, Teacher and Clinician forms	.70–.90
ITSEA (Carter & Briggs-Gowan, 2000) and BITSEA (Briggs-Gowan & Carter, 2001)	Harcourt	12–36 months	Normed locally; T scores for 4 domains and 17 subscales, 3 index scores	Externalizing, Internalizing, Dysregulation, Competence	ITSEA 20–30 minutes BITSEA 10 minutes	ITSEA .80 to .90 BITSEA Problem Behavior .82 Competence .72

adult-oriented, office-based services funded through third-party insurance reimbursements and managed Medicaid resources. Services are not preventive but focus on only those young children with the most severe social–emotional problems that meet criteria for severe diagnoses and are less amenable to improvement. Services remain ensconced in state and county agency "silos" and are intractable to much-needed systems reforms and integration.

Perhaps the most optimistic light being shed on this systemic problem derives from the System of Care (SOC) initiatives funded by the Substance Abuse and Mental Health Services Administration (SAMHSA). Nevertheless, while promoting some systems integration, SOC still focuses on children and families with the most severe needs and requires traditional diagnoses for access to services.

True systems reform initiatives have four major distinguishing attributes: emphasis on prevention and early intervention; access, coordination, collaboration, and consistency to integrate the "unsystem"; links among the adult- and child-serving agencies; and a commitment to field validation and evidence-based practices in community settings. The most innovative and groundbreaking systems reform efforts eschew traditional services and sources of funding and are community-based "natural experiments." These local initiatives form a "system of early care" (SOEC) approach.

Ten core principles and practices are common to SOEC initiatives:

1. Early identification of risk status for flexible access to services.
2. Continuum of prevention and intervention supports.
3. Family-centered and culturally competent practices.
4. Community-based, in vivo supports only in home and classroom program settings.
5. Integrated care coordination and multiple points of system entry across various agencies to coordinate and synchronize comprehensive interdisciplinary services.
6. Integrated transagency care plans for both child and family services.
7. Focus on strengths or assets rather than deficits and disorders—building social–emotional and behavioral foundations for resiliency and early school success.
8. Mentoring to foster uniform competencies, credentialing, and use of best practices in early childhood for interdisciplinary professionals.
9. Common computer and Web interfaces across agencies to share client, program, and outcomes data.
10. Ongoing impact and outcomes evaluation for quality improvements.

HEALTHYCHILD: EVIDENCE-BASED SOEC EXAMPLE

HealthyCHILD is a contractual venture with school districts, Head Start, and early intervention programs that was originally funded in its model development and experimental-control group, field-validation phase by the U.S. Department of Education, Office of Special Education and Rehabilitative Services (OSERS) in 1994–1998. The HealthyCHILD model and research outcomes have been described in refereed articles (Bagnato et al., 2004; Bagnato, 1999). The HealthyCHILD model coordinates transagency education, medical, and behavioral health supports through a prevention–intervention continuum for young children who are at developmental risk and who have developmental delays or disabilities and behavioral disorders.

What Is HealthyCHILD?

HealthyCHILD is a partnership among Children's Hospital, the UCLID Center at the University of Pittsburgh, all types of school- and community-based early childhood programs (e.g., Head Start, early intervention, early care and education), and primary care physicians to deliver medical and behavioral health care support to young children (ages 0–8) by providing teachers, caregivers, parents, and administrators with consultation, intervention, mentoring/education, and technical assistance. HealthyCHILD is unique in that it provides on-site consultation and support on-site within the child's classroom, and sometimes in the home. HealthyCHILD specializes in the needs of children with challenging or atypical behaviors, developmental delays or disabilities, and acute and chronic medical concerns (e.g., asthma, seizures, genetic syndromes, diabetes).

What Is the HealthyCHILD Developmental Health Care Team?

The operational feature of the HealthyCHILD model is a mobile team composed of interdisciplinary health care professionals who are both generalists and specialists. The full team is composed of a pediatric nurse, developmental school psychologist, developmental/behavioral health care consultant, an interagency liaison, the child's teacher, the child's parent(s), other team members, and graduate student fellows within the UCLID Center. A developmental pediatrician offers consultation to the team.

What Services Does HealthyCHILD Deliver?

HealthyCHILD services are based on individual child and classroom needs. Services include direct classroom consultation about children, professional development training and mentoring of staff, technical assistance, observational assessment, direct service, diagnosis, referral, and parent–professional team meetings based on program needs assessment.

What Is the Major Focus of HealthyCHILD?

HealthyCHILD supports have four major objectives: (1) promoting children's success in all types of early care and education settings including Head Start, early intervention, early care and education classrooms, and family child care; (2) increasing the skills of teachers and caregivers through both preventive and supportive health care strategies; (3) providing consultative and direct services to children with a range of behavioral health concerns and acute and chronic medical conditions; (4) identifying the impact of the child's health care needs on performance and early learning in the early childhood setting.

What Specific Help Do Teachers, Caregivers, and Parents Get from HealthyCHILD?

- On-site, in vivo training in health care issues in the classroom or home setting.
- Ongoing classroom visits and consultations by developmental consultants regarding changes in classroom climates that will improve child health, development, behavior, and adjustment.
- Modeling of health care strategies for teachers, caregivers, and parents.
- Written Developmental Healthcare Plan of individual goals and strategies to meet the physical and behavioral needs of referred children.
- Written consultation summary report with diagnosis to gain access to behavioral health and mental health wrap-around services.
- Liaisons with primary care physicians.
- Collaborative meetings between parents, agency staff, and school personnel.
- Support at transition meetings to advise on children's entry into kindergarten and first grade.
- Linkages with community resources, various health and human service agencies (e.g., early intervention, wrap-around mental health), and public schools.
- Provision of written resources about developmental health care.

Figure 10.2 presents a schematic of the operational elements of the SOEC plan for HealthyCHILD. The COLT, or Collaborative Leadership

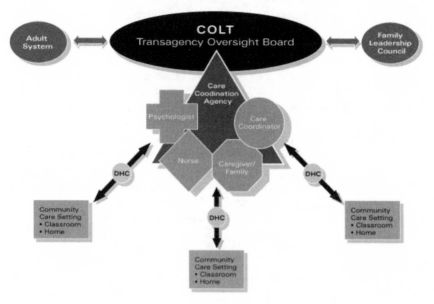

FIGURE 10.2. HealthyCHILD System of Early Care (SOEC) model.

Team, includes representatives from all stakeholders who can make consensus decisions that enable their staff to collaborate in unique ways to meet the needs of children and families. A care coordinator partners with the parents and family to champion the integration of comprehensive services and delivery in local community contexts. The most visible member of the HealthyCHILD team is the developmental health care consultant (DHC), who provides on-site consultation, mentoring, and support to teachers, providers, and parents about prevention strategies for behavioral and medical needs (asthma, universal health precautions, environmental arrangements). Our data show that 80% of problems can be managed using the prevention approach. Individualization is required for 20% of the children's needs; in these instances, various members of the mobile team, notably the nurse and psychologist, with physician consultation, provide intensive supports by writing individualized developmental health care plans and modeling such strategies for caregivers. HealthyCHILD encompasses most of the 10 elements that make up innovative and effective SOEC initiatives. The HealthyCHILD model, strategies, and practices are supported by a decade of evidence-based research.

BEST-PRACTICE GUIDEPOINTS

♦ Learn, understand, and apply the philosophy and principles of services without labels and developmentally appropriate practices when dealing with early problems in self-regulation described in DC: 0–3.

♦ Engage parents and professionals in collaborating and contributing observations and informed judgments about children's social and self-regulatory behavior using TABS and complementary instruments.

♦ Use TABS to qualify children for early intervention services and supports as well as behavioral support through wrap-around services.

♦ Resist efforts to apply psychopathological labels to infants, toddlers, and preschoolers before documenting their response to intervention.

♦ Use measures designed specifically to document the progressive acquisition of social skill and self-regulatory behaviors by children during participation in early childhood intervention programs.

♦ Partner with cooperating human service agencies and early care and education programs to institute *prevention* programs involving ongoing consultation and support to parents and teachers on-site about ways to build social and self-control behaviors in children.

BEST-PRACTICE EVIDENCE

American Academy of Pediatrics. (2001). Developmental surveillance and screening of infants and young children. *Pediatrics, 108*(1), 194.

Bagnato, S. J. (1996). Psychology in education as developmental healthcare: A proposal for fundamental change and survival. In R. Talley, T. Kubiszyn, M. Brassard, & R. J. Short (Eds.), *Making psychology in schools indispensable: Critical issues and emerging perspectives* (pp. 159–164). Washington, DC: American Psychological Association.

Bagnato, S. J. (1998). Do actions speak louder than words? The case of the disappearance of social communication oddities: A research profile. *Seminars in Speech and Language, 19*(1), 31–39.

Bagnato, S. J. (1998). Book reviews: Diagnostic Classification: 0–3, Diagnostic classification of mental health and developmental disorders of infancy and early childhood. *Journal of Psychoeducational Assessment, 16*(1), 69–71.

Bagnato, S. J. (1999). *Collaborative developmental healthcare support in inclusive early childhood programs: The efficacy and outcomes of the HealthyCHILD model (1994–1998).* Washington, DC: Children's Hospital of Pittsburgh, U.S. Office of Education, Office of Special Education and Rehabilitative Services, and the Jewish Healthcare Foundation.

Bagnato, S. J. (2000). *HealthyCHILD developmental healthcare support in early childhood settings: Final CCRD Report.* Harrisburg, PA: Commonwealth of Pennsylvania, Department of Public Welfare.

Bagnato, S. J. (2003). *System of early care: Building family-centered healthcare partner-*

ships and supports for young children in everyday settings: Position statement, proposed model, and workscope. Pittsburgh, PA: Allegheny County Children's Cabinet, Department of Human Services.

Bagnato, S. J., Blair, K., Slater, J., McNally, R., Matthew, J., & Minzenberg, B. (2004). Developmental healthcare partnerships in inclusive early childhood settings: The HealthyCHILD model. *Infants and Young Children, 17*(4), 301–317.

Bagnato, S. J., Minzenberg, B., Blair, K., Silex-Fireman, K., & McNally, R. (1998). Developmental healthcare partnerships in inclusive early childhood settings: The HealthyCHILD model. *Infants and Young Children, 17*(4), 301–317.

Bagnato, S. J., & Neisworth, J. T. (2000). Normative detection of early regulatory disorders and autism: Empirical confirmation of DC: 0–3. *Infants and Young Children, 12*(2), 98–109.

Bagnato, S. J., Neisworth, J. T., Salvia, J., & Hunt, F. (1999a). *TABS Manual for the Temperament and Atypical Behavior Scale: Early childhood indicators or developmental dysfunction.* Baltimore: Brookes.

Bagnato, S. J., Neisworth, J. T., Salvia, J., & Hunt, F. (1999b). *Temperament and Atypical Behavior Scale: Early childhood indicators or developmental dysfunction.* Baltimore: Brookes.

Bates, J. E. (1989). Concepts and measures of temperament. In G. A. Kohnstamm, J. E. Bates, & M. K. Rothbart (Eds.), *Temperament in childhood* (p. 4). New York: Wiley.

Bricker, D., & Squires, J. (1999). *Ages and Stages Questionnaire: A parent-completed. child-monitoring system.* Baltimore: Brookes.

Briggs-Gowen, M. J., & Carter, A. S. (2002). *Brief Infant–Toddler Social and Emotional Assessment (BITSEA).* San Antonio, TX: Harcourt.

Carter, A. S., & Briggs-Gowan, M. J. (2000). *Infant Toddler Social Emotional Assessment (ITSEA).* San Antonio, TX: Harcourt.

DeGangi, G. A. (1991). Assessment of sensory, emotional and attentional problems in regulatory disordered infants: Part 1. *Infants and Young Children, 3*(1), 1–8.

Durand, M., & Crimmons, D. B. (1991). *Motivational Assessment Scale.* Topeka, KS: Monaco & Associates.

Fox, L., Dunlap, G., Hemmeter, M. L., Joseph, G. E., & Strain, P. S. (2003). The Teaching Pyramid: A model for supporting social competence and preventing challenging behavior in young children. *Young Children, 58*(4), 48–52.

Gilliam, W. S., & Shahar, G. (2006). Prekindergarteners expulsion and suspension: Rates and predictors in one state. *Infants and Young Children, 19*(3), 228–245.

Gresham, F., & Elliott, S. (1991). *Social Skills Rating System.* Circle Pines, MN: American Guidance Service.

Hanson, L., Deere, K., Lee, C., Lewin, A., & Seval, C. (2001). *Key principles in providing integrated behavioral health services for young children and their families: The Starting Early Starting Smart experience.* Washington, DC: Casey Family Programs and the U.S. Department of Health and Human Services, Substance Abuse and Mental Health Services Administration.

Kauffman Early Education Exchange. (2001). *Set for success: Building a strong foundation for school readiness based on the social–emotional development of young children.* Kansas City, MO: Ewing Marion Kauffman Foundation.

Knitzer, J. (2000a). Early childhood mental health services: A policy and systems development perspective. In J. P. Shonkoff & S. J. Meisels (Eds.), *Handbook of early childhood intervention* (2nd ed., pp. 416–438). Cambridge, UK: Press Syndicate of the University of Cambridge.

Knitzer, J. (2000b). *Using mental health strategies to move the early childhood agenda and promote school readiness*. New York: Carnegie Corporation of New York and the National Center for Children in Poverty.

Martin, R. P. (1988). *Temperament Assessment Battery for Children*. Austin, TX: PRO-ED.

Melaville, A., & Blank, M. J. (1991). *What it takes: Structuring interagency partnerships to connect children and families with comprehensive services*. Washington, DC: Education and Human Services Consortium.

Merrell, K. W. (1994). *Preschool and Kindergarten Behavior Scales*. Austin, TX: PRO-ED.

Miller, J. A., Bagnato, S. J., Dunst, C. J., & Mangis, H. (2005). Psychoeducational interventions in pediatric neuropsychiatry. In C. E. Coffey & R. A. Brumback (Eds.), *Textbook of pediatric neuropsychiatry* (2nd ed., pp. 701–714). Washington, DC: American Psychiatric Press.

Neisworth, J. T., & Bagnato, S. J. (1995). Neurobehavioral markers for early regulatory disorders. *Infants and Young Children, 8*(1), 8–17.

Salisbury, C. (2003). Integrating education and human service plans: The interagency planning and support project. *Journal of Early Intervention, 26*(1), 59–75.

Shonkoff, J. P., & Phillips, J. P. (Eds.). (2000). *From neurons to neighborhoods: The science of early childhood development*. Washington, DC: National Academy Press.

Sparrow, S., Balla, D., & Cicchetti, D. (1998). *Vineland Social–Emotional Early Childhood Scales*. Circle Pines, MN: American Guidance Service.

Squires, J., Bricker, D., Twombly, E., & Yockelson, S. (2001). *Ages and Stages Questionnaire: Social–Emotional. A parent-completed, child-monitoring system*. Baltimore: Brookes.

Stroul, B. A. (2002). *System of care: A framework for system reform in children's mental health* (Issue brief). Washington, DC: Georgetown University Child Development Center, National Technical Assistance Center for Children's Mental Health.

Zero to Three. (1994). *Diagnostic Classification of Mental Health and Developmental Disorders of Infancy and Early Childhood, Revised Edition*. Arlington, VA: Zero to Three/National Center for Clinical Infant Programs.

CHAPTER 11

◆ ◆ ◆

How Should We Forecast and Plan for Kindergarten Transition and Early School Success?

◆

with KIMBERLY A. BLAIR

BEST-PRACTICE ISSUES

◆ Is it necessary to plan children's transition to kindergarten?

◆ Why must we evaluate young children's development prior to the transition to kindergarten?

◆ Should published early learning standards and teacher expectations guide assessments for kindergarten entry?

◆ What domains should be assessed in determining the needs of young children prior to kindergarten?

◆ What are the best methods for assessing and monitoring young children's progress as they make the transition to elementary school?

◆ How do we conduct a comprehensive assessment that will provide the information necessary to plan for successful learning in kindergarten?

Lucas is repeating the first grade. His teachers report that he demonstrates strong math skills but struggles with acquiring basic reading

---

Kimberly A. Blair, PhD, is Assistant Professor in the Department of Psychiatry at the University of Pittsburgh School of Medicine.

and writing skills. According to the results of a speech and language assessment conducted the spring prior to entering kindergarten, Lucas demonstrated significant delays in expressive and receptive language skills. At that time, Lucas began receiving early intervention speech and language services two times per week. When Lucas entered kindergarten that fall, there had been very little attention paid to his transition to kindergarten, including how his language difficulties would impact his early learning. Special education services continued to consist entirely of pull-out speech and language therapy twice per week, primarily focusing on articulation issues.

Throughout kindergarten and his first time in the first grade, Lucas failed to develop reading skills normally. His continued difficulties learning to read contributed to the development of comorbid social–emotional difficulties. After a second time in the first grade failed to produce significant improvements, Lucas was referred for a complete psychoeducational assessment. This evaluation resulted in the expansion of his special education services. The results of that assessment confirmed a language-based learning disability far more involved than the articulation problems for which he had been receiving early intervention. Moreover, Lucas demonstrated superior nonverbal reasoning skills, explaining his strength in mathematics. Not only did Lucas lose two years of development by not being provided adequate supports for developing reading skills, his retention in the first grade had also slowed the progress he should have been making in his area of academic strength—mathematics.

Adequate planning for transitioning young children from early intervention services to school-age services is crucial to the early academic success of children with disabilities. Academically, careful planning can mean the difference between success and failure. As we see with Lucas, academic failure can also have implications for social–emotional adjustment as well as one's motivation to learn. How could support from early intervention and school staff have better helped Lucas to be successful in kindergarten?

HOW SHOULD PLANNING A CHILD'S TRANSITION TO KINDERGARTEN BE APPROACHED?

The transition to kindergarten for a child with special needs is a multifaceted process that requires not only an understanding of the child's own unique strengths and needs but also an appreciation of the multiple contextual influences that contribute to a child's early school success. Thus, in planning the transition between early childhood programs and kindergarten, the expectations of the school environment and the child's experiences within the family, peer group, and community setting should also be considered. Pianta and Kraft-Sayre (2003) describe a *developmental approach* to transition that incorporates the skills of the child, the influence on the child of experiences with family, peers, school, and community settings, the interactions between key settings and individuals, and the way each of these processes change over time. Given these multiple influences on children's early school success, it will be important to consider the strengths and needs of the child as a function of the expectations of the school environment and implement a transition plan that incorporates the interconnected and interdependent family, school, peer, and community factors that influence the child's development and transition process over time.

Have a Plan

For young children about to enter kindergarten, it is important for schools to have developed a comprehensive transition plan to facilitate the process. All young children, including those with and without special needs, will benefit from a well-coordinated, smooth transition from early childhood programs to kindergarten. To accomplish this task, transition activities should include planning at a systems level for all transitioning children, as well as include specific activities designed to facilitate the kindergarten transitions of children with special needs.

Team Building

At the systems level, Pianta and Kraft-Sayre (2003) outline nine steps to successful kindergarten transition and provide specific tools for facilitating progress with these steps. This approach is based on the developmental model for transition described above. They argue that their approach is useful for community planning and school-level planning and it is recommended that transition planning take place at both levels. I provide only a brief summary of their model here, but readers are encouraged to seek out the original source for more detailed description of their transition model and resources for implementation.

The first step in planning for kindergarten transition is to establish collaborative teams (Pianta & Kraft-Sayre, 2003). At the community level, a transition team composed of community leaders, teachers, early education teachers, and school and family-level administrators coordinates and organizes transition programs implemented at the school level across the community. This committee works to identify transition needs, and current practices and resources, allocates resources, and directs policy. At the school level, teachers and parents work together to adapt and implement transition programs based on the need of their individual school. The second step in a transition program is to identify a transition coordinator at each team level described above who will facilitate and lead transition plans and activities (Pianta & Kraft-Sayre, 2003).

Needs Assessment and Transition Planning

Steps 3 through 7 describe how to develop transition plans. Step 3 in Pianta and Kraft-Sayre's (2003) model for successful kindergarten transition involves organizing team meetings and conducting a needs assessment where each team member contributes his or her own perspective on the transition needs of the school based on area of expertise. Subsequently (Step 4), the team generates a large list of ideas for transition activities, so that programs, schools, and teachers can individualize their practices based on the needs of the children and families in the community. Step 5 is to create a transition timeline that incorporates activities beginning long before the first day of kindergarten. Pianta and Kraft-Sayre (2003) recommend that the transition process begin as early as the fall of the preschool year and focus on building relationships, with more typical transition activities such as school visits beginning in the spring of the preschool year. Through the summer, the focus should be on promoting peer relationships with traditional transition activities such as open houses and back-to-school nights that can be scheduled in the late summer. After the timeline is crafted, Pianta and Kraft-Sayre recommend that time be spent identifying required, resources, and planning individual activities.

Once the plan is developed, and prior to implementation, Step 6 requires that the transition teams consider any barriers to the successful execution of the plan. These barriers might include any factors that may prevent or discourage the active participation of any of the team members, bar parent participation, or limit school resources. As soon as any barriers are identified, Step 7 suggests that school and community teams revise timelines and activities accordingly.

Implementation and Monitoring

Now that there is an established timeline, it is time to implement the transition plan. Pianta and Kraft-Sayre (2003) recommend that at Step 8 the large list of transition activities generated in the planning process be developed into a transition practices menu that will facilitate the connections between the child, family, school, peer group, and community. The selection of transition activities should be based on the needs not only of the schools but also of individual children and families. Once the plan is implemented, ongoing assessment, evaluation, and revision of the plan (Step 9) are necessary in order to determine what needs are not being met, which strategies work well, and which do not. Feedback should be sought from the multiple stakeholders in the kindergarten transition process and can be done through interviews, checklists, and logs. Adjustments and changes should be made as needed to help the transition planning and implementation process.

Young Children with Special Needs

Children with disabilities require special planning, as there are special needs that should be considered that are unique to each child. Transition supports and procedures for students with special needs are required by federal and state special education law to guard all children with disabilities from discrimination. These laws require that educators fill roles that may not be necessary outside of the context of special education. The systemwide plan for kindergarten transition should include provisions and transition activities that are child-specific, including transition activities specific to the child with special needs.

School personnel serve specific functions in the process of transitioning children from early intervention programs to kindergarten. These functions include teachers serving as information liaisons, supporting families, advocating for systems improvements that support transition services for children with disabilities, and creating continuity in expectations, curriculum, and instruction across general and special education programs. As information liaison, educators coordinate a complex process of transferring services from one context to another. This requires that they be knowledgeable about the programs the children are coming from as well as the programs they are transitioning into. As part of this role, educators can observe one another's programs and meet and collaborate concerning the needs of the child, including the transfer of records and development of individualized education plans (IEPs).

Throughout the transition process, there should be a support system for families. This can be accomplished through open lines of communication, and by providing information about differences between sending and receiving programs, the rationale for policies and practices concerning transition, and the rights and responsibilities of families and schools. Schools should also work with families to clarify the skills that will be essential for the child's success in the new program and facilitate family involvement in the transition process by providing opportunities for family and child to visit and learn about the new school and soliciting parental support for the transition process planned for each child.

WHAT IS THE PURPOSE OF ASSESSMENT PRIOR TO THE TRANSITION TO KINDERGARTEN?

The primary objective of the prekindergarten evaluation is to identify the child's developmental, cognitive, academic, and social strengths and weaknesses. A comprehensive assessment of the child's well-developed and least well-developed skills will provide the information necessary to (1) make diagnostic or eligibility decisions in order to recommend appropriate support services; and (2) develop effective IEPs based on the child's needs.

WHAT SHOULD WE ASSESS TO DETERMINE THE NEEDS OF YOUNG CHILDREN PRIOR TO KINDERGARTEN ENTRY?

Before we can answer this question, we must ask ourselves, "What will be expected of our preschoolers in their next school environment?" As young children transition to kindergarten from preschool programs, expectations as dictated by formal early learning standards should be considered. A number of organizations have established educational goals for beginning kindergarten. The National Education Goals Panel (NEGP), Head Start, and many individual state boards of education have established early learning goals for early childhood programs to ready children for kindergarten.

National Education Goals Panel

Established by the president and 50 state governors in 1990, the NEGP signaled a national effort to identify the expectations of early childhood programs for preparing children to be "ready to learn" when they enter kindergarten. This panel of experts in early childhood education defined what types of skills were required to be successful in kindergarten across five broad dimensions. Although the NEGP identified the types of skills that are related to "school readiness," the cultural and individual variability in children's early development was emphasized so each child should not be expected to exhibit a specific set of skills and abilities prior to entering kindergarten.

The NEGP suggested five broad skill areas (physical well-being and motor development, social and emotional development, language development, cognition and general knowledge, and approaches to learning) necessary for children's early school success. The NEGP describes physical well-being as including the gross motor skills, fine motor skills, sensorimotor skills, and oral motor skills necessary to perform age-appropriate tasks and physical competencies. Self-efficacy, appropriate emotional expression, empathy, and having social skills necessary to cooperate with peers, as well as form and sustain reciprocal friendships, are the hallmarks of age-appropriate social–emotional development. "Approaches to learning" refers to motivational, attitudinal variables and cognitive learning styles when approaching problems, specifically, behaviors such as curiosity about new tasks and challenges, initiative, task persistence, attentiveness, and imagination. The language domain includes vocabulary as well as receptive, expressive, and pragmatic skills. Also included are emergent literacy competencies such as literature and print awareness, story sense, and early writing skills. Cognition and general knowledge are most commonly associated with schooling and include abilities such as representational thought, problem solving, mathematical knowledge, social knowledge, and imagination. These domain areas were meant to be suggestive, not definitive and the NEGP called for the further definition of the specific, measurable skills associated with these domains.

Head Start Performance Standards

Head Start leads the field in terms of quality of early learning standards. While Head Start's performance standards traditionally have focused on comprehensive, family-based approaches to early education that outline the experiences necessary to support children's development across physical, social, emotional, and cognitive domains, a more recent emphasis has been on supporting early language and literacy. The Head Start School Readiness and Coordination Act of 2003 focuses on greater support for early language and preliteracy development by requiring language-rich environments, teachers well trained in language and emergent literacy, and appropriate curricula and assessment. The act also requires local Head Start agencies to work on aligning early education services with the expectations for kindergarten readiness established by local educational agencies.

State Standards

Although many states determine kindergarten readiness by age, the current federal early childhood initiative calls on states to invest in early education in order to ensure that children are ready to learn when they enter kindergarten. As part of this initiative, states have been encouraged to develop early learning guidelines that align with state K–12 standards. Many states have developed or are developing outcome standards for early childhood programs. Pennsylvania's newly developed Early Learning Standards include standards for language, literacy, math, creative arts, motor skills, personal/social skills, and approaches to learning. Unfortunately, though many states include in their standards language and literacy skills, social–emotional skills and approaches to learning standards receive the less attention.

WHAT DO KINDERGARTEN TEACHERS WANT TO KNOW ABOUT YOUNG CHILDREN AS THEY ENTER THEIR CLASSROOMS?

Contrary to early learning standards established at the state and national level, many kindergarten teachers appear to have different priorities in terms of the kinds of skills young children should learn before entering kindergarten. Kindergarten teachers have their own ideas about what skills are important to teach young children for success in kindergarten and these expectations are not always consistent with the formal standards set by government entities. Kindergarten teachers tend to place heightened value on developing social and behavioral skills, whereas formal policy standards tend to favor early academic skill development.

Several studies have found that kindergarten teachers often place more value on the social–behavioral underpinnings of early learning than on the more academically based skills. Piotrkowski, Botsko, and Matthews (2000) found that kindergarten teachers considered both basic knowledge (i.e., knows ABCs, colors, counts to 10) and advanced knowledge (i.e., knows days of the week, cuts simple shapes with scissors, recognizes words that rhyme, reads a few simple words, counts to 50 or more, colors inside the lines) as less essential to early school success than the level of young children's interest and engagement. Specifically, teachers expressed serious concerns regarding the ability to communicate, get along with others, and follow directions.

Lin, Lawrence, and Gorrell (2003) also found that overall, kindergarten teachers place a higher priority on preparing children to satisfy the social demands of school than on early academic skills. These teachers indicated serious concerns about kindergarten behaviors that centered on children's ability to express themselves, follow directions, and share. In this study, teachers also had moderately high expectations for young children to exhibit self-regulation abilities in the kindergarten classroom, indicating concerns about specific task orientation and self-regulatory behaviors such as sitting still, finishing tasks, and problem solving that can be highly supportive of academic accomplishment. Alternatively, very few teachers named several key academic items as being very important or essential, including counting to 20 or more, knowing most of the alphabet, naming colors and shapes, and using a pencil.

The school readiness expectations of kindergarten teachers may have important implications for understanding what those teachers do in their classrooms to be ready for children and the expectations they have for their success. According to Rimm-Kaufman, Pianta, and Cox (2000), teachers report that a high proportion of their students have problems following directions, lack academic skills, and have difficulty working independently. Kindergarten teachers' expectations that these competencies should already be developed in early learning programs reflect the shift from the socially oriented preschool goals to the academically oriented goals of kindergarten (Rimm-Kaufman, Pianta, & Cox, 2000). Young children transitioning to kindergarten without proper attention paid to both academic and social learning skills are at a greater risk for early school failure as their teachers may expect a particular level of social ability necessary for academic learning to take place. Children receiving early intervention services may be further challenged given that they must successfully cope with the expectations of both general and special education teachers (Lane, Pierson, & Givener, 2003). Therefore, understanding what kindergarten teachers' expectations are has important implications for children enrolled in general and special education as it relates to transitioning and providing successful inclusive experiences for students with special needs.

What Does the Typical Child Know at School Entry?

The Early Childhood Longitudinal Study—Kindergarten (ECLS-K) is one of the few studies of its kind to systematically measure and monitor young children's learning and development over time. Results from the ECLS-K have outlined early findings related to what the skills of America's kindergarteners typically are at school entry. In literacy, they have found that most kindergarten children are able to recognize upper- and lowercase letters of the alphabet by name but cannot read basic words by sight and do not yet demonstrate knowledge of letters representing beginning and ending sounds of simple words. Most kindergarten children recognize most or all single-digit numbers, count to 10, and identify simple geometric shapes; however, very few can read two-digit numbers, identify ordinal positions of objects, recognize numbers in a sequence, or do simple math calculations. Behaviorally, most kindergarteners are able to get along with other children, are eager to learn new things, pay attention reasonably well, and persist in completing tasks. However, a sizable minority do exhibit behavior that may impede learning: one-quarter are "never" or "sometimes" eager to learn and one-third have difficulty paying attention.

WHAT DOMAINS SHOULD WE ASSESS TO DETERMINE THE NEEDS OF YOUNG CHILDREN PRIOR TO KINDERGARTEN?

The expectations of the next school environment established by formal early learning standards and teachers indicate several key competencies that should be assessed in order to plan for a child's successful transition from preschool to kindergarten. It seems clear that these competencies include but also transcend simple preacademic skills such as counting and reciting ABCs and includes those behavioral tendencies that are highly supportive of academic achievement. These competencies include: (1) basic academic readiness skills, (2) social skills and self-regulatory criteria such as attention span and ability to focus, and (3) approaches to learning such as initiative and persistence. Therefore, a kindergarten transition assessment should not only include a comprehensive assessment of developmental functioning and family contextual factors but also assess those competencies that reflect early school success: basic academic skills, social and self-regulatory skills, and approaches to learning.

WHAT ARE THE BEST METHODS OF EVALUATING YOUNG CHILDREN TO PLAN FOR EARLY SCHOOL SUCCESS?

There are unique issues involved in evaluating young children that make it difficult to use traditional assessment tools in the identification of academic strengths and learning difficulties. These issues concern the utility and appropriateness of traditional evaluation procedures as well as the unique behavioral challenges that are encountered in early childhood. Given some of the limitations described in Chapter 2, assessing a child's basic academic readiness skills, social and self-regulatory skills, and approaches to learning through traditional assessment procedures does not always leave one with confidence in their results. Moreover, many traditional measures do not inform treatment options well.

I advocate an approach to the kindergarten transition assessment that incorporates authentic formal and informal assessments, detailed observations of the child's functional skills in the classroom, and information provided by those individuals that know the child best, their parents and teachers. Additionally, best practice is to conduct a comprehensive evaluation that incorporates the expertise of personnel from multiple disciplines where appropriate, including speech–language, occupational, and physical therapists, early childhood, special education, and school age teachers, psychologists, reading specialists, administrators, counselors, social workers, nurses, and physicians.

HOW DO WE CONDUCT A COMPREHENSIVE ASSESSMENT THAT WILL FACILITATE PLANNING FOR SUCCESSFUL LEARNING IN KINDERGARTEN?

It has been argued that the most valid and useful evaluations of young children incorporate the use of authentic assessment techniques. However, as children progress through elementary school there is less availability of appropriate authentic assessments and fewer opportunities to conduct the ongoing assessments as classroom instruction becomes more structured and teacher-driven. Additionally, school districts often require formal, standardized assessments both for determining eligibility for special education and for monitoring annual yearly progress. Given these circumstances, it is recommended that an evaluation for kindergarten transition also incorporate authentic assessment techniques. Table 11.1 provides some examples of authentic, curriculum-based measures and other norm-referenced, yet curriculum-consistent measures that can be used in an authentic-friendly manner. A comprehensive evaluation will include the following: developmental and educational histories provided by the child's family, preschool teachers, and school records; classroom observations that provide contextual information regarding the child's development across all developmental domains; standardized and authentic assessments of cognitive abilities that include both language and problem solving; assessments of basic preacademic skills; behavior rating scales completed by the child's parents and preschool teacher to provide information about social behavior and self-regulation; and assessments of a child's approaches to learning.

Developmental and Educational History

With young children, it is crucial to involve parents and teachers in the assessment process—those individuals who know the child best. When interviewing parents, teachers, and children, crucial information needs to be obtained. The comprehensive developmental history obtained from parents should include an assessment of early behavior, family needs, and parent stress, in addition to the standard developmental milestones, medical history, and family history. Teachers will provide valuable information regarding the child's progress and functioning in the classroom setting. It will also be important to review educational records, particularly those that provide information on past levels of functioning and effective intervention strategies.

Classroom Observations

Observations are very important when working with young children. It is important to look for how a child behaves individually, with peers, and with adults. Children should be observed in a variety of settings in order to understand and identify the most difficult problems. In the assessment process it is important to be aware of the importance of play during early childhood. Play becomes a dominant mechanism through which learning occurs. Not only does play provide opportunities for practicing emerging cognitive skills, including cause-and-effect thinking, perspective taking, and exploration, it also provides young children with the opportunity for social–emotional learning. Young children during playtime will practice social roles and social skills, develop relationships, and express feelings that often cannot yet be expressed through words. Observing a child's ability to function successfully in the early child care setting often provides the richest information about current skills and future educational needs.

Cognitive and Language Abilities

Cognitive abilities encompass a wide range of abilities that include such skills as problem solving, conceptual knowledge, memory, visual processing, and comprehension. An assessment of cognitive abilities in young children can be completed using authentic assessments (see Table 11.1), standardized developmental assessments, or traditional intellectual ability tests. Even though a young child's cognitive abilities can be adequately assessed using authentic assessments, school districts will often require a traditional intelligence test as part of the diagnostic battery administered to children to determine eligibility for special education. Traditional IQ tests tend to cover a broad range of cognitive abilities associated with the theoretical basis under which they were developed. Although individual tests are developed from different theoretical approaches and may present different subtypes of cognitive abilities, the most common approach assesses cognitive ability in terms of two general areas—nonverbal and verbal reasoning. If a skills-based approach to interpretation is used rather than a global IQ score, results may provide information that points to the child's cognitive strengths and weakness, which then can be used to develop intervention plans and make diagnostic decisions.

Language development is a major goal of early childhood and a child's language ability is highly predictive of academic achievement. Language delays are often the first identified and can be associated with future learning disabilities in reading and writing. Therefore, it is frequently appropriate to obtain a more in-depth language assessment that includes both receptive and expressive language. It is important for members of the multidisciplinary team to coordinate evaluations, as assessments of language can be done by psychologists or speech–language therapists. The assessment of language skills is crucial in the transition to kindergarten as it can lead to identification of potential problems associated with language-based learning disabilities. Often overlooked, listening comprehension (receptive language) and oral expression (expressive language) are two areas of specific learning disabilities identified by the Individuals with Disabilities Education Act (IDEA). As with Lucas at the beginning of this chapter, continued language interventions at this early stage in a child's schooling can mean future difficulties acquiring reading skills will be planned for or avoided altogether.

Preacademic Skills

Another component of a comprehensive evaluation is the measurement of early academic achievement. Preacademic achievement includes but is not limited to numbers and counting, knowing letters and reciting the alphabet, and naming colors and shapes. It may also include the understanding of basic concepts (direction/position, quantity, comparisons, etc.). This component simply measures what academic skills the child has acquired—it does not necessarily indicate the child's ability to acquire these skills.

Social Behavior and Self-Regulation

As described earlier, kindergarten teachers are most interested in those social behaviors that can be supportive of academic accomplishment and may indicate a child's ability to function successfully in a more structured school setting. Teachers are concerned about kindergarten behaviors that center on children expressing themselves, following directions, and sharing, as well as specific task orientation and self-regulatory behaviors such as sitting still and finishing tasks.

Current methods of evaluating young children for the types of behaviors described above rely almost exclusively on the reports of parents and caregivers. Measures that are commonly used for evaluating the social and emotional well being of young children include parent and teacher/caregiver behavior rating scales, interviews, and behavioral observations. A variety of behavioral rating scales are available for use with young children entering kindergarten and many of these scales not only evaluate maladaptive skills such as hyperactivity, aggression, and attention problems but also assess positive social development and social skills.

Approaches to Learning

"Approaches to learning" refers to the range of attitudes, habits, inclinations, and dispositions that reflects the methods through which children become involved in learning and develop strategies by which to pursue it. The fostering of positive approaches to learning cannot be emphasized enough, as they are at the core of both social–emotional development and cognitive advancement and encompass the growth of learning behaviors such as curiosity, creativity, independence, cooperativeness, and persistence, which serve to drive each child's learning and development.

In contrast to the assessment of cognition and language, there are few tools that specifically measure a child's approaches to learning as a single dimension. The best approach to making judgments in this domain is to reflect on the child's behavior as observed in the classroom and during assessment, and in the reports of parents and teachers.

TABLE 11.1. Authentic, Curriculum-Consistent Measures

Name	Publisher (Date)	Types of scores	Domains/subdomains	Administration	Reliability	Comments
Battelle Developmental Inventory: 2nd edition	Riverside (2004)	Norm-referenced; Standard scores for domains; Scaled scores for subdomains	• Personal/Social (Adult interaction, Self-concept and social growth, Peer interaction) • Adaptive (Personal responsibility, Self-care) • Motor (Fine motor, Perceptual motor, Gross motor) • Communication (Expressive communication, Receptive communication) • Cognitive (Perceptual discrimination/conceptual development, Reasoning and academic skills, Attention and memory)	Individually administered, teacher observation, parent interview; 10–30 minutes for screener, 1 to 2 hours complete	.90 to .99	Requires supervised training; parental input needed to complete some items.
Developmental Assessment of Young Children	PRO-ED (1998)	Norm-referenced; Standard scores for domains; General developmental quotient	• Cognition • Communication • Social-emotional development • Physical development • Adaptive behavior	Teacher observation; 10–20 minutes per subtest	.94 to .99	
Developmental Observation Checklist System	PRO-ED (1994)	Norm-referenced; Provides quotients, NCE scores, age equivalents, and percentiles	• Language • Motor • Social • Cognitive	Parent/teacher observation; 30 minutes to complete, 15–20 to score	.85 to .94	Includes additional instructions for children with special needs
Learning Accomplishment Profile	Kaplan Early Learning/ PACT House (1992)	Diagnostic norm-referenced and criterion-referenced versions available; Provides percentile	• Fine Motor (Writing, Manipulation) • Language (Comprehension, Naming) • Gross Motor (Body Movement, Object Movement)	Individually administered; 45 to 90 minutes		

Instrument	Publisher (date)	Scoring	Areas assessed	Administration/Time	Reliability	Comments
		ranks, age equivalent scores, and normal curve equivalents	• Cognitive (Counting, Matching) • Pre-Writing • Language • Self-Help • Personal-Social • Social-Emotional	Teacher report; 5–8 minutes per scale	.91 to .98	
Basic School Skills Inventory—3rd edition	PRO-ED (1998)	Norm-referenced; Provides standard scores, percentiles, and age and grade equivalents	• Spoken Language • Reading • Writing • Mathematics • Classroom Behavior • Daily Living Skills • Overall Skill Level			
Bracken Basic Concepts Scale—Revised	Psychological Corporation (1998)	May be used for norm-referenced, criterion-referenced, or curriculum-based assessments; Provides standard scores, percentile ranks, and age equivalent for each of the composites, and a scaled score for each of the subtests	• Colors • Letters • Numbers—Counting • Sizes • Comparisons • Shapes • Direction-Position • Self-Social Awareness • Texture-Material • Quantity • Time-Sequence	Individually administered; 30–45 minutes	.88 to .94	Criterion-referenced Spanish edition available
Kaufman Survey of Early Academic and Language Skills (K-SEALS)	AGS (1993)	Norm-referenced; Provides standard scores, percentile ranks, and age equivalents	• Vocabulary • Numbers–Letters and Words • Articulation Survey • Early Academic and Language Skills Composite • Language Scales (Expressive Skills, Receptive Skills) • Early Academic Scales (Number Skills, Letter and Word Skills)	Individually administered; 15–20 minutes	.88 to .94	

CONCLUSIONS

The transition to kindergarten can be difficult for all young children, but especially for those with special needs. Successful transitioning by young children from early intervention services to school-age services is crucial to the early academic success of children with disabilities and it is therefore important for school systems to spend time developing a systematic transition process. When considering the transition of individual children, it will be important to complete comprehensive assessments to identify strengths and needs in order to make appropriate identifications for eligibility and to plan individualized interventions. The identification of strengths and needs should be obtained through comprehensive evaluations, which are guided by learning expectations for kindergarten, as dictated by early learning standards and teacher expectations. Comprehensive assessments should be multidisciplinary, multimethod, and multi-informant. Due to the limitations of traditional assessments with young children, an authentic approach is recommended. In those circumstances where standardized, traditional testing is required, it is strongly suggested that authentic assessments be used as well.

BEST-PRACTICE GUIDEPOINTS

♦ Develop a detailed, systemwide plan for the transition of children from early intervention to kindergarten/school-age programs.

♦ Conduct comprehensive assessments to obtain necessary information for eligibility determination and educational planning just prior to kindergarten.

♦ Use authentic assessment methods and procedures.

♦ Authentic assessments should be used in conjunction with traditional assessments, if they are required.

♦ Include comprehensive information that is based on state/federal outcome benchmarks and teacher expectations.

♦ Emphasize performance information on social and behavioral competencies as much as information on cognitive and academic competencies.

BEST-PRACTICE EVIDENCE

Bagnato, S. J., & Neisworth, J. T. (1991). *Assessment for early intervention: Best practice for professionals.* New York: Guilford Press.

Fowler, S. A., Schwartz, I., & Atwater, J. (1991). Perspectives on the transition from preschool to kindergarten for children with disabilities and their families. *Exceptional Children, 58*(2), 136–145.

Head Start Act, 42 U.S.C. § 9836 641(a)(l)(B) (2003). Retrieved on February 8, 2005 from *www.theorator.com/bills108/hr2210.html*

Head Start Bureau. (1992). *Head Start program performance standards* (DHHS Publication No. ACF92-31131). Washington, DC: U.S. Department of Health and Human Services.

Jewett, J., Tertell, L., King-Taylor, M., Parker, D., Tertell, L., & Orr, M. (1998). Four early childhood teachers reflect on helping children with special needs make the transition to kindergarten. *Elementary School Journal, 98*(4), 329–338.

Kagan, S. L., Moore, E., & Bredekamp, S. (Eds.). (1995, June). *Reconsidering children's early development and learning: Toward common views and vocabulary*. Washington, DC: National Education Goals Panel.

Lane, K. L., Pierson, M. R., & Givener, C. C. (2003). Teacher expectations of student behavior: Which skills do elementary and secondary teachers deem necessary for success in the classroom? *Education and Treatment of Children, 26*(4), 413–430.

Lane, K. L., Pierson, M., & Givener, C. (2004). Secondary teacher's views on social competence: Skills essential for success. *Journal of Special Education, 38*(3), 174–187.

La Paro, K. M., Pianta, R. C., & Cox, M. (2000). Teachers' reported transition practices for children transitioning into kindergarten and first grade. *Exceptional Children, 67*(1), 7–20.

Lin, H., Lawrence, F. R., & Gorrell, J. (2003). Kindergarten teachers' views on children's readiness for school. *Early Childhood Research Quarterly, 18*(2), 225–237.

National Association of Early Childhood Specialists in State Departments of Education. (2000). *STILL unacceptable trends in kindergarten entry and placement*. Washington, DC: Author.

Pianta, R. C., Cox, M. J., Taylor, L., & Early, D. (1999). Kindergarten teachers' practices related to the transition to school: Results of a national survey. *Elementary School Journal, 100*(1), 71–86.

Pianta, R. C., & Kraft-Sayre, M. (2003). *Successful kindergarten transition: Your guide to connecting children, families, and schools*. Baltimore: Brookes.

Pianta, R. C., Kraft-Sayre, M., Rimm-Kaufman, S., Gercke, N., & Higgins, N. (2001). Collaboration in building partnerships between families and schools: The National Center for Early Development and Learning's Kindergarten Transition Intervention. *Early Childhood Research Quarterly, 16*(1), 117–132.

Piotrkowski, C. S., Botsko, M., & Matthews, E. (2000). Parents and teachers' beliefs about children's school readiness in a high-need community. *Early Childhood Research Quarterly, 15*, 537–558.

Rimm-Kaufman, S. E., Pianta, R., & Cox, M. (2000). Teachers' judgments of success in the transition to kindergarten. *Early Childhood Research Quarterly, 15*(2), 147–166.

Rous, B., & Hallam, R. A. (1998). Easing the transition to kindergarten: Assessment of social, behavioral, and functional skills in young children with disabilities. *Young Exceptional Children, 1*(4), 16–27.

Saluja, G., Scott-Little, C., & Clifford, R. M. (2000). Readiness for school: A survey of state policies and definitions. *Early Childhood Research and Practice, 2*(2). Retrieved February 8, 2005, from http://ecrp.uiuc.edu/v2n2/saluja.html

Scott-Little, C., Kagan, S. L., & Frelow, V. S. (2003). Creating the conditions for success with early learning standards: Results from a national study of state-level standards for children's learning prior to kindergarten. *Early Childhood Research and Practice, 5*(2). Retrieved December 11, 2005 from http://eric.ed.gov/ERICDOCS/data/ericdocs2/content_storage010000000b/80/23/80/32.pdf.

West, J., Denton, K., & Germino-Hausken, E. (2000). America's kindergarteners: Findings from the Early Childhood Longitudinal Study, kindergarten class 1998–99, Fall 1998. *Education Statistics Quarterly, 2*(1), 7–13.

CHAPTER 12

◆ ◆ ◆

How Can Authentic Program Evaluation Document Early Childhood Intervention Outcomes?

◆

BEST-PRACTICE ISSUES

◆ Why are experimental–control group designs rarely used to evaluate early childhood intervention programs?

◆ How can authentic curriculum-based measures be used for program evaluation research?

◆ Why is measuring child outcomes insufficient for program evaluation?

◆ How can programs measure the child's developmental ecology?

◆ What applied metrics can be used to summarize program impact?

◆ Can researchers control for maturation in program evaluation without use of a control group?

Professionals who believe in and operate early childhood intervention programs must document change. Parents and professionals continually evaluate. They make judgments about how well a child is doing, the quality of teaching or parenting, the utility of assessment, staff morale, and other program aspects. Indeed, program evaluation of some sort goes on implicitly if not explicitly, and informally if not formally.

At its worst, formal program evaluation is sometimes regarded as a perfunctory task. When the evaluation procedures and outcomes have little utility for the staff or parents and are disconnected from program content, it is easy to understand the view of evaluation as a bureaucratic routine. Unfortunately, many evaluative efforts and materials do fail to provide any constructive information and are useless for subsequent decision making.

At its best, however, evaluation is an integral part of the program and is valued for the information it provides regarding the status and improvement of enrolled children, benefit to families, and the quality of staff and program operations. When the appropriate measurement tools and procedures are used, program evaluation documents the hard work of the staff, progress of the children, satisfaction of the parents, and the overall quality of effort. Doing a program evaluation is much like having a physical examination: perhaps it's a little anxiety producing, but it is intended to offer a checkup and suggestions for improvement. Likewise, a program "checkup" should yield a status report and suggestions for improvement. Evaluation need not be arduous and complicated, or abound with statistics. To be most unobtrusive, evaluation processes should be infused into typical work routines—it is an ongoing process, not an isolated event.

This chapter offers a roadmap and guidepoints for making program evaluation sensible, useful, and positive; it illustrates strategies that program administrators and interdisciplinary practitioners can use to document the complex interrelationships among program aspects and child success and to conduct credible, applied program evaluation research that will balance reality and rigor.

IS THERE AGREEMENT ABOUT HOW TO EVALUATE EARLY CHILDHOOD INTERVENTION OUTCOMES?

There clearly exists an increased urgency and emphasis on accountability in all human service fields, including medicine, mental health, and education. Within education, No Child Left Behind (NCLB) is the most notable example of the accountability movement; NCLB has stimulated efforts to create state and national standards and benchmarks for proficiency and success. Within early intervention, the Office of Special Education Programs (OSEP) has funded the Early Childhood Outcomes Center (ECO) at SRI International to develop and field-validate national criteria to document the benefits of early intervention services for children and families. Similarly, Head Start has mandated the National Reporting System (NRS) to document outcomes. Most states have created early learning standards by which prekindergarten progress and potential for early school success are gauged.

Nevertheless, despite this "fast track" approach, there is little agreement on the best ways to evaluate the impact and outcomes of early childhood intervention programs; moreover, most of these programs occur in diverse community settings and should be regarded properly as "natural experiments."

Traditionalists argue for randomized experimental control group designs as the "gold standard." However, such conventional experimental designs have high internal validity but low external validity and have yielded few feasible interventions in community settings. On the other hand, community-based researchers argue for flexible designs, evaluation methodologies, and statistical techniques to accommodate fluid changes in nonlaboratory conditions. Yet, alternative methods are criticized for a lack of internal validity and sufficient rigor to draw conclusions about impact and outcomes, let alone efficacy (proof that the intervention produced the results). It has been best stated that conventional designs answer the "Can it work?" question under controlled conditions, while alternative designs answer the questions: "Does it work? for whom? and in what setting?" in the more natural and less controlled settings that are most usually found in early childhood intervention programs.

ADVANTAGES OF ALTERNATIVE OR "AUTHENTIC" PROGRAM EVALUATION METHODS FOR REAL-WORLD RESEARCH

I believe that alternative modes of evaluation, or "authentic program evaluation research methods," provide the most practical ways for early childhood intervention programs to document the quality, impact, and outcomes of their instruction, care, services, and supports for all children and families. Authentic and alternative methods have the following advantages:

- Use collaboration (participatory action research) to match evaluation research methods with community-based program needs and missions.
- Engage the community as research partners to "own" the evaluation as their legacy, and to integrate methods into typical work routines.
- Avoid the ethical dilemma of exclusion of children for research purposes.
- Document the specific features of programs that best predict outcomes.
- Use natural caregivers as the best informed assessors of child status and progress in everyday routines rather than strangers.
- Employ descriptive data profiling methods for formative evaluation to improve intervention practices and program quality.
- Apply multivariate and multiple regression techniques to analyze predicted and expected summative research outcomes.

WHY MUST WE EVALUATE
EARLY CHILDHOOD INTERVENTION OUTCOMES?

In busy programs, staff often question the value and effort needed for program evaluation, especially when the measurement methods and process are not integrated into typical everyday work routines. There are seven distinct purposes for program evaluation:

1. Describe and quantify program features.
2. Highlight successful program practices.
3. Improve weak program practices.
4. Demonstrate individual child and family progress.
5. Demonstrate success across groups of children and families.
6. Align program missions and standards with expected outcomes.
7. Document program quality, impact, and outcomes to funders/stakeholders for self-advocacy.

When done properly and practically, program evaluation and outcomes research will enable administrators and staff to show how good they are at what they do. Fundamentally, ongoing program evaluation research is vital for program improvement and survival.

WHAT IS "AUTHENTIC" PROGRAM EVALUATION?

Authentic program evaluation is the systematic gathering of ongoing information from everyday routines about the changing interrelationships among programmatic aspects and the characteristics of children and families so as to improve program quality and to document impact and success toward attaining program missions and standards. Authentic program evaluation is distinguished by the following attributes:

- Use of natural observations in everyday settings and activities to record child status and progress
- Use of caregivers as primary assessors
- Links among the content of assessment methods, curricular goals and objectives, and expected overarching outcomes (e.g., state and national standards, program missions)
- Comprehensive and ecological focus across multiple variables: child, family, and program
- Ongoing data collection time-points (e.g., September, January, May) to create developmental "growth curve" skill attainment profiles on individual children and groups

- Portable MIS database archiving and record-keeping infused into staff's daily work routines; increasing use of Palm Pilot and PC table assessment formats for more naturalistic appraisal of children and programs
- Formative feedback to parents and professionals about both children's development and program features for program improvement
- Summative statistical analyses to describe child outcomes and to predict program impact.

Two Parallel Phases of Authentic Program Evaluation

All high-quality program evaluation research has two phases that operate in parallel or tandem. *Formative evaluation* provides ongoing feedback to teachers, parents, and administrators about the progress of individual children, groups, and families, and about program changes so that program improvements can be implemented. *Summative evaluation and research* aggregates and statistically analyzes data about individual and group progress at the end of a preestablished period of instruction, care, and intervention in order to estimate program impact and to determine which program practices might account for these benefits.

The best program evaluation is optimistic about how programs can foster the developmental success of children and families; it is based on the concept expressed in the following admonition: *The best predictor of future behavior is a past behavior history; yet, small increments of progress during early childhood intervention begin to create a new history that can predict a new future for all children and families.*

ESSENTIAL COMPONENTS OF A COMPREHENSIVE AUTHENTIC PROGRAM EVALUATION SYSTEM FOR EARLY INTERVENTION

A comprehensive program evaluation system attempts to measure and estimate the interrelationships among multiple elements of each child's *developmental* ecology. At a minimum, such an authentic evaluation system surveys status and progress for three primary categories of outcome variables:

1. *Child:* Developmental, early learning, social–behavioral, and early school success.
2. *Program:* Quality and intensity of the early childhood program and its interventions, care routines, services, and supports.
3. *Parent/family:* Parenting behavior, parental and family stress, and social support.

Child

Most often, accountability rests on how well children fare as a result of their participation in a program. Child progress may be seen as a *product*, while program arrangements and procedures are considered *process*. Of course, program administrators and staff usually strive to use the process in a way they believe will yield the optimal products (e.g., progress in children's development). Often, however, program activities are driven more by a theory, set of principles, or expedience than by outcome data. As an instance, a program may have goals and procedures for "fostering creativity," but never evaluate this worthwhile goal. Clearly, then, *a first responsibility is to clarify child goals and objectives so that they are subject to evaluation.* Until this criterion is met, child attainment cannot be objectively assessed either through norm or criterion-based instruments. Table 12.1 poses the types of questions that are often the focus of early childhood intervention program evaluation research.

Authentic Curriculum-Embedded Instruments

Programs usually employ an organized and teachable series of (typically developmental) objectives that make up the *curriculum*. Often a program will "sort of" have a curriculum that, upon inspection, is little more than a list of major developmental landmarks, perhaps along with some program-specific goals. Such loosely organized quasi curricula are akin to sketchy blueprints: they do not provide much guidance and will not focus efforts toward predetermined outcomes.

Programs should be urged to adopt one or more of the high quality curricular systems and curriculum-embedded instruments available. It may

---

TABLE 12.1. Examples of Frequently Posed Child Outcome Questions for Program Evaluation Research

- What percentage of children have met state standards for the acquisition of age-appropriate early literacy skills?
- What percentage of children have moved from delay to non-delay status in any developmental domain?
- Do children at developmental risk (at program entry) show significant developmental progress that outpaces their maturational expectations?
- Do children with challenging or atypical social behaviors show significant increases in social skills and associated decreases in problem behaviors?
- What percentage of children showed specific acquisitions of curricular skills over a 12-month period of program participation?
- Did children with severe disabilities at least maintain their general developmental rates while showing specific improvements in some developmental objectives?
- What percentage of children with developmental delays showed progress on at least 80% of their IFSP and IEP objectives over a 12-month period?

---

be the responsibility of the psychologist or other interdisciplinary professional to discuss with program staff and administrators the virtues of a structured curriculum so that criterion- or curriculum-based child assessment and program evaluation can take place. Similarly, curriculum-referenced measures that also have national norms are complementary forms of measurement that can help appraise both individual child progress and comparison to peers.

Assuming that the program is using one or more curricula, child program progress is best appraised through curriculum-based assessment (CBA) involving embedded measures such as the ARPS: Assessment, Evaluation, and Programming System (Bricker, 2002). Indeed, it can be said with some truth that the curriculum is the heart of the program.

CBA is the most relevant, direct, and sensitive measure of the program's influence on the child's performance. Many curricula provide ways to monitor attainment of curricular objectives. For purposes of *program* evaluation, the curricular progress of enrolled children can be summarized and averaged. The average performance of children within the curriculum can be extremely helpful in gauging the general impact of the program. Sometimes, program staff also wish to detect the possible *differential* impact of the program on the several domains of development included in most curricula (e.g., cognitive, motor, social, language). So, for example, the average attainment in motor skills may be compared with the average attainment in the cognitive, social, and communication areas. When great discrepancies are revealed, this has implications for strengthening program efforts in the weaker developmental domains.

Curriculum based child program evaluation need not be complicated. As mentioned, numerous curricula are commercially available and choice among curricula will depend on factors such as child characteristics and match with program missions and objectives. From the standpoint of program evaluation, age inclusiveness is an especially important curriculum characteristic. Curricula that span several years provide continuity and lend themselves to pre- and posttest assessment. Use of one CBA measure at the beginning and a different one at the end of the year because a child has moved beyond the first one creates special evaluation problems. Fortunately, curriculum developers are sensitive to this issue and have produced curriculum packages that are continuous (0–5 years of age) and can accommodate longitudinal monitoring and evaluation.

Authentic Curriculum-Referenced Measures

As discussed previously, authentic CBA measures also include "curriculum-referenced" instruments that are compatible with most curricula used in early childhood intervention programs because their item content is generic but similar to the content of the curriculum objectives, yet with less finely graded skill sequences. Two examples of such referenced measures are the Developmental Observation Checklist System (DOCS; Hresko et al., 1984) and the Adaptive Behavior Assessment System II (ABAS; Harrison & Oakland, 2003). Both measures are nationally standardized scales that yield standard scores to profile child status and progress.

Program

Improvements in child and family status are certainly cardinal aspects to be evaluated. Program evaluation encompasses recording of program efforts, as well as program-related effects. It is often quite important to know how much time and effort are involved working with parents, toilet training a child, or providing speech–language therapy or other specified services. An accounting of the program's intensity should accompany the reported effects. What it took to bring about a goal is important information to parents, staff, and agency administrations. Sometimes evaluation of staff effort will reveal that inordinate time and work are entailed in bringing about minor changes. Often, the effort should be shifted to a more productive program aspect. In this regard, some curricula require much more work to implement than is reasonable for a busy staff. Analysis of staff activities will help to detect various time and effort "sinkholes."

An early childhood education program is a composite of its missions, clients, staff, and physical environment, as well as its curriculum. Too often program evaluation fails to include appraisal of those aspects of the program that can indirectly or even directly affect child and family services. The extent and quality of child integration, staff morale, and child study team functioning, and the acceptability of program objectives and methods are examples of factors that can seriously influence program effectiveness.

Issues such as the breadth of program goals, the intensity and duration of services, and the detection of unintended effects are valuable to examine through program evaluation. Use of multiple measures and inclusion of child, family, and program ecology components can go a long way in providing a more complete picture of program effects. I remind the reader of the poor showing evidenced by Head Start programs when IQ was used as a primary evaluation criterion. When grade level advancement, reduced enrollment in special education, improved peer relations, and other dependent variables were examined, the evaluation picture was much more positive.

Two dimensions of *program ecology* are briefly discussed in this section: program quality and program intensity. Table 12.2 surveys sample evaluation questions pertinent to program ecology. For each question, a Time 1 to Time 2 measure can be taken to assess stability or change in that aspect. Sometimes program circumstances, such as availability of learning

TABLE 12.2. Examples of Family-Related Evaluation Questions

- How many and what types of family goals were written into IFSP/IEP?
- How many goals and objectives were attained?
- What changes occurred in family expressed needs?
- Did the reported stress levels of parents decrease?
- What changes occurred in support services provided?
- Did the quality of home environments change?
- Were there changes in parent–child interactions?
- Were there "spillover" effects detected or reported with siblings or other family members?

materials and space, are excellent at the beginning of the year but deteriorate after several months and full enrollment. Likewise, extent of social inclusion can certainly shift through time.

Programmatic dimensions have been largely ignored in early childhood intervention research. Researchers have presumed that separating groups of study children based on the type of program in which they were enrolled was sufficient. Increasing interest is focusing on documenting specific programmatic aspects that are likely related to child outcome (e.g., quality, intensity, type of services).

New-generation early intervention studies conducted in natural settings without control groups or randomization use sophisticated regression techniques that rely on measures of such programmatic aspects to examine possible predictive relationships between positive child outcomes and the type, quality, and intensity of services and supports that may be responsible for the successful outcomes.

Program Quality

There are many evaluation questions related to program operations. Perhaps the most frequently measured dimension is program quality, which is most often linked with state and national accreditation (e.g., NAEYC). Evaluation must begin with several agreed-upon major questions; as the year begins, other concerns can be added. It is also important to note that available instruments can contain numerous items that cover many of the questions posed by programs. To illustrate, the Early Childhood Environment Rating Scale—Revised (ECERS; Harms & Clifford, 1998) includes 37 items that appraise personal care routines, furnishings and display, language reasoning experiences, fine and gross motor activities, creative activities, social development, and adult needs. The ECERS uses a 7-point rating scale, yields a profile, and can be used to suggest targets to refine and improve program circumstances. Similarly, the Caregiver Interaction Scale (CIS; Arnett, 1989a) is an efficient way to estimate adult care and teaching skills, including sensitivity to child cues, use of appropriate language levels, and provision of prompts and positive consequences.

Program Intensity

Evaluation of program service delivery typically has been limited to a simple listing or number of services provided. Stating that children received speech and language services or that occupational therapy was provided to a certain number of children is an inadequate evaluation. This is much like early research in special education, when reports only stated that children were enrolled in special or regular classes—without specification of what was "special." The *intensity* of services (e.g., number of hours, sessions, focus of intervention, extent of inclusion) is crucial information for evaluating program efficiency, impact, and for helping professionals to detect relationships between intervention variables and outcome, especially in early intervention. The System to Plan Early Childhood Services (SPECS; Bagnato & Neisworth, 1990) includes a program specifications component (P-Specs) that provides a relatively easy way to quantify the extent of program activities, yielding a profile of the intensity of program services. P-Specs is used to quantify these various early intervention programmatic and service elements in the following categories: early intervention, adaptive services, behavior therapy, speech/language therapy, occupational therapy, physical therapy, vision services, hearing services, medical support, and transition support (see the P-Specs example in the final section of the chapter, on authentic assessment in action).

Parent/Family

The major mission of early intervention is, of course, to optimize children's development by minimizing social barriers through increased opportunities and expanding each child's functional capabilities. Contemporary empirical research as well as logic, however, shows us that child development is not simply maturational—it is the result of interactions with physical and social contexts experienced by the child. When the importance of the child's environment is recognized, assessment must be expanded to include appraisal of the "ecology" of the child, including the family/parenting circumstances and quality of the preschool environment. *Program evaluation must capture some context-based information.* Measures of changes in parent ratings of their child's development, of the acceptability of the child's program, of improved family functioning, of the team's cohesiveness, and of the program arrangements are examples of valuable ecological measures.

It can be said that early intervention and assessment are focused on child progress, but within a developmental context that includes the family, home, and programmatic circumstances.

Child development specialists and educators have for some time reported that early intervention effects go beyond the child and that family involvement is crucial for optimizing short- and long-term intervention impact.

As almost any educator knows, some families are easy to work with and some definitely are not! Further, children at risk or with delays or disabilities may very well come from families that do not resemble old fashioned nuclear families. A single-parent (usually the mother), low-income foster family with several siblings is not unusual. Frequently, the grandmother or even an older sibling may be a major if not primary caregiver. High levels of stress and distress, poor nutritional practices, sporadic employment, and other difficulties often vex families with special needs preschoolers. The complexities and obstacles associated with these families can understandably produce much professional avoidance behavior. But troubled families are the very ones that need the most help to offset the debilitating circumstances that distort and delay child development. In addition to the logical arguments, public law, and continued research, professional ethics dictate that early intervention programs address the family context. Since family program participation is now a mandate, family-relevant measures must be routinely included in program evaluation.

Like children, families are idiosyncratic and there is no predetermined set of evaluation questions and measures that "fits all."

Consider the following to illustrate evaluation at the family level. Perhaps the mother of a 4-year-old has asked for help to improve parenting skills, or a social worker has observed this need. The Home Observation for Measurement of the Environment (HOME; Caldwell & Bradley, 1984) could be employed at Times 1 and 2. The HOME assesses qualities of parent–child interaction and can act as a criterion-referenced tool to provide parenting objectives. Those skills apparently lacking can become individualized family service plan (IFSP) objectives; attainment of the parenting skills can then be assessed and improvements included in program evaluation reports. Improvements across several families might be separately documented as well as summed.

As another illustration, many families of children with handicaps experience great stress that interferes with family life and caregiving. The Parenting Stress Index (3rd ed.) (PSI; Abidin, 1990) has proved to be a useful gauge of family stress levels. Many PSI items (e.g., those dealing with mood, sense of competence, child activity level) can become targets for the IFSP or for counseling recommendations.

Similarly, the Family Needs Survey (Bailey & Simeonsson, 1988) enables parents to report their family's priorities so that the IFSP can incorporate these. Program evaluation efforts, then, would document whether or not services had been effectively delivered over a time period to address the family's goals.

The Parent Behavior Checklist (PBC; Fox, 1998) is a parent self-report measure that focuses on three aspects of parenting behavior: expectations, nurturing, and discipline. It can be used to document changes through normative comparisons in these dimensions when parents are involved in their child's program and in family support services.

The program evaluators must first help to identify the major family questions/concerns prior to selecting instruments. Repeated use of the instruments can help to register the changed status of the family and reflect favorably on the program. Table 12.3 poses many measurable questions regarding parent and family concerns and attributes in early childhood intervention programs.

TABLE 12.3. Examples of Program-Related Evaluation Questions

- Is the staff–child ratio satisfactory with respect to requirements?
- Is the staff–child ratio adequate to deliver the program?
- Are staff qualifications satisfactory, especially with respect to the inclusion of children with special needs?
- Are staff inservice activities scheduled and/or completed?
- Is staff inservice training helpful as judged by the staff?
- Has inservice training noticeably improved staff/program operations?
- Are IEPs/IFSPs available for all enrolled children with special needs?
- Are the IEPs/IFSPs useful "working documents" or are they perfunctory?
- Does the program have an overall curriculum that meets the needs of enrolled children and staff capabilities?
- Are proper ancillary services available to the children who need them?
- Are ancillary services coordinated and delivered satisfactorily?
- Is child progress monitored and recorded?
- Is the intensity of services recorded and does it change?
- Is the child service team cohesive and collaborative in its assessment and reporting activities?
- Are program goals and procedures acceptable to parents and staff?
- Are assessment reports useful for program planning?
- Are child transitional services in place and effective when a child is sent to a new program?
- Are follow-up procedures and information in place for children who have left the program?

WHAT ARE THE STEPS FOR IMPLEMENTING AN AUTHENTIC PROGRAM EVALUATION OUTCOMES MODEL IN EARLY CHILDHOOD PROGRAMS?

While much pressure exists to document child outcomes, programs need not despair. A series of collaborative decisions by administrators and staff can enable programs to implement a framework for authentic program evaluation infused into everyday work routines; such a model will make outcomes evaluation an integrated activity that occurs on an ongoing basis rather than a separate event requiring an extra expense of energy and cost. Programs should follow these steps to implement an authentic program evaluation model:

1. *Choose a core curriculum system and related child outcome measures.* Through collaborative decision making, program administrators, teachers, team members, and parents can reach consensus about the core curriculum and integrated assessment system to adopt in the program. This decision is based on many factors related to the type of program, its missions, its objectives and standards, and the mix of children with varying degrees of capabilities who are included in the program settings. The curriculum-embedded assessment helps to accomplish many purposes including appraisal of functional skills and deficits, identification of individual goals for program planning, and the monitoring of individual goal attainment.

In addition, the team can select complementary—often norm-referenced—measures to describe child status and progress and to provide other normative comparisons, and especially to fulfill some state and local requirements regarding the assessment of early learning and proficiency in early literacy. Select measures that are both authentic and curriculum referenced to accomplish this purpose.

2. *Select measures for related outcomes (family, program quality, program intensity).* The team should select measures that describe and classify associated dimensions of the child's "developmental ecology." At a minimum, these include measures of program quality, program or service intensity, and parent/family functioning. By including such dimensions, programs set the stage for conducting program evaluation research that can estimate program impact by demonstrating a statistical relationship or prediction (hierarchical linear modeling) among programmatic attributes and child progress and success.

3. *Set a data collection timeline: Time 1, Time 2, Time 3.* For ease, simplicity, and alignment with typical program work routines, programs should establish time points for collecting child performance and related data which are understandable. For example, the following two or three

time points often coincide with other program requirements (program entry, IEP/IFSP reviews, end-of-year transitions): September–October–January/February–May/June. The 2-month clusters provide enough time for the teachers, staff, and parents to collect multisource data on the child.

4. *Train to ensure complete and accurate data collection by teachers and caregivers.* One of the most damaging mistakes that programs make is to begin the child assessments before completing rigorous training and mentoring of the teachers and staff. Without ongoing training (initial, booster, and follow-up checks), observation forms and checklists will be full of errors, mostly in terms of overlooked items or misinterpreted items. Without training, the data will be unreliable and therefore invalid for the intended purpose.

5. *Enter data into a computerized management information system database.* In the modern era, programs must use a computerized management information system (MIS) to enter, aggregate, summarize, and export child data for statistical analysis. In addition, with advances in technology, many assessment systems are beginning to rely upon Palm Pilot or Tablet PC formats to record data in vivo and then to immediately import it into the MIS through a Web-based interface.

6. *Provide formative teacher feedback on child performance.* Research demonstrates that assessment for program evaluation is much more meaningful and reinforcing for teachers if they receive summaries of the data for each child or group that translates into objectives for program planning (Bagnato, Suen, Brickley, Smith-Jones, & Dettore, 2002). This is the sine qua non of CBA. A program can use an MIS system to generate individual letters or reports written in the "child's voice" to establish "getting there" items or next step skills as objectives for instruction and care.

7. *Apply summative metrics to describe individual and group progress and provide a basis for statistical analysis of program impact.* Various applied metrics are available for programs to use to describe the status and progress of children and to estimate program impact. The following section outlines several of these curricular and norm-referenced metrics.

WHAT ARE PRACTICAL METRICS FOR PROFILING INDIVIDUAL AND GROUP CHILD PROGRESS TO ESTIMATE PROGRAM IMPACT?

Curriculum-Based Applied Metrics

Curriculum-based evaluation is arguably the most relevant and direct way to estimate child progress on program objectives associated with program participation and missions. When goals, objectives, and other measurable criteria are stated, a real program for child attainment is created. We may, of course, debate the value of the program (or specific child) objectives.

Assuming, however, that a program adopts a reasonable developmental curriculum or other set of agreed upon objectives, criterion-referenced evaluation has unquestioned content validity and accountability.

Several metrics and procedures are available for summarizing criterion-related progress, including (1) number of criteria mastered, (2) percent mastery of curricular objectives, (3) goal attainment scaling, and (4) the Curricular Efficiency Index (CEI).

Number of Objectives Achieved

A simple yet important kind of information is the total number of curricular objectives reached by each child. These totals can be summed across children to yield a group total. Totals can also be summed for each curricular domain. Most curricula include ways to check off mastery and record totals for each domain and across domains.

Percent Objectives Achieved

Absolute number of achieved objectives does not include any imperative information. Most teachers wish to know where a child is in the program curriculum at entry. Again, many curricula include ways to probe approximate levels of mastery at the onset of the program. A percentage can be computed with the estimated number of objectives already attained over the total number of objectives within the curriculum appropriate to that child's age. A 4-year-old may show uneven mastery across domains or, in the case of general developmental delay, an even profile. At Time 2, a percentage can again be calculated that will reveal actual progress compared with possible progress.

Goal Attainment Scaling

The Goal Attainment Scaling (GAS; Kiresuk, Smith, & Cardillo, 1994) technique has predominantly been used in adult programs but offers strong advantages for early intervention evaluation (Simeonsson, Huntington, & Short, 1982). Essentially, it involves identification of individual child goals and the specification of five levels of possible attainment for each along a continuum of worst to best or minimal to maximum outcomes. This is akin to task analysis or instructional analysis procedures of describing performance progress wherein, for example, the behavior occurs but only with maximum prompting and support, then with reduced support, and so forth. until it is performed independently under typical circumstances. A progression or scale is thus constructed and attainment can be tracked along the scale. With GAS, however, progress toward individualized goals can be compared across children and programs. The technique also includes the option of differentially weighting the goals to reflect presumed importance or difficulty. The weights are determined by clinical judgment and should probably be determined in concert with parents.

GAS scores can be derived at any time during intervention. Child attainment can be compared between Time 1 and Time 2. Also, attainment might be compared with predicted outcomes.

GAS combines the advantages of intervention-based goal planning and normative measurement. A standardized score is computed, with a mean of 50 and SD of 10. The GAS score is calculated by use of a formula. Because they are transformed, GAS scores are comparable across children, goals, and programs. In this sense, the technique combines features of normative and curriculum-based assessment.

Consider the display of a goal attainment scale for a preschooler (Figure 12.1). The attainment of the child can be compared with initial attainment level and with levels at later times.

Curricular Efficiency Index

The CEI is a convenient way to summarize the curricular progress of children based upon the curriculum content itself. The CEI makes applied use of discrete objectives within age ranges of the developmental curriculum as an index of functional skill attainment. The CEI can be used with individual or group data but uses curriculum-based objectives (raw scores) rather than norm-referenced standard scores or age scores.

In its simplest form for summarizing group progress, the formula for CEI is

$$CEI = \frac{\text{Mean number of curricular objectives achieved by all children}}{\text{Months in the program}}$$

(The numerator refers to the total number of objectives achieved by all children divided by the number of children.) Use of this simple formula will yield a value that shows the average number of objectives attained per month by a group. But in the simple form, the CEI does not compare progress with what *could* or *should* be achieved—to do this, some standard for comparison must be used. The curricular progress of preschoolers with special needs can be compared against two standards: (1) the expected (typical) achievement of curricular goals as indicated in the curriculum; and (2) the progress of same-age peers using the same curriculum and preferably enrolled in the same inclusive program (a local norm).

The first standard—normal expectation as structured by the curriculum—refers to the use of the number of objectives available within an age range in the curriculum employed. If there are 40 motor objectives expected of 4-

Scale attainment levels	Scale 1: Expresses, communicates (w1 = 5)	Scale 2: Social orientation (w2 = 2)	Scale 3: Attention span (w3 = 3)	Scale 4: Play behavior (w4 = 4)	Scale 5: Frustration response (w5 = 3)
−2 Most unfavorable treatment outcome thought likely	Communicates needs/wants by use of upper extremities, reaches for/pushes away with hands (I)	Turns away from social approach, no response to persons present (I)	Attends to tasks for less than 30 sec. (I)	Plays with toy/object less than 30 sec., throws it when finished (I)	Gives up if only slightly frustrated, 1 or 2 attempts, cries if pushed. (I)
−1 Less than expected success with treatment	Will have command of 10 signs, difficult to elicit	Intermittent response to social approach and persons present less than half the time	Attends to tasks for 1 min. if receives reward and social reinforcement	Plays with toy/object for 30 sec., puts down when finished half of time (A)	Gives up if only slightly frustrated, will try again if pushed without crying
0 Expected level of treatment success	Will have command of 10 signs and will use them when reminded	Consistently responds to social approach, shows awareness of others present less than half of time (A)	Attends to task for 1 min. when receives much social reinforcement (A)	Plays with toy/object for 30 sec., puts down when finished 100% of time	Gives up only after several attempts (5–6) (A)
1 More than expected success with treatment	Will have command of 10 signs and use them consistently whenever appropriate (A)	Consistently responds to social approach and shows appropriate awareness of others present	Attends to task for 1 min. with little or no reinforcement needed	Plays with toys/object for up to 1 min.	Will persist through a good number of tries (8–10) before giving up
2 Best anticipated success with treatment	Will have command of and consistently use 15–20 signs	Consistently responds to social approach, initiates social interaction with familiar others	Attends to task for as long as is appropriate in situation, switches to new task as presented	Plays with toys/object for as long as 3 min.	Will use varied and imaginative ways to achieve the end before giving up

w = weights; I = initial performance; A = attained level.

FIGURE 12.1. Example of a goal-attainment scale. From Simeonsson, Huntington, and Short (1982). Copyright 1982 by PRO-ED. Reprinted by permission.

271

year-olds within a year of development, then that figure may be used to divide into the average number of motor objectives achieved within a year by program children. Thus, if the group average for the year in motor development were 30 objectives, this number divided by 40 would produce an index of .75 or a rate of 75% expected by the curriculum developers. This sort of comparison can be done within each domain as well as with the total across the entire curriculum. Use of the CEI in this way presumes *full-year programming*, since the objectives included in most developmental curricula are based on a full year of development. When the program is less than a year, the normally expected number of objectives can be adjusted. A 6-month program, for example, could not expect even normally developing youngsters to master a full developmental year of objectives.

Use this CEI formula to compare the actual with expected curricular attainment by a group:

$$CEI = \frac{\text{Mean number of objectives attained by an individual child or group}}{\text{Number of objectives expected within a 12-month span on the curriculum}}$$

It is best to employ the above CEI formula in a summative fashion, near the end of a program cycle. The information generated can be informative to staff, parents, and related agencies. A total CEI should be calculated to summarize overall curricular progress. This total CEI is in addition to separate CEIs for each curricular domain.

Cross-domain comparison is especially important when the mission is to encourage balanced, "whole child" development. It is true, of course, that participating children may have special difficulties with certain developmental domains (e.g., language), but a low comparative CEI should alert staff to bolster efforts in that domain.

The second CEI standard for comparison uses a kind of "local norm" and offers information on the relative progress of preschoolers with special needs versus peers (combined typically developing and delayed) within a program. This CEI is best used for evaluation within inclusive programs where group comparisons are feasible and representative. It is often the case, for instance in Head Start, that inclusive programs may include five or six special needs youngsters within a total group of about 20 children.

Using a local norm group—the child's classroom peers—the formula for the CEI is

$$CEI = \frac{\text{Mean number of objectives attained by individual child}}{\text{Mean number of objectives attained by peers in local classroom}}$$

Comparing progress with an "in-house norm" has distinct advantages since many variables are held constant (i.e., same curriculum, room, teacher). However, the "normalcy" of the peers and other factors may limit interpretation of relative attainment.

Table 12.4 demonstrates curricular progress and goal attainment for an 18-month-old toddler with cerebral palsy on the Carolina Curriculum for Infants with Special Needs (Johnson-Martin & Attermier, 2004). Note that her Intervention Efficiency Index (IEI), CEI, and developmental quotient (DQ) all capture her substantial gains during 12 months of early intervention services; both her IEI and CEI document a progress profile that is within the low average to average range during her 12-month period of intervention. This rate shows significant progress beyond her rate at entry into the program (DQ = 63). The following calculations show progress on these indexes discussed in previous sections (see page 275 for description of IEI).

- Developmental Rate (DQ) = T1= 11.3/18= 63%

- Developmental Rate (DQ) = T2= 22.6/30= 75%

- IEI = $\dfrac{22.6 - 11.3 = 11.3 \text{ months}}{12.0 \text{ months}}$
  IEI = .94 × 100 = 94%

- CEI = $\dfrac{8 \text{ actual goals achieved}}{9 \text{ expected goals}}$
  CEI = .88 × 100= 88%

TABLE 12.4. Illustration of the Curricular Efficiency Index for an 18-Month-old Toddler with Cerebral Palsy on the Carolina Curriculum Assessment Log and Developmental Progress Chart

Age	Curriculum sequences: Imitation–sound and gestures	Date 1 (CA = 18)	Date 2 (CA = 30)
3 mo	Uses consistent signals for hunger, distress	2	2
	Vocalizes 5+ sounds	2	2
	Laughs	2	2
6 mo	Vocalizes 3+ feelings	1	2
9 mo	Vocalizes repetitive combos	1	2
15 mo	Uses 3+ words/signs to label	0	2
18 mo	Says/signs "No," with meaning	0	2
	Uses 7+ words/signs to label	0	1
24 mo	Uses 15+ words/signs to label	0	1
	Developmental age scoring =	11.3 mo (8 × 1.41)	22.6 mo (16 × 1.41)

Note. CA = chronological age.

Norm-Based Applied Metrics

When program evaluators use norm-referenced scores, they have the advantage of being able to note Time 1–Time 2 changes in the position of enrolled children relative to a norm group. Since normative scores are corrected for chronological age, increases in a child's normative position show that he or she is more than keeping up with the norm group. Four types of comparative scores are widely used: developmental age (DA), ratio DQ, percentile (or percentile rank), and standard scores (or deviation scores, including T-scores, z-scores, and normal curve equivalents).

Developmental Age

A DA is the average age at which 50% of children in the norm or standardization group attained a given raw score. The attraction of this score type is its ease of interpretation (e.g., a 3-year-old child's motor performance is like that of a 4-year-old in the norm group). "He's acting like a 2-year-old child" is understood by parents and is much more appreciated by them than statistics and confidence intervals. However, for evaluation reports, the reader should be cautioned against stretching the interpretation of changes in DA since developmental age increments are not of equal intervals and cannot be mathematically manipulated as would an equal interval scale.

Developmental Quotient

Like the old ratio IQ formula, DQ is obtained by dividing a child's DA by his CA (chronological age) and multiplying by 100. A child who is maintaining a "normal" status will obtain a DQ of 100. But as with IQ ([MA/CA] × 100), there are limits to the interpretation of DQs when averaged across children or in comparing them pre– and posttest.

Again, because of unequal intervals, a child who shows a DQ of 50 cannot be said to be developing at only half the normal rate. A change from a DQ of 80 to 120 cannot be interpreted as a 50 percent increase in rate. However, in the absence of a normative standard score for young children with disabilities, the ratio DQ used as a an applied or "clinical" metric provides a relatively accurate and communicable estimate of status and progress. The ratio DQ functions as a type of "rate of development indicator" and can be used most often with curriculum-based measures that do not have norms but which do derive developmental age levels. Nevertheless, despite its technical limitations, like DA, the ratio DQ is understood by most parents and should be considered for reporting except where more accurate and formal interpretations are needed.

Percentiles

Like DA, percentiles are not based on equal intervals. Movement from a 50th to 60th percentile, for example, requires a smaller raw score increase than one near the end of a distribution, for example, from the 80th to 90th percentile. Thus, as with DQ, a doubling of percentile rank cannot be interpreted as "twice as good" since interpretation is distorted by the unequal interval nature of the ranks. However, like DQ, percentile rankings are easily communicated and carry useful meaning.

Deviation Standard Scores

Norm-based instruments use the standard score (SS) derived from the national standardization sample to interpret performance. A standard score has mean and standard deviations that are the same across age groups, usually a mean of 100 and *SD* of 15. Score distributions and increments are adjusted to fit the properties of a normal curve; this permits comparative interpretation. An SS of –1 *SD* would mean performance that is equal to or exceeded by 85% of the normally distributed scores. Because they are scores that have been transferred to normal curve equivalents, standard scores can be compared from Time 1 to Time 2 and can be used to evaluate progress even when different measures are used.

Intervention Efficiency Index

The IEI (Bagnato & Neisworth, 1980) is an applied metric used to express gains in developmental competencies during the time of participation in the program. The IEI makes applied use of developmental months gain within a sequential period of intervention as an index of progress associated with the program. Thus, the IEI functions as a general estimate of rate of developmental progress as a function of intervention. The IEI is computed as follows with an example:

$$\frac{\text{Developmental age gain in months (DA2 – DA1)}}{\text{Time in program (expressed in months)}}$$

$$\frac{\text{DA2 – DA1}}{\text{Time in intervention}} \times 100$$

30 months – 15 months = 15 months/12 months = 1.25

IEI = 125%

Time in program is usually expressed in months, producing an index of gain per month of participation. For example, a typical or theoretical "average" rate of progress would be 1 month of gain for each month of program participation. Thus, the child with a delay who shows 24 months of progress in a 12-month period would be demonstrating an IEI of 2.00 (2 months gain for each month in the program) or double the expected rate (200%). For purposes of program evaluation, a child's absolute gain must be interpreted with respect to time in program. As with other indices of changes, a number of problems are associated with the IEI if it is viewed as being a pure measure of program impact. The child's rate of development at program entry, the assumption of developmental rate constancy while in a program, and other issues limit the IEI for more exacting purposes. However, the IEI is a way to evaluate *gains relative to duration of program participation*. It is a practical way to summarize children's progress while in (but not necessarily due to) an early intervention program. An overall IEI can be computed as well as separate IEIs for each developmental domain (e.g., cognitive, language, social, motor, self-care). When children evidence quite different IEIs within the same program, it is possible that the program is differentially effective for different types of disabilities; this may produce implications for increased service intensity or other program adjustments.

Expected–Actual Progress Solution: Gain Exceeding Maturation

In most instances, natural community experiments involving innovative early childhood intervention programs do not use the presumed "gold standard," a randomized experimental control group design. Instead, programs rely on a repeated-measures approach in the program that enrolls all children. Thus, since no control group is possible (or desired, due to ethical concerns about exclusion from reasonably beneficial opportunities), researchers need a way to estimate program or intervention "effects."

Perhaps one of the most innovative solutions to this dilemma is the combination of curricular and norm-referenced metrics buttressed by statistical analyses in order to document the extent to which individual and group progress exceeds maturational expectations. Bagnato and colleagues (2002) adapted and improved a metric by McCall, Ryan, and Green (1999), the "constructed comparison group," to estimate the extent to which each child outpaces maturational expectations in early childhood intervention studies. The Expected–Actual Progress Solution (EAPS; Bagnato, Suen, & Sangha, 2006) charts expected developmental trajectories or longitudinal developmental progress curves on children in large databases.

Within the Heinz Pennsylvania Early Childhood Initiative (ECI; Bagnato et al., 2002), infants, toddlers, and preschoolers were continuously enrolling for early care and education and support services over a 6-year period of time. Capitalizing on this natural phenomenon, researchers and program staff trained teachers to conduct authentic assessments on all children during the first 1–2 weeks after they entered each of the 25 neighborhood ECI programs. These entry-level assessments formed the baseline on mean DOCS raw scores for all entering 6-month-olds, 1-year-olds, 2-year-olds, 3-year-olds, 4-year-olds, and 5-year-olds. Thus, the EAPS used these entry or baseline assessments to form an "expected" developmental growth curve encompassing children of all ages (see Figure 12.2). Theoretically, these levels are unaffected by intervention since they were gathered before specific program participation began. Therefore, the expected developmental growth curve outlines the progress trajectory that would be expected for this group of nearly 1,000 preschoolers who were raised in poverty without benefit of high-quality program involvements up to that point. Then, future progress assessments can be compared to this local norm or "constructed comparison group." The comparison then enables researchers to control for age-related effects and to estimate the amount of progress attributable to intervention beyond maturation. The EAPS establishes preintervention attainment levels on children at each age point from 1 year to 6 years based on their assessment levels at program entrance. Only raw score data is used in the EAPS calculations. Raw scores on, for example the DOCS, provide greater item precision, and a wider range of variability through smaller increments of gain can be detected. Moreover, it is arguable that with atypical samples of children, strict comparisons to the norm group are not justified and use of standard scores merely standardizes performances that children with delays cannot meet.

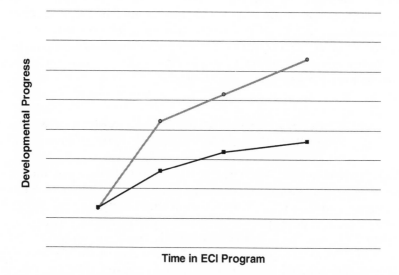

FIGURE 12.2. Impact of ECI on child developmental progress exceeding maturational expectations: theoretical scheme.

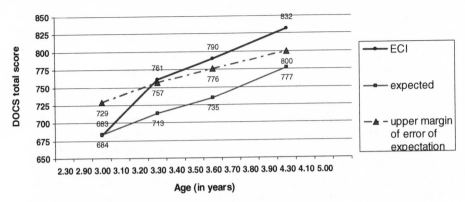

FIGURE 12.3. Statistical impact of ECI program participation on child developmental progress for 843 high-risk children: Expected–Actual Progress Solution (EAPS). Regression formula for the EAPS: Predicted DOCS raw score = –163.18 + 1.286 (Age) – 0.000437 (Age)2 (Bagnato et al., 2002).

Figure 12.2 presents the schematic that illustrates how an expected–actual developmental growth curve is constructed. Figure 12.3 shows the resulting EAPS for ECI based on a regression formula. Note that the graph plots both the expected trajectory and the actual performance pattern on the average raw scores of the DOCS for the children who have participated in ECI. In addition, the 95% confidence interval is plotted between the expected and actual performance curves. Developmental progress levels above the 95% confidence interval indicate that the children in ECI demonstrated developmental skill attainments that outpaced maturational expectations. This regression equation controls for age and thus defines progress that outpaces maturation. ECI was effective in promoting developmental progress for the children who participated.

HOW DOES AUTHENTIC PROGRAM EVALUATION RESEARCH WORK "IN ACTION"?: THE PAPII

The Commonwealth of Pennsylvania, Department of Education, Bureau of Special Education, instituted a model program to encourage and document the impact and success of an inclusion initiative for young children with mild to moderate developmental delays in early childhood programs operated by 23 school districts. The Pennsylvania Preschool Integration Initiative (PAPII) enrolled approximately 2,000 children. I use the results of PAPII to illustrate various program evaluation research strategies that can portray outcomes in early intervention programs.

The program evaluation research measures selected for PAPII examine various issues, from the differential rates of curricular progress within various developmental domains to concerns about reductions in parent-identified levels of family stress, to changes in the "intensity" of amount of specialized effort program staff exerts for special needs children. Matched with these issues and indicators are examples of relevant measures and metrics that will help to answer pertinent administrative questions and concerns to guide ongoing program review and necessary changes in program practices. *Program evaluation is an important check-and-balance, quality assurance operation.* Program evaluation answers larger questions about changes in groups of children and parents as well as general changes in the physical and social environment and procedures of the program itself as it attempts to address child and family needs. Well-conceived program evaluation methods can begin to answer questions about the efficacy of the program and its practices (i.e., the expertise and hard work of its staff).

This final section offers a brief illustration of the contents and results of the evaluation of an integrated preschool program. Tables 12.5–12.8 address four major direct service and administrative issues: the curricular progress of enrolled children, reductions in child social behavior problems, reductions in the stress levels of parents and families, and changes in the amount and intensity of services provided to children by the early intervention staff.

The illustrative preschool program enrolled 30 nondevelopmentally delayed (NDD) and 25 developmentally delayed (DD) children (average chronological age at program entry = 57 months) within five integrated

TABLE 12.5. Curricular Progress of PAPII Children on the Battelle Developmental Inventory during 7 Months of Participation in an Inclusive Preschool Program

	NDD					DD				
Domain	DA1	DQ1	DA2	DQ2	IEI	DA1	DQ1	DA2	DQ2	IEI
Self-Regulation	42	74	51	80	1.29	36	62	45	69	1.29
Personal–Social	49	86	59	92	1.43	43	74	51	78	1.14
Adaptive	49	86	55	86	0.86	46	79	49	75	0.43
Gross Motor	49	86	55	86	0.86	46	79	49	75	0.43
Fine Motor	46	81	56	88	1.43	41	71	51	78	1.43
Motor	48	84	55	86	1.00	42	72	50	77	1.14
Receptive Language	50	88	62	97	1.71	39	67	56	86	2.43
Expressive Language	45	79	56	88	1.29	35	60	45	69	1.43
Communication	45	39	51	80	0.86	35	60	45	69	1.43
Cognitive	51	89	61	95	1.43	42	72	51	78	1.43
Total Development	47.2	82.8	56.2	88	1.26	39.8	68.6	49.2	75.4	1.33

Note. NDD = Nondevelopmentally delayed; DD = Developmentally delayed; DA = Developmental age; DQ = Developmental quotient or ratio; IEI = Intervention Efficiency Index.

classrooms (approximately 11 children per classroom). The program evaluation effort was conducted over a 7-month period of intervention. Child, family, and program ecology components were targeted for evaluation. The program evaluation included convergent information to demonstrate that children and families benefitted substantially from program participation. Table 12.5 shows that NDD and DD children benefitted equally from the program. In fact, curricular progress data suggest that some children classified as NDD actually showed evidence of being at risk for developmental difficulties at program entry in personal–social skills and expressive language skills. The DD group showed notable gains in all domains with measurable increases in personal–social, fine motor, communication, and cognitive/conceptual skills. Both groups showed accelerated rates of progress during the 7-month intervention period (IEI rates on total development = 1.26 and 1.3, respectively).

Similar beneficial changes in child social behavior were evident also (see Table 12.6). The group of NDD children showed no clinically significant behavior problems compared to same-age peers; some concern, however, was initially expressed by teachers and parents concerning the anxious behaviors. Preschoolers in the DD group showed reductions in observed levels of anxiety and general behavior problems. Evidence of hyperactive and distractible behavior remained after 7 months of intervention. This most probably reflected the continuing developmental immaturity of the children and the need for the program to continually emphasize prerequisite behaviors in the IEP and IFSP goals.

Parents reported significant changes in how they viewed themselves and their family's ability to cope after participating in parent support groups, behavior management counseling, and classroom participation with their children (see Table 12.7). Some parents of NDD children participated also. Stress levels for DD parents dropped substantially from 84% to 59% during the intervention period.

TABLE 12.6. Reductions in Child Social Behavior Problems on the Preschool and Kindergarten Behavior Scale after 7 Months of Inclusive Preschool Programming

| | NDD | | | | DD | | | |
| | Pre | | Post | | Pre | | Post | |
Factor	Teacher	Parent	Teacher	Parent	Teacher	Parent	Teacher	Parent
Antisocial/Aggressive	50	70	50	70	80	81	70	81
Anxiety/Somatic	65	80	65	80	92[a]	87	80	88
Attention/Overactive	40	46	40	44	90[a]	75	90[a]	71
Total Behavior	40	70	30	60	90[a]	84	80	84

[a]90th percentile or above = elicited cutoff for clinical behavior problems.

TABLE 12.7. Reductions in Parent/Family Stress Levels
on the Parenting Stress Index during Program Participation

Factor	NDD group parents		DD group parents	
	Pre (%ile)	Post (%ile)	Pre (% ile)	Post (%ile)
Child Stress	20	22	86	61
Parent Stress	38	31	92	62
Total Stress	30	30	84	59
Life Stress	41	38	91	60

Finally, staff and administrators, in reviewing the 7-month intervention period and planning allocation of staff and resources for the following year, were interested in overall changes in the level of intensity of program support services. These included such factors as hours of speech–language and occupational therapy services, the number of children transitioning into diagnostic or regular kindergarten settings, the number of children diagnosed with specific developmental disabilities, the types of adaptive technology (e.g., computers, communication systems, microswitch toys) needed for children, and the number of children needing medical consultation. Table 12.8 outlines the changes in program intensity on the SPECS system that incorporate these considerations. In general, DD children show substantially fewer program intensity needs in several areas including specialized early education services, occupational therapy, hearing services, and transition services.

With these data, program administrators and staff can plan for next year and alter the program to continue its fine record of effective service delivery to children and families.

TABLE 12.8. Changes in the Intensity of Needed Program Services
on the Program Specifications (P-Specs) Scale over a 7-Month Period
of Intervention

Program option	Program intensity levels			
	NDD		DD	
	Pre (%)	Post (%)	Pre (%)	Post (%)
Early education	10	5	60	45
Adaptive services	0	0	30	25
Behavior therapy	20	15	65	45
Speech–language therapy	20	10	75	50
Physical therapy	0	0	35	20
Occupational therapy	0	0	65	40
Vision services	0	0	25	5
Hearing services	5	5	45	15
Medical services	0	0	10	5
Transition services	5	5	70	50

BEST-PRACTICE GUIDEPOINTS

♦ Choose a core curriculum as a uniform roadmap for measuring child status and progress.

♦ Choose complementary measures of child, program, and family/parent attributes that will document program impact.

♦ Base choice of measures on factors related to program missions, expected outcomes/standards, and types of children participating.

♦ Train teachers, staff, and parents as reliable and valid observers and assessors of children.

♦ Set practical time points for ongoing assessments.

♦ Invest in an MIS that will enable the responsive profiling and analysis of child and program outcomes.

BEST-PRACTICE EVIDENCE

Abidin, R. R. (1983). *Parenting Stress Index, Third Edition.* Simi Valley, CA: Psychological Publications.

Arnett, J. (1989). Caregivers in day-care centers: Does training matter? *Journal of Applied Behavioral Psychology, 10*(4), 541–552.

Arnett, J. (1989a). *Caregiver Interaction Scale.* Unpublished. Retrieved on January 10, 2007 from http://www.mschildcare.org/resources/caregiverinteractionscale.html.

Bagnato, S. J., Grom, R., & Haynes, L. (2004). Alternative designs for community-based research: Pittsburgh's Early Childhood Initiative (ECI). *Evaluation Exchange, 9*(3), 6–8.

Bagnato, S. J., & Neisworth, J. T. (1980). Intervention efficiency index (IEI): An approach to preschool program accountability. *Exceptional Children 46*(4), 264–269.

Bagnato, S. J., & Neisworth, J. T. (1990). *The System to Plan Early Childhood Services (SPECS).* Circle Pines, MN: American Guidance Service.

Bagnato, S. J., Suen, H., Brickley, D., Smith-Jones, J., & Dettore, E. (2002). Child developmental impact of Pittsburgh's Early Childhood Initiative (ECI) in high-risk communities: First-phase authentic evaluation research. *Early Childhood Research Quarterly, 17*(4), 559–589.

Bagnato, S. J., Suen, H., & Sangha, A. (2006). *The Expected–Actual Progress Solution: Creating a constructed comparison group to control for maturation in early childhood intervention studies.* Unpublished manuscript.

Bailey, D. E., & Simmeonsson, R. J. (1988). *Family Needs Survey.* Frank Porter Graham Child Development Center, University of North Carolina

Bricker, D. (2002). *AEPS: Assessment, Evaluation, and Programming System for Infants and Young Children* (2nd ed.). Baltimore: Brookes.

Caldwell, B. M., & Bradley, R. H. (1984). *Home observation for measurement of the environment.* Little Rock: University of Arkansas.

Fox, R. A. (1994). *Parent Behavior Checklist.* Formerly published by PRO-ED, Austin,TX. Currently available from the author (Robert.fox@marquette.edu).

Gilliam, W. S., & Leiter, V. (2003). Evaluating early childhood programs: Improving quality and informing policy. *Zero to Three, 23*(6), 6–13.

Harms, T., Clifford, R. M., & Cryer, D. (1998). *Early Childhood Environment Rating Scale—Revised.* New York: Teachers College Press.

Harrison, P., & Oakland, T. (2003). *Adaptive Behavior Assessment System, Second Edition.* San Antonio, TX: The Psychological Corporation.

Hresko, W. P., Miguel, S. A., Sherbenou, R. J., & Burton, S. D. (1984). *Developmental Observation Checklist System.* Austin, TX: PRO-ED.

Jason, L., Keys, C., Suarex-Balcazar, Y., Taylor, R., & Davis, M. (2004). *Participatory community research: Theories and methods in action.* Washington, DC: American Psychological Association.

Kiresuk, T. J., Smith, A., & Cardillo, J. E. (1994). *Goal attainment scaling: Applications, theory, and measurement.* Hillsdale, NJ: Erlbaum.

McCall, R. B., Ryan, C. S., & Green, B. L. (1999). Some non-randomized constructed comparison groups for evaluating age-related outcomes of intervention programs. *American Journal of Evaluation, 2*(20), 213–226.

Reynolds, A. J. (2004). Research on early childhood interventions in the confirmatory mode. *Children and Youth Services Review, 26*(1), 15–38.

Simeonsson, R. J., Huntington, G., & Short, R. (1982). Individual differences and goals: An approach to the evaluation of child progress. *Topics in Early Childhood Special Education, 1*(4), 71–80.

Yoshikawa, H., Rosman, E., & Hsueh, J. (2002). Resolving paradoxical criteria for the expansion and replication of early childhood care and education programs. *Early Childhood Research Quarterly, 17*(1), 3–27.

Synopsis and Conclusions
What Are the Essential Best-Practice Guidepoints for Authentic Assessment of Preschool Children?

◆

Chapter 1. What Are the Professional Standards for Assessment for Preschool Children?

The early childhood fields have championed competencies for teachers and other interdisciplinary professionals in "best practices" for the care and teaching of all young children. Developmentally appropriate measurement—authentic assessment—of young children is a core professional practice. The standards reflect the unique needs of young children, particularly those who are at developmental risk or have developmental delays or disabilities. The standards reflect the unique qualities of effective early childhood intervention programs. Assessment is one of the foundations for effective and high-quality programs for young children.

Essential Guidepoints

- Professionals and families collaborate in planning and implementing assessment.
- Assessment is individualized and appropriate for the child and family.
- Assessment provides useful information for intervention.
- Professionals share information in respectful and useful ways.
- Professionals meet legal and procedural requirements and meet recommended practice guidelines.

Chapter 2. How Can Authentic Assessment Prevent the Mismeasure of Young Children?

Authentic assessment is the developmentally appropriate alternative to conventional tests and testing practices. Conventional testing and its requirements are misaligned with typical early childhood behavior and are divorced from the child's natural developmental ecology: conventional testing is decontextualized. In contrast, authentic assessment relies on the structured observations of familiar caregivers in the child's life to collect ongoing information about real-life skills captured in real-life settings. Authentic assessment complements young children and their programs best; authentic assessment represents early childhood best. "Misrepresenting children by mis-measuring them denies children their rights to beneficial expectations and opportunities" (Neisworth & Bagnato, 2004, p. 198).

Essential Guidepoints

- Eliminate tabletop testing procedures with contrived test kits.
- Use authentic assessment methods and procedures to accomplish all early childhood intervention purposes, including eligibility determination.
- Share assessment responsibilities with a team of parents/caregivers and professionals working together.
- Orchestrate assessments across several people, places, and times rather than one session.
- Select a common curriculum-based instrument to unify interdisciplinary and interagency teamwork within and between programs.
- Select instruments that have some "universal" attributes and can sensitively monitor child progress. Incorporate portable, computer-based technologies to make assessments more natural, efficient, and practical.

Chapter 3. What Are the Foundations for Authentic Assessment of Typical and Atypical Early Development?

Early childhood professionals must have a basic and applied understanding of early child development. They must be able to simultaneously experience and observe how the child's interaction with toys and people in daily activities provides evidence of various levels of competency, and use these observations in problem solving; this understanding must become nearly "intuitive" based upon a practical knowledge of stages of typical and atypical development.

Essential Guidepoints

- Use a Piagetian framework to observe and understand developmental stages and progressions for all children.
- Analyze and use a comprehensive developmental curriculum to operationalize the stages of early development.
- Use a sequenced developmental curriculum to document observations about typical and atypical developmental progressions.

Chapter 4. What Are the Best Contexts for Authentic Assessment?

Natural settings and routines in the home, preschool, and community are the real-life contexts for authentic assessment. The continuum of measurement contexts enables early childhood professionals to choose the best contexts and associated arrangements to observe the child's optimal skills. While observations of naturally occurring skills are preferred, many children, especially those with mild to severe developmental disabilities, require "analogue" contexts in order to fully sample their capabilities. Professionals can "set the stage" for a fully representative sample of behavior by helping the child to display competencies through the best choice of toys, settings, arrangements, and interactions.

Analogue Contexts for Typical Preschoolers

- Desensitize fears.
- Expect inattention.
- Reduce distractions.
- Give simple, active directions.
- Use real toys.
- Use child-sized furniture.
- Work and play together.
- Alternate easy and difficult tasks.
- Ensure multiple sessions and times.
- Model, prompt, and reward new behaviors.

Analogue Contexts for Preschoolers at Risk and with Mild Delays

- Rearrange natural home and preschool settings.
- Provide extra structure with toys and activities.
- Emphasize optimal positioning.
- Play but be in charge.
- Acquaint child with peers and adults first.

- Include parents and favorite toys and games.
- Maintain a reassuring and positive manner.
- Allow breaks.
- Reward through praise and favorite activities.
- Alternate work and play.
- Use active, concrete directions.
- Model prerequisite behaviors.
- Set limits as needed

Analogue Contexts for Preschoolers with Moderate and Severe Disabilities

Sensory Impairments
- Appraise vision and hearing.
- Consult with specialists.
- Use multisensory materials and methods.
- Exaggerate gestures, expressions, and voice.
- Use universally designed content and disability-specific norms

Developmental Retardation
- Limit stereotypical behaviors.
- Use response-contingent toys.
- Emphasize social interactions.

Neuromotor Impairments
- Team with PT/OT, teacher, and parent.
- Stress individual positioning.
- Use adaptive equipment and accommodations.
- Discover best response modes.

Affective/Behavior Disorders
- Use a formal observational protocol.
- Limit self-stimulatory behaviors.
- Emphasize nonverbal and reciprocal tasks.
- Appraise parent–child and child–peer social interactions.

Chapter 5. Can Professionals "Test without Tests" for Authentic Assessment?

People are walking and talking assessment instruments—observers of child behavior. With training, mentoring, and the right tools, early childhood professionals and parents can become reliable and valid observers and assessors of children's capabilities. At its most basic level, authentic assessment is a process of "testing without tests" by "shopping for skills." Developmental observation schedules contain sequences of naturally occurring skills that structure the observations of professionals and parents; with such observation formats, they can be attuned to observing and recording everyday functional competencies—the everyday "intelligent behavior" of young children during their typical work and play.

Essential Guidepoints

- Recognize that instances of intelligent behavior or problem solving (e.g., finding the correct toy at the bottom of the toy box, steering a shopping cart around obstacles, getting objects out of reach) can be readily observed and recorded in natural daily routines instead of in contrived test tasks.
- Be sensible in grouping competencies that can be observed in certain settings to increase ease and efficiency.
- Engage parents in the gathering of authentic performance information about their children in daily routines at home.
- Establish analogue, but natural situations within the home or classroom using typical toys and objects and peer pairings in which hard-to-observe and inconsistent behaviors can be prompted or occasioned.

Chapter 6. How Does Authentic Curriculum-Based Assessment Work?

Successful early childhood intervention programs use developmental curricula as their roadmaps for teaching and caring for children. Increasingly, publishers are producing developmental curricula that include technically adequate developmental observation schedules (curriculum-embedded); compatible measures—many with national norms—are available that link with such curricula (curriculum-referenced). Both types of measures rely on authentic assessment procedures. Professionals in successful programs must be well versed in the choice and ongoing use of authentic curriculum-based measures for the benefit of their children and their programs.

Essential Guidepoints

- Select appropriate curricula and scales by developmental age; severity of disability; program characteristics; age and domain coverage; parent involvement; focus on inclusion; progress evaluation elements; and field-derived evidence base.
- Structure parent–professional collaboration with curriculum-based assessment.
- Map a child's individual program with a developmental curriculum.

- Focus on *functional goals* within multiple developmental domains.
- Evaluate the developmental sequences and functional skill hierarchies.
- Monitor skills acquisition regularly during intervention.
- Evaluate overall progress in multiple domains by comparing beginning-of-year and end-of-year levels of attainment.

Chapter 7. Can Clinical Judgments Guide Parent–Professional Team Decision-Making for Early Intervention?

Parents and professionals make "clinical" or informed judgments repeatedly about their children; they are both unavoidable and valuable. With structure, informed opinions can help early childhood teams to make accurate, collaborative, and beneficial decisions about the functional capabilities and programmatic needs of children, particularly those with atypical development and behavior.

Essential Guidepoints

- Use clinical judgment systems to detect capabilities in children that are inconsistent or low threshold in their expression.
- Rely upon clinical judgment systems to unify and facilitate parent–professional team decisions about child characteristics and specific programmatic and intervention needs.
- *Operationally define* the attributes to be judged.
- Use *rating formats* to guide and structure how specific attributes are classified by various people.
- Select exemplary *clinical judgment scales* to standardize the decision making.
- Ensure that individuals providing clinical judgments have undergone *training* in the use of the clinical judgment instrument and decision-making process.
- Generate *consensus decision making* via a structured process of resolving differences in clinical judgments and reaching agreement on child/family needs.

Chapter 8. How Can We Effectively Assess for Severe Disabilities?

Young children with severe disabilities and atypical behavior present unique challenges for early childhood specialists. Many young children with severe impairments are still described by psychologists and others as *untestable.* No child is untestable; many professionals do not know how to assess properly for severe disabilities. Authentic and curriculum-based assessment procedures are available so that one can implement an integrated and linked approach to intervention based upon a functional approach.

Essential Guidepoints

- Use a functional and adaptive approach to assess the strengths and limitations of children with severe disabilities.
- Rely on both parents working together with specific professionals (e.g., physical therapist, speech–language pathologist) in a natural setting to best assess the child's functional competencies.
- Focus the assessment process on identifying functional goals and strategies for intervention.
- Emphasize an ecological assessment of the child's and family's environment as the core of best practices with severe disabilities.
- Implement a process of conducting frequent observational assessments based on sequential curricular competencies to document small increments of change in the child's behavior.

Chapter 9. How Can We Do Functional Behavioral Assessment with Preschoolers?

Many preschool children have challenging and unusual behaviors that require in-depth assessment of the environment and the child to determine the circumstances that are maintaining atypical behavior and inhibiting development. Functional behavioral assessment procedures can be tailored for the preschool child so that the child's strengths can be maximized.

Essential Guidepoints

- Recognize that challenging behavior (oppositional, stereotypical, self-abuse, etc.) is often amplified and maintained by the child's circumstances.
- Aspects of the child's setting can become "triggers" that set off undesirable behaviors.
- Research has helped us classify four main functions of challenging behavior: gaining attention, accessing tangible reinforcers, escaping from demands, and sensory self-stimulation.
- Functional behavior assessment procedures allow us to identify the triggers and consequences that support challenging behavior.
- The goal of a functional behavior assessment is to find the function of the unwanted behavior so that a developmentally appropriate

alternative can be taught—a socially acceptable behavior that serves the same function or purpose for the child.

Chapter 10. What Are Proper Approaches to Detect, Classify, and Intervene for Temperament and Self-Regulatory Behavior Problems in Young Children?

Young children are not adults; problems with young children's behavior must not be viewed from an adult perspective as a form of psychopathology or mental disease. The early childhood fields require more developmentally appropriate schemes for classifying social behavior difficulties so they are more amenable to effective intervention in natural settings. The concepts of extremes of temperament and problems in acquiring self-control skills are aligned with the philosophy and practices of the early childhood fields. Authentic assessment approaches for early temperament and self-regulation are available.

Essential Guidepoints

- Learn, understand, and apply the philosophy and principles of "services without labels" and developmentally appropriate practice when approaching the early problems in self-regulation embodied in the DC: 0–3.
- Use the TABS to qualify children for early intervention services and supports as well as behavioral support through wrap-around services.
- Resist efforts to apply psychopathological labels to infants, toddlers, and preschoolers before documenting their response to intervention.
- Use measures designed specifically to document the progressive acquisition of social skill and self-regulatory behaviors by children during participation in early childhood intervention programs.

Chapter 11. How Should We Forecast and Plan for Kindergarten Transition and Early School Success?

With the push for state and national standards and universal preschool to promote early school success, the transition to kindergarten has gained new prominence. Links between preschool and kindergarten curricula and expectations are being fostered. The transition to school must be systematic, collaborative, and supportive for the child, the parents, and the teachers. Early childhood professionals can work with their school colleagues to ensure a healthy transition that builds upon children's preschool successes.

Essential Guidepoints

- Develop a detailed, systemwide plan for the transition of children from early intervention to kindergarten/school-age programs.
- Conduct comprehensive assessments to obtain necessary information for eligibility determination and educational planning just prior to kindergarten.
- Include comprehensive information that is based on state/federal outcome benchmarks and teacher expectations.
- Emphasize performance information on social and behavioral competencies as much as information on cognitive and academic competencies.

Chapter 12. How Can Authentic Program Evaluation Document Early Childhood Intervention Outcomes?

Effective and successful early childhood intervention programs use ongoing measurement and evaluation research to improve their quality and practices. Authentic program evaluation enables early childhood professionals to integrate evaluation and research into everyday work routines. Effective programs can show clear evidence of their impact and outcomes for children and families.

Essential Guidepoints

- Choose a core curriculum as a uniform roadmap for measuring child status and progress.
- Choose complementary measures of child, program, and family/parent attributes that will document program impact.
- Base choice of measures on factors related to program missions, expected outcomes/standards, and types of children participating.
- Train teachers, staff, and parents as reliable and valid observers and assessors of children.
- Set practical timepoints for ongoing assessments.
- Invest in a management information system that will enable the responsive profiling and analysis of child and program outcomes.

Neisworth, J. T., & Bagnato, S. J. (2004). The mismeasure of young children: The authentic assessment alternative. *Infants and Young Children, 17*(3), 198–212.

APPENDIX A

♦ ♦ ♦

NAEYC's Code of Ethical Conduct

♦

The *NAEYC Code of Ethical Conduct* offers guidelines for responsible behavior and sets forth a common basis for resolving the principal ethical dilemmas encountered in early childhood care and education. The primary focus of the Code is on daily practice with children and their families in programs for children from birth through 8 years of age. The Code was initially developed by NAEYC and approved by the Governing Board in 1989. Revisions to the Code were adopted in 1992, 1997, and 2005.

The last revision process, leading to the 2005 version of the Code, resulted in the addition of new ideals and principles that primarily address issues regarding child assessment and accountability, as well as respect and support for diversity. **Ideals** (I) reflect exemplary practice (our aspirations), and **Principles** (P) describe practices that are required, prohibited, or permitted. The principles guide conduct and assist practitioners in resolving ethical dilemmas. Both ideals and principles are intended to direct practitioners to those questions that, when responsibly answered, can provide the basis for conscientious decision-making.

The ideals that reflect the field's ethical standing on child assessments include:

I-1.6—To use assessment instruments and strategies that are appropriate for the children to be assessed, that are used only for the purposes for which they were designed, and that have the potential to benefit children.

I-1.7—To use assessment information to understand and support children's development and learning, to support instruction, and to identify children who may need additional services.

I-4.5—To work to ensure that appropriate assessment systems, which include multiple sources of information, are used for purposes that benefit children.

The principles that reflect the field's ethical standing on child assessments include:

P-1.5—We shall use appropriate assessment systems, which include multiple sources of information, to provide information on children's learning and development.

P-1.6—We shall strive to ensure that decisions such as those related to enrollment, retention, or assignment to special education services, will be based on multiple sources of information and will never be based on a single assessment, such as a test score or a single observation.

P-2.6—As families share information with us about their children and families, we shall consider this information to plan and implement the program.

P-2.7—We shall inform families about the nature and purpose of the program's child assessments and how data about their child will be used.

P-2.8—We shall treat child assessment information confidentially and share this information only when there is a legitimate need for it.

P-4.5—We shall be knowledgeable about the appropriate use of assessment strategies and instruments and interpret results accurately to families.

NAEYC and NAECS/SDE Position Statement

Early Childhood Curriculum, Assessment, and Program Evaluation

BUILDING AN EFFECTIVE, ACCOUNTABLE SYSTEM IN PROGRAMS FOR CHILDREN BIRTH THROUGH AGE 8

A Joint Position Statement of the
National Association for the Education of Young Children (NAEYC) and the
National Association of Early Childhood Specialists in State Departments of Education (NAECS/SDE)

Introduction

High-quality early education produces long-lasting benefits. With this evidence, federal, state, and local decision makers are asking critical questions about young children's education. What should children be taught in the years from birth through age eight? How would we know if they are developing well and learning what we want them to learn? And how could we decide whether programs for children from infancy through the primary grades are doing a good job?

Answers to these questions—questions about *early childhood curriculum, child assessment, and program evaluation*—are the foundation of this joint position statement from the National Association for the Education of Young Children (NAEYC) and the National Association of Early Childhood Specialists in State Departments of Education (NAECS/SDE).

The Position

The National Association for the Education of Young Children and the National Association of Early Childhood Specialists in State Departments of Education take the position that policy makers, the early childhood profession, and other stakeholders in young children's lives have a shared responsibility to

• construct comprehensive systems of curriculum, assessment, and program evaluation guided by sound

early childhood practices, effective early learning standards and program standards, and a set of core principles and values: belief in civic and democratic values; commitment to ethical behavior on behalf of children; use of important goals as guides to action; coordinated systems; support for children as individuals and members of families, cultures, and communities; partnerships with families; respect for evidence; and shared accountability.

• implement curriculum that is thoughtfully planned, challenging, engaging, developmentally appropriate, culturally and linguistically responsive, comprehensive, and likely to promote positive outcomes for all young children.

• make ethical, appropriate, valid, and reliable assessment a central part of all early childhood programs. To assess young children's strengths, progress, and needs, use assessment methods that are developmentally appropriate, culturally and linguistically responsive, tied to children's daily activities, supported by professional development, inclusive of families, and connected to specific, beneficial purposes: (1) making sound decisions about teaching and learning, (2) identifying significant concerns that may require focused intervention for individual children, and (3) helping programs improve their educational and developmental interventions.

• regularly engage in program evaluation guided by program goals and using varied, appropriate, concep-

Adopted November 2003

tually and technically sound evidence to determine the extent to which programs meet the expected standards of quality and to examine intended as well as unintended results.

• provide the support, professional development, and other resources to allow staff in early childhood programs to implement high-quality curriculum, assessment, and program evaluation practices and to connect those practices with well-defined early learning standards and program standards.

Recommendations

Curriculum

Implement curriculum that is thoughtfully planned, challenging, engaging, developmentally appropriate, culturally and linguistically responsive, comprehensive, and likely to promote positive outcomes for all young children.

Indicators of Effectiveness

• *Children are active and engaged.*

Children from babyhood through primary grades—and beyond—need to be cognitively, physically, socially, and artistically active. In their own ways, children of all ages and abilities can become interested and engaged, develop positive attitudes toward learning, and have their feelings of security, emotional competence, and linkages to family and community supported.

• *Goals are clear and shared by all.*

Curriculum goals are clearly defined, shared, and understood by all "stakeholders" (for example, program administrators, teachers, and families). The curriculum and related activities and teaching strategies are designed to help achieve these goals in a unified, coherent way.

• *Curriculum is evidence-based.*

The curriculum is based on evidence that is developmentally, culturally, and linguistically relevant for the children who will experience the curriculum. It is organized around principles of child development and learning.

• *Valued content is learned through investigation, play, and focused, intentional teaching.*

Children learn by exploring, thinking about, and inquiring about all sorts of phenomena. These experiences help children investigate "big ideas," those that are important at any age and are con-

nected to later learning. Pedagogy or teaching strategies are tailored to children's ages, developmental capacities, language and culture, and abilities or disabilities.

• *Curriculum builds on prior learning and experiences.*

The content and implementation of the curriculum builds on children's prior individual, age-related, and cultural learning, is inclusive of children with disabilities, and is supportive of background knowledge gained at home and in the community. The curriculum supports children whose home language is not English in building a solid base for later learning.

• *Curriculum is comprehensive.*

The curriculum encompasses critical areas of development including children's physical well-being and motor development; social and emotional development; approaches to learning; language development; and cognition and general knowledge; and subject matter areas such as science, mathematics, language, literacy, social studies, and the arts (more fully and explicitly for older children).

• *Professional standards validate the curriculum's subject-matter content.*

When subject-specific curricula are adopted, they meet the standards of relevant professional organizations (for example, the American Alliance for Health, Physical Education, Recreation and Dance [AAHPERD], the National Association for Music Education [MENC]; the National Council of Teachers of English [NCTE]; the National Council of Teachers of Mathematics [NCTM]; the National Dance Education Organization [NDEO]; the National Science Teachers Association [NSTA]) and are reviewed and implemented so that they fit together coherently.

• *The curriculum is likely to benefit children.*

Research and other evidence indicates that the curriculum, if implemented as intended, will likely have beneficial effects. These benefits include a wide range of outcomes. When evidence is not yet available, plans are developed to obtain this evidence.

Assessment of Young Children

Make ethical, appropriate, valid, and reliable assessment a central part of all early childhood programs. To assess young children's strengths, progress, and needs, use assessment methods that are developmentally appropriate, culturally and linguistically responsive, tied to children's daily activities, supported by professional development, inclusive of families, and connected to specific, beneficial purposes:

(1) making sound decisions about teaching and learning, (2) identifying significant concerns that may require focused intervention for individual children, and (3) helping programs improve their educational and developmental interventions.

Indicators of Effectiveness

• *Ethical principles guide assessment practices.*

Ethical principles underlie all assessment practices. Young children are not denied opportunities or services, and decisions are not made about children on the basis of a single assessment.

• *Assessment instruments are used for their intended purposes.*

Assessments are used in ways consistent with the purposes for which they were designed. If the assessments will be used for additional purposes, they are validated for those purposes.

• *Assessments are appropriate for ages and other characteristics of children being assessed.*

Assessments are designed for and validated for use with children whose ages, cultures, home languages, socioeconomic status, abilities and disabilities, and other characteristics are similar to those of the children with whom the assessments will be used.

• *Assessment instruments are in compliance with professional criteria for quality.*

Assessments are valid and reliable. Accepted professional standards of quality are the basis for selection, use, and interpretation of assessment instruments, including screening tools. NAEYC and NAECS/SDE support and adhere to the measurement standards set forth in 1999 by the American Educational Research Association, the American Psychological Association, and the National Center for Measurement in Education. When individual norm-referenced tests are used, they meet these guidelines.

• *What is assessed is developmentally and educationally significant.*

The objects of assessment include a comprehensive, developmentally, and educationally important set of goals, rather than a narrow set of skills. Assessments are aligned with early learning standards, with program goals, and with specific emphases in the curriculum.

• *Assessment evidence is used to understand and improve learning.*

Assessments lead to improved knowledge about children. This knowledge is translated into improved

curriculum implementation and teaching practices. Assessment helps early childhood professionals understand the learning of a specific child or group of children; enhance overall knowledge of child development; improve educational programs for young children while supporting continuity across grades and settings; and access resources and supports for children with specific needs.

• *Assessment evidence is gathered from realistic settings and situations that reflect children's actual performance.*

To influence teaching strategies or to identify children in need of further evaluation, the evidence used to assess young children's characteristics and progress is derived from real-world classroom or family contexts that are consistent with children's culture, language, and experiences.

• *Assessments use multiple sources of evidence gathered over time.*

The assessment system emphasizes repeated, systematic observation, documentation, and other forms of criterion- or performance-oriented assessment using broad, varied, and complementary methods with accommodations for children with disabilities.

• *Screening is always linked to follow-up.*

When a screening or other assessment identifies concerns, appropriate follow-up, referral, or other intervention is used. Diagnosis or labeling is never the result of a brief screening or one-time assessment.

• *Use of individually administered, norm-referenced tests is limited.*

The use of formal standardized testing and norm-referenced assessments of young children is limited to situations in which such measures are appropriate and potentially beneficial, such as identifying potential disabilities. (See also the indicator concerning the use of individual norm-referenced tests as part of program evaluation and accountability.)

• *Staff and families are knowledgeable about assessment.*

Staff are given resources that support their knowledge and skills about early childhood assessment and their ability to assess children in culturally and linguistically appropriate ways. Preservice and in-service training builds teachers' and administrators' "assessment literacy," creating a community that sees assessment as a tool to improve outcomes for children. Families are part of this community, with regular communication, partnership, and involvement.

Program Evaluation and Accountability

Regularly evaluate early childhood programs in light of program goals, using varied, appropriate, conceptually and technically sound evidence to determine the extent to which programs meet the expected standards of quality and to examine intended as well as unintended results.

Indicators of Effectiveness

• *Evaluation is used for continuous improvement.*

Programs undertake regular evaluation, including self-evaluation, to document the extent to which they are achieving desired results, with the goal of engaging in continuous improvement. Evaluations focus on processes and implementation as well as outcomes. Over time, evidence is gathered that program evaluations do influence specific improvements.

• *Goals become guides for evaluation.*

Evaluation designs and measures are guided by goals identified by the program, by families and other stakeholders, and by the developers of a program or curriculum, while also allowing the evaluation to reveal unintended consequences.

• *Comprehensive goals are used.*

The program goals used to guide the evaluation are comprehensive, including goals related to families, teachers and other staff, and community as well as child-oriented goals that address a broad set of developmental and learning outcomes.

• *Evaluations use valid designs.*

Programs are evaluated using scientifically valid designs, guided by a "logic model" that describes ways in which the program sees its interventions having both medium- and longer-term effects on children and, in some cases, families and communities.

• *Multiple sources of data are available.*

An effective evaluation system should include multiple measures, including program data, child demographic data, information about staff qualifications, administrative practices, classroom quality assessments, implementation data, and other information that provides a context for interpreting the results of child assessments.

• *Sampling is used when assessing individual children as part of large-scale program evaluation.*

When individually administered, norm-referenced tests of children's progress are used as part of program evaluation and accountability, matrix sampling is used (that is, administered only to a systematic sample of children) so as to diminish the burden of testing on children and to reduce the likelihood that data will be inappropriately used to make judgments about individual children.

• *Safeguards are in place if standardized tests are used as part of evaluations.*

When individually administered, norm-referenced tests are used as part of program evaluation, they must be developmentally and culturally appropriate for the particular children in the program, conducted in the language children are most comfortable with, with other accommodations as appropriate, valid in terms of the curriculum, and technically sound (including reliability and validity). Quality checks on data are conducted regularly, and the system includes multiple data sources collected over time.

• *Children's gains over time are emphasized.*

When child assessments are used as part of program evaluation, the primary focus is on children's gains or progress as documented in observations, samples of classroom work, and other assessments over the duration of the program. The focus is not just on children's scores upon exit from the program.

• *Well-trained individuals conduct evaluations.*

Program evaluations, at whatever level or scope, are conducted by well-trained individuals who are able to evaluate programs in fair and unbiased ways. Self-assessment processes used as part of comprehensive program evaluation follow a valid model. Assessor training goes beyond single workshops and includes ongoing quality checks. Data are analyzed systematically and can be quantified or aggregated to provide evidence of the extent to which the program is meeting its goals.

• *Evaluation results are publicly shared.*

Families, policy makers, and other stakeholders have the right to know the results of program evaluations. Data from program monitoring and evaluation, aggregated appropriately and based on reliable measures, should be made available and accessible to the public.

Creating Change through Support for Programs

Implementing the preceding recommendations for curriculum, child assessment, and program evaluation requires a solid foundation. Calls for better results and greater accountability from programs for children in preschool, kindergarten, and the primary grades have not been backed up by essential supports for teacher recruitment and compensation, professional preparation and ongoing professional development, and other ingredients of quality early education.

The overarching need is to create an integrated, well-financed system of early care and education that has the capacity to support learning and development in all children, including children living in poverty, children whose home language is not English, and children with disabilities. Unlike many other countries, the United States continues to have a fragmented system for educating children from birth through age eight, under multiple auspices, with greatly varying levels of support, and with inadequate communication and collaboration.

Many challenges face efforts to provide all young children with high-quality curriculum, assessment, and evaluation of their programs. Public commitment, along with investments in a well-financed system of early childhood education and in other components of services for young children and their families, will make it possible to implement these recommendations fully and effectively.

This document is an official position statement of the National Association for the Education of Young Children and the National Association of Early Childhood Specialists in State Departments of Education.

Index